CROHN'S DISEASE

Edited by **Sami Karoui**

Crohn's Disease
Edited by Sami Karoui

Published by InTech
Janeza Trdine 9, 51000 Rijeka, Croatia

Publishing Process Manager Alida Lesnjakovic

Technical Editor Teodora Smiljanic

Cover Designer InTech Design Team

Additional hard copies can be obtained from orders@intechopen.com

Crohn's Disease, Edited by Sami Karoui
p. cm.
ISBN 978-953-307-811-3

For EU product safety concerns:
IN TECH d.o.o., Prolaz Marije Krucifikse Kozulić 3, 51000 Rijeka, Croatia,
info@intechopen.com or visit our website at intechopen.com.

Meet the editor

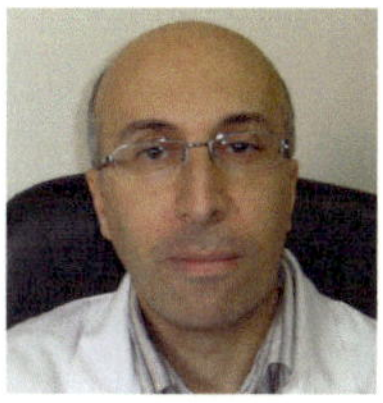

Sami Karoui was born in Tunis in 1968. He studied at the Faculty of Medicine of Tunis, and he continued his study of Gastroenterology and Hepatology at the University Hospital in Tunis. He received his diploma in Gastroenterology in 1998, and he has been working in the Department of Gastroenterology A (La Rabta Hospital – Tunis) and in the Faculty of Medicine of Tunis since 2008 as professor of Gastroenterology and Hepatology.

Contents

Preface

Crohn's disease (CD) is a lifelong disease arising from interaction between genetic and environmental factors. The precise aetiology of CD is unknown, and therefore, a causal treatment is not yet available. During the last few years, there have been many advances concerning etiopathogeny, diagnosis tools, and management of CD.

Inflammatory bowel disease, and particularly CD, results from an inappropriate inflammatory response to intestinal microbes in a genetically susceptible host. The intestinal lamina propria contains a complex population of immune cells that balance the requirement for immune tolerance of luminal microbiota with the need to defend against pathogens and the excessive entry of luminal microbiota. The hallmark of active CD is a pronounced infiltration into the lamina propria of innate immune cells (neutrophils, macrophages, dendritic cells, and natural killer T cells), and adaptive immune cells (B cells and T cells). Increased numbers and activation of these cells in the intestinal mucosa elevate local levels of TNF alpha, interleukin 1 ß, interferon γ, and cytokines of the interleukin-23-Th17 pathway. CD is associated with a Th1 T cell mediated response, characterized by enhanced production of interferon γ and TNF α. IL-12 and possibly IL-23 govern the Th1 cell differentiation, but optimal induction and stabilization of polarized Th1 cells would require additional cytokines.

Genetic factors are intimately involved in the pathogenesis of CD. To data, CARD15/NOD2 in the only confirmed CD susceptibility gene identified. There are a number of other likely candidates of genes and loci that have been described, although details remain less clear, and their roles less well characterized. Potential application of genetic testing in CD is a prediction of disease susceptibility, choice and response to therapy, and disease prevention with specific interventions. More recently, associations with CD have been established for ATG16L1 and immunity-related GTPase M Protein, two genes involved in autophagy.

Clinical features of CD vary depending on the location, behaviour, and severity of disease, as well as extra-intestinal manifestations and medication. The diagnosis is confirmed by clinical evaluation, and a combination of endoscopic, histological, radiological, and/or biochemical investigations. Ileocolonoscopy with multiple biopsy specimens is well established as the first line procedure for the diagnosis of CD. In some cases, the diagnosis can be difficult, confounding by ileocoecal tuberculosis, yersiniosis, and ulcerative colitis is a case of involvement of the colon. Histological, bacteriological, and some biochemical markers can help the clinicians to establish the right diagnosis and to prescribe the optimal treatment.

The main goals of therapy in CD are to induce a clinical remission and then maintain that remission over time. Secondary management goals include mucosal healing, maintaining the quality of life of patients, restoring nutritional balance, preventing the complications of the disease, and timing surgical therapy to minimize the morbidity of the disease. Specific therapy of CD depends upon disease severity, location, and complications. In fact, current practice guidelines recommend using a sequential approach to treatment according to the severity of the clinical presentation and associated complications. Categories of severity are based on the type and acuity of symptoms, as well as response to medications, and include mild to moderate, moderate to severe, and severe to fulminant disease. Sulfasalazine and Mesalamine can still be considered first-line therapies for selected patients with mildly to moderately active CD. Studies have conclusively shown the benefit of corticosteroids in induction of remission in patients with CD. Patients unable to discontinue corticosteroids should be considered for alternative therapies such as azathioprine, methotrexate, or infliximab. Anti-TNF α antibodies and Natalizumab were both superior to a placebo in inducing remission and in preventing relapses in luminal CD patients.

Dr Sami Karoui
Department of Gastroenterology A
La Rabta Hospital, Tunis
Tunisia

Part 1

Advances in Etiopathogeny of Crohn's Disease

1

Alteration of the Crypt Epithelial-Stromal Interface by Proinflammatory Cytokines in Crohn's Disease

Amira Seltana, Manon Lepage and Jean-François Beaulieu
Université de Sherbrooke
Canada

1. Introduction

The intestinal epithelium is a very dynamic tissue, being completely renewed over a 3-5 day period in the human. Epithelial cells in the intestine lie on a specialized layer of extracellular matrix material referred to as the basement membrane (BM). Intestinal epithelial cell interactions with BM molecules such as collagens, laminins, fibronectin and tenascin regulate crucial functions of the normal intestinal epithelial renewal process such as cell adhesion, migration, signalization and gene expression as well as anoikis. BM molecules can be secreted by epithelial cells but a number of them are exclusively synthesized and deposited by the subepithelial myofibroblasts. In this chapter, we will review alterations at the epithelial-stromal interface in Crohn's disease (CD) with a specific emphasis on epithelial cell and myofibroblast susceptibility to proinflammatory cytokines in the crypt region.

2. Epithelial BM molecules in the normal human intestine

The epithelial BM of the human intestine has been found to contain all the major components specific to most basement membranes as well as a number of non-exclusive BM components. There is good evidence that both types of BM components play an active role in intestinal epithelial cell biology through their interaction with specific cell membrane integrin and non-integrin receptors, which mediate cell adhesion, migration, cell cycle and gene expression. Current knowledge about epithelial BM composition in the normal human intestine is summarized below. More detailed information on BM molecules and their receptors in the intestine can be found elsewhere (Beaulieu 1997a, Beaulieu 2001, Lussier et al. 2000, Ménard et al. 2006, Teller&Beaulieu 2001).

2.1 Exclusive and non-exclusive BM components

As illustrated in Figure 1, exclusive BM components include the type IV collagens and laminins. These macromolecules are complex protein families composed of various sub-units. Detailed analysis of various genetic forms of type IV collagens and laminins revealed the presence of at least two distinct types of type IV collagen heterotrimers based on the expression of the $\alpha1(IV)/\alpha2(IV)$ and $\alpha5(IV)/\alpha6(IV)$ chains (Beaulieu 1992, Beaulieu et al.

1994, Simoneau et al. 1998) and the 4 main laminins, LM-111, LM-211, LM-332 and LM-511 (Beaulieu 1992, Beaulieu&Vachon 1994, Teller et al. 2007).

A second interesting feature of the intestinal epithelial BM is the presence of a relatively large number of non-exclusive BM components, such as fibronectin, tenascin-C, osteopontin and type VI collagen that have been found to be integral epithelial BM components (Aufderheide&Ekblom 1988, Beaulieu et al. 1991, Beaulieu 1992, Groulx et al. 2011, Simon-Assmann et al. 1990b) although they can be found also in the underlying interstitial matrix (Fig.1).

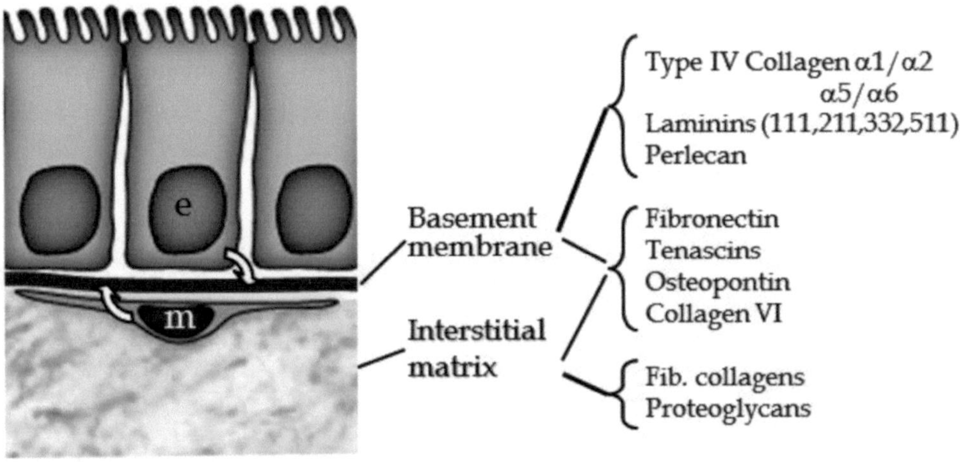

Fig. 1. The intestinal epithelial BM. The BM, which is located at the interface between the epithelial cells (e) and the subepithelial myofibroblasts (m), contains BM-specific macromolecules (e.g. type IV collagens and laminins) as well as non-exclusive BM components (e.g. tenascin-C and type VI collagen). Both types of components can originate from the epithelial cells and/or the subepithelial myofibroblasts (white arrows).

The third interesting phenomenon relative to the epithelial BM in the intestine is the dual tissular origin of the BM components. Indeed, while the type IV collagen α5(IV) and α6(IV) chains as well as type VI collagen are expressed at least in part by epithelial cells, the major type IV collagen chains α1(IV) and α2(IV) are exclusively of stromal origin (Beaulieu et al. 1994, Groulx et al. 2011, Simon-Assmann et al. 1990a, Simoneau et al. 1998, Vachon et al. 1993), presumably synthesized by the subepithelial myofibroblasts (Fig. 1). Analysis of the tissular origin of the laminins also revealed dual epithelial/stromal origin for laminins LM-111 and LM-332 (epithelial), LM211 (stromal) and LM511 (both) (Perreault et al. 1998, Teller et al. 2007).

2.2 Spatial and temporal BM microenvironments

Spatial and temporal patterns of expression for BM components in the intact intestinal epithelium have been very informative in evaluating the potential role of individual macromolecules in the regulation of cell functions, most notably cell growth and differentiation, under a normal environment. Indeed, during development, the process of endodermal differentiation into a functional epithelium coincides with the morphogenesis of the villi and the crypts in both the small and large intestines. In the mature intestine, the epithelial renewing units consist of spatially well-separated proliferative and differentiated cell populations. Furthermore, the renewing units differ along the proximal-distal gradient, the crypt-to-villus axis of the small intestine being replaced by a gland-to-surface epithelial axis in the colon (Beaulieu 1997b, Ménard&Beaulieu 1994, Ménard et al. 2006) (Fig. 2).

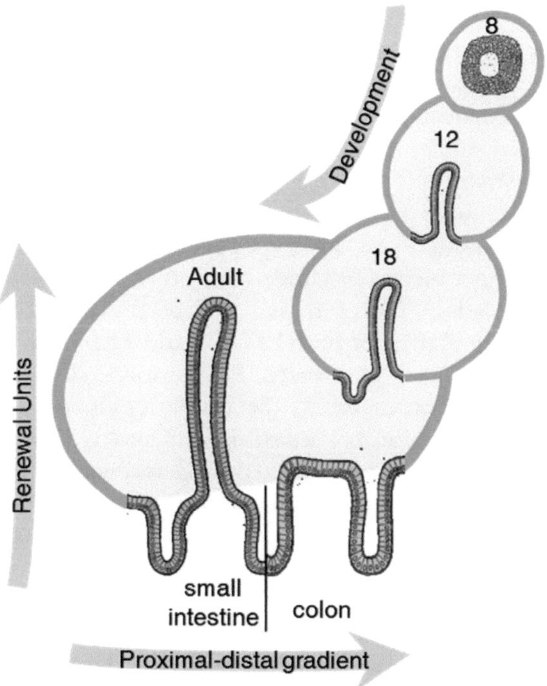

Fig. 2. Development and characteristics of the epithelium in the human small and large intestines. The human intestine develops relatively early during ontogeny. Villi develop between 9 and 11 weeks of gestation while crypts form around 16 weeks so that typical adult-like crypt-villus architecture is already established in the small intestine at mid-gestation (18 to 20 weeks). Similar crypt-villus architecture is transitorily present in the developing colon up to mid-gestation. However, at birth, the villi have disappeared and the typical adult gland-to-surface epithelial architecture has been established (proximal-distal gradient). At maturity, the proliferative cell populations responsible for the renewing of the epithelium are located in the lower ⅔ of the small intestinal crypts and the lower ½ of the colonic glands. The functional cells of these renewing units are located on the villus and the surface epithelium of the small and large intestines, respectively (Adapted from (Teller&Beaulieu 2001).

3. Alterations of epithelial BM composition in CD

Alterations of epithelial BM composition have been reported in various intestinal pathologies (Belanger&Beaulieu 2000, Teller&Beaulieu 2001). Although none of these alterations has yet been demonstrated to be the primary defect in any intestinal disease, they are not exclusively secondary to the disruption of the epithelial-stromal interface. In colorectal cancers for instance, laminin alterations are thought to play an active role in invasion (Lohi 2001). Alteration in the distribution and/or expression of BM molecules were also observed in other intestinal pathologies such as tufting enteropathy (Goulet et al. 1995) and chronic inflammatory bowel conditions (Bouatrouss 1998). The alterations in the epithelial BM composition in the context of inflammatory bowel disease pathogenesis and as potential disease indicators will now be discussed.

3.1 BM components in the crypts of inflamed specimens from CD patients

Although clinically distinct, chronic inflammatory bowel diseases such as CD and ulcerative colitis share common histopathological features including mucosal inflammation, villous atrophy, crypt hypertrophy and epithelial cell injury (Chadwick 1991).

In CD, an important redistribution of laminins was observed at the epithelial-stromal interface of inflamed specimens as compared to non-inflamed specimens from the same patients (Bouatrouss et al. 2000). First, the crypt specific laminin, LM-211, was found to be essentially absent from the mucosa. Second, two other laminins, LM-332 and LM-511, remained strongly expressed in the epithelial BM of the atrophied and inflamed villi. However, a significant upregulation of both LM-332 and LM-511 expression was observed in the lower crypts of inflamed CD specimens. Furthermore, a significant reduction in the levels of tenascin-C was also observed in the crypt region of inflamed CD specimens (Francoeur et al. 2009). Incidentally, the intestinal mucosa is among the few sites where tenascin-C remains expressed in adulthood (Belanger&Beaulieu 2000). Interestingly, in ulcerative colitis, most of the epithelial BM surrounding the glands has been found to be devoid of immunoreactive laminin (Schmehl et al. 2000) and tenascin-C (Francoeur et al. 2009) in actively affected colonic tissues. Also, alterations in laminin and tenascin-C expression were not observed in celiac disease (Korhonen et al. 2000), an immune-mediated intestinal pathology that is also characterized by villus atrophy and crypt hyperplasia (Maki&Collin 1997), suggesting that the redistribution of laminins and tenascin-C in CD could be related to the chronic inflammatory condition.

From these studies, it can be concluded that important alterations in epithelial BM molecule expression occur in the intestinal mucosa of patients with inflammatory bowel diseases. The fact that these alterations appear to be mainly confined to the crypts in these diseases, as summarized for CD in Fig. 3, suggests that compositional changes in the crypt epithelial BM may be of functional importance in the pathogenesis of these afflictions.

3.2 Effects of proinflammatory cytokines on human intestinal epithelial crypt cells

One of the landmarks of inflammatory bowel conditions such as CD is the chronic imbalance between immunoregulatory and proinflammatory cytokines (Bouma&Strober 2003, Fiocchi 1997a, MacDonald&Monteleone 2006, Sartor 2006). Among the cytokines most frequently found to be elevated in the inflamed CD mucosa are interleukin-1β and 6 (IL-1β and IL-6), tumor necrosis factor α (TNFα) and interferon γ (IFNγ). Because they represent the main component of the intestinal barrier, epithelial cells have been one of the nonimmune cell types most extensively studied in inflammatory bowel diseases. While morphological and functional alterations in epithelial integrity were described several years ago (Dvorak&Dickersin 1980, Hollander 1993), more recent work has provided evidence that these changes are primarily mediated by cytokines released from adjacent inflammatory cells as well as from the epithelial cells themselves (Abraham&Medzhitov 2011, Dionne et al. 1999, Fiocchi 1997b, McKay&Baird 1999, Podolsky 2000).

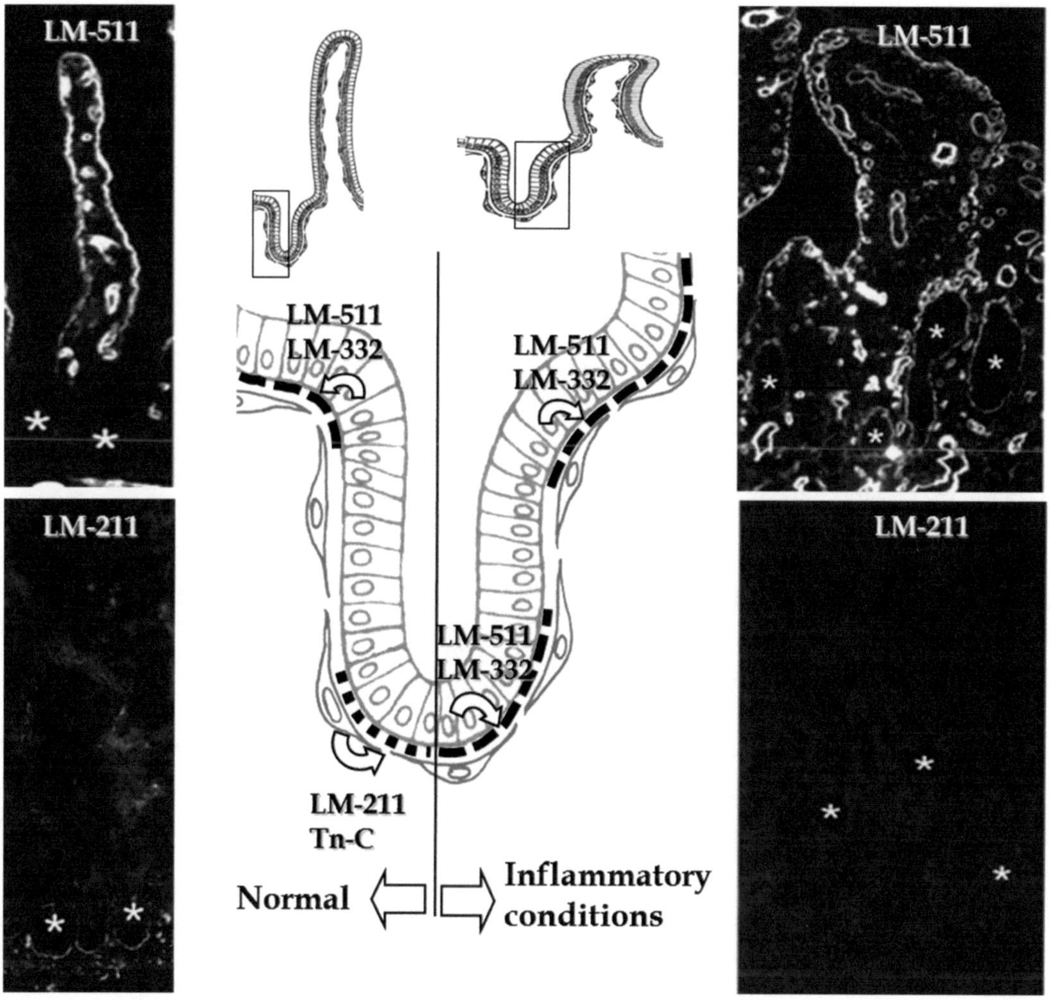

Fig. 3. Alterations of epithelial BM composition in the human intestinal mucosa under normal vs inflammatory conditions. In the normal small intestine (left), laminins LM-322 and LM-511 are found in the BM of the villus epithelial cells while laminin LM-211, is found in the BM of crypt epithelial cells. Tenascin-C (Tn-C) is found in the epithelial BM of both the crypts and villi. LM-332 and LM-511 of the epithelial BM are mainly produced by epithelial cells (E) while LM-211 and Tn-C are synthesized by the sub-epithelial myofibroblasts (SEMF). In inflamed CD specimens (inflammatory conditions), laminins LM-332 and LM-511 remain expressed by epithelial cells of the atrophied villi while in the crypts, the other laminin, LM-211, as well as most of the Tn-C at the epithelial BM are lost and replaced by the neo-expression of laminins LM-332 and LM-511. Functionally, these events are associated with pro-inflammatory cytokines which a) stimulate LM-332 and LM-511 production by crypt epithelial cells and b) induce apoptosis and de-differentiation of the sub-epithelial myofibroblasts (see sections 3.2 and 3.3 and Fig. 4 for more details).

Considering that changes in BM composition under inflammatory conditions are mainly observed in the lower part of the crypt (Fig. 3), our laboratory investigated the effect of proinflammatory cytokines on laminin expression in human intestinal epithelial cells using the well-characterized human intestinal epithelial crypt (HIEC) cell line as an experimental cell model representative of the human intestinal lower crypt (Benoit et al. 2010, Pageot et al. 2000, Quaroni&Beaulieu 1997). Individually, all tested cytokines including IL-1β, IL-6, TNFα and IFNγ as well as transforming growth factor β (TGFβ) exerted relatively modest effects on laminin LM-332 and LM-511 production in HIEC cells. However in combination, a synergistic effect of TNFα and IFNγ was observed on both laminin LM-332 and LM-511 production at protein and transcript levels (Francoeur et al. 2004). TNFα and IFNγ synergy has also been reported in various intestinal epithelial cell models for chemokine production (Warhurst et al. 1998), alteration in epithelial barrier properties (Wang et al. 2006), and acquisition of susceptibility to Fas-induced apoptosis (Begue et al. 2006, Ruemmele et al. 1999). The TNFα/IFNγ combination was also found to synergistically induce caspase-dependent apoptosis in HIEC cells (Francoeur et al. 2004). Interestingly, caspase inhibitors completely prevented TNFα/IFNγ-induced apoptosis but did not influence the induction of laminin expression indicating that the two events occurred independently.

The contribution of TGFβ in the synergistic effects of TNFα/IFNγ on laminin production was investigated in light of the fact that levels of TGFβ have been reported to be elevated in the mucosa of CD patients (Babyatsky et al. 1996) and that this multifunctional cytokine can exert a crucial function on intestinal epithelial wound healing (Podolsky 2000), in part through its ability to stimulate extracellular matrix molecule expression (Verrecchia&Mauviel 2002). Indeed, in rodent intestinal crypt cells, the promotion of epithelial healing by specific cytokines such as IL-1β, IFNγ and TGFα was found to act under a bioactive TGFβ dependent mechanism (Dignass&Podolsky 1993). However, TGFβ was found to be significantly less potent than the TNFα/IFNγ combination in human intestinal crypt cells on laminin production suggesting a TGFβ-independent mechanism (Francoeur et al. 2004).

In summary, the two proinflammatory cytokines TNFα and IFNγ synergistically induce the expression of the specific BM molecules, laminin LM-332 and LM-511, in human intestinal crypt cells. The synergistic effect of the TNFα/IFNγ combination on laminin production was found to be independent of the effect of these cytokines on cell apoptosis and appears to be controlled by an apparent TGFβ-independent mechanism.

3.3 Effects of proinflammatory cytokines on human pericryptal subepithelial myofibroblasts

Along with the epithelial cells, myofibroblasts are another important nonprofessional immune mucosal cell type for which evidence supports a participation in the pathogenesis of inflammatory bowel diseases (Fiocchi 1997b, Macdonald&Monteleone 2005). The myofibroblast is an intermediate cell type between the smooth muscle cell and the fibroblast that is characterized by alpha smooth muscle actin (αSMA) and vimentin expression (Gabbiani 2003). While there is evidence that intramucosal myofibroblasts can be involved in CD (Vallance et al. 2005), it is the intestinal subepithelial myofibroblasts present immediately subjacent to the epithelial BM (Powell et al. 2005) in the form of a pericryptal sheath that have been the primary focus of attention in the pathogenesis of inflammatory bowel diseases. Because of their vicinity to the basal surface of epithelial cells, they are potential targets for bacteria and their products deposited in the subepithelial compartment when the epithelial barrier is disrupted. In turn, when stimulated, myofibroblasts can release various cytokines and chemokines (Fiocchi 1997b, Powell et al. 1999, Powell et al. 2005) and extracellular matrix molecules (Riedl et al. 1992) suggesting that intestinal subepithelial myofibroblasts can participate in the innate immune response (Otte et al. 2003, Saada et al. 2006). Furthermore, the subepithelial myofibroblast represents a key component of epithelial-stromal interactions in the intestine (Ménard et al. 2006, Powell et al. 2005), which can regulate both basic and healing epithelial cell functions through the secretion of paracrine factors such as the Wnts, BMPs, and TGFβ, which target epithelial cells (Ménard et al. 2006, Powell et al. 2005), the release of proteinases (Kruidenier et al. 2006, McKaig et al. 2003) and the production of extracellular matrix molecules that contribute to the epithelial BM such as laminin LM-211 and tenascin-C (Beaulieu 1997a, Perreault et al. 1998, Riedl et al. 1992, Teller et al. 2007, Vachon et al. 1993).

Analysis of subepithelial myofibroblast characteristics in inflamed small intestinal mucosa of CD patients revealed a number of alterations in the crypt region (Francoeur et al. 2009). First, a disappearance of αSMA positive cells was observed in a large proportion of the crypts while in others, the αSMA cellular staining was abnormally thick and co-stained by desmin suggesting a reorganization/redifferentiation into smooth muscle cells. Characterization of the pericryptal myofibroblastic sheath in the colonic mucosa from patients with various pathologic conditions including CD, ulcerative colitis, acute infectious colitis and noninfectious colitis confirmed the disappearance of αSMA positive cells (also desmin negative) in the inflamed mucosa from inflammatory bowel diseases but not in other pathological conditions. Analysis of the expression of tenascin-C, which is exclusively produced by the myofibroblasts and muscle cells of the human intestine (Belanger&Beaulieu 2000) in the crypt epithelial BM revealed a close correlation between myofibroblast disappearance (loss of normal αSMA staining) and loss of tenascin-C staining (Francoeur et al. 2009). The significant reduction of αSMA positive cells in the pericryptal region concomitant with a disappearance of tenascin-C (Francoeur et al. 2009) and laminin LM-211 (Bouatrouss et al. 2000) suggested that pericryptal myofibroblasts are lost in the inflamed mucosa of CD patients.

To test this hypothesis, we used various preparations of myofibroblastic cells isolated from the human intestinal mucosa (Pinchuk et al. 2007, Teller et al. 2007, Vachon et al. 1993) as experimental cell models. Myofibroblasts are known to respond to various inflammatory signals (Otte et al. 2003, Saada et al. 2006) and have been shown to be altered in inflammatory bowel diseases (Fiocchi 1997b, Powell et al. 1999, Powell et al. 2005). For instance, mesenchymal cells isolated from the inflamed mucosa show higher levels of collagen production than their normal counterparts. We thus investigated the possibility that a loss of pericryptal myofibroblasts occurs in the inflamed regions of CD mucosa by testing myofibroblast susceptibility to the same panel of proinflammatory cytokines used above for epithelial cells (section 3.2). Individually, IL-1β, IL-6, TNFα and IFNγ as well as TGFβ exerted little or no effect on the growth and survival of intestinal myofibroblasts. However, cytokine combinations containing TNFα and IFNγ induced significant caspase-dependent apoptosis, suggesting that this mechanism may account for the loss of myofibroblasts in the inflamed CD mucosa. While not yet reported for myofibroblasts, the synergistic effect of TNFα/IFNγ on various functions has been described in other cell types, namely intestinal epithelial cells (Begue et al. 2006, Francoeur et al. 2004, Ruemmele et al. 1999, Wang et al. 2006, Warhurst et al. 1998).

Interestingly, the pro-apoptotic effect of pro-inflammatory cytokines was only observed with myofibroblasts isolated from normal mucosa, myofibroblasts isolated from inflamed mucosa being apoptosis-resistant (Francoeur et al. 2009). Distinct intrinsic properties of myofibroblasts isolated from inflammatory bowel disease vs non-inflammatory bowel disease patients remains to be elucidated but is not without precedent (Lawrance et al. 2001). The contribution of bone marrow-derived myofibroblasts in the regenerative process in inflammatory bowel disease (Andoh et al. 2005, Brittan et al. 2007) may explain the resistance to cytokine-mediated apoptosis.

The high levels of TGFβ in the inflamed mucosa may need to be further investigated considering its anti-inflammatory effect in inflammatory bowel diseases (Fiocchi 2001) and its promoting effect on myofibroblast differentiation (Simmons et al. 2002). Indeed, although not directly tested on myofibroblasts for apoptosis, TGFβ was found to significantly enhance αSMA expression in intestinal myofibroblasts while all other cytokines reduced αSMA expression. Interestingly, TGFβ completely reversed the down-regulation of αSMA expression triggered by individual proinflammatory cytokines but failed to prevent the αSMA down-regulation induced by the TNFα/IFNγ combination, suggesting a dedifferentiation mechanism (Francoeur et al. 2009).

In summary, these studies showed that the myofibroblasts of the intestinal pericryptal sheath are a target for proinflammatory cytokines in active inflammatory bowel diseases. The disappearance of laminin LM-211 and tenascin-C in the pericryptal region of the inflamed CD mucosa appears to be a direct consequence of the alteration of the myofibroblastic sheath. While proinflammatory cytokines appear to be responsible for the net reduction of the number of pericryptal myofibroblasts, the mechanisms involved include caspase-dependent apoptosis and dedifferentiation toward a fibroblastic phenotype.

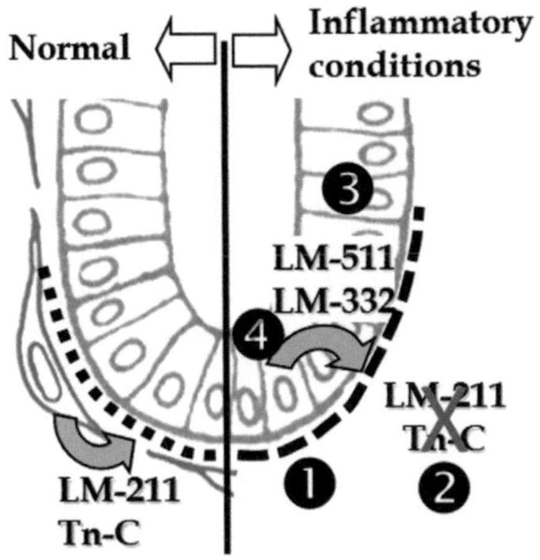

Fig. 4. Functional alterations of human intestinal epithelial-stromal components resulting from the synergistic effects of TNFα and IFNγ. The TNFα/IFNγ combination was found to trigger myofibroblast caspase-dependent apoptosis and myofibroblast dedifferentiation, which results in the disappearance of a significant portion of the pericryptal sheath (1) and, concomitantly, the loss of two extracellular matrix molecules specifically synthesized by these cells: laminin LM-211 and tenascin-C (Tn-C) (2). The TNFα/IFNγ combination was found to also elicit caspase-dependent apoptosis in epithelial crypt cells (3) as well as induction of the expression of the laminins LM-332 and LM-511 (4), two laminins normally not expressed in the lower crypt. Expression of LM-511 may compensate for the disappearance of LM-211.

4. Conclusions

It is becoming more and more evident that under inflammatory conditions, the intestinal immune response relies on a complex interplay between immune and nonprofessional immune cells (Fiocchi 1997b, Macdonald&Monteleone 2005). Proinflammatory cytokines, namely TNFα and IFNγ in combination, were shown to induce human intestinal crypt epithelial cell apoptosis and altered expression and distribution of laminins LM-332 and LM-511 in the crypts (Francoeur et al. 2004), two events that contribute to the disruption of epithelial cell homeostasis (Bouatrouss et al. 2000, Teller&Beaulieu 2001). As summarized in Fig. 4, the proinflammatory conditions that prevail in the intestinal mucosa of patients affected with inflammatory bowel diseases also disrupt the pericryptal sheath, as shown by the loss of myofibroblasts and altered expression of laminin LM-211 and tenascin-C (Francoeur et al. 2009). Taken together, these data suggest that the entire epithelial-stromal interface is affected in the intestine under proinflammatory conditions.

5. Acknowledgements

The authors wish to thank the other members of the laboratory for discussion, namely Drs Caroline Francoeur and Yamina Bouatrouss who were particularly involved in the original work and Elizabeth Herring for proofreading the manuscript.

The work was supported by grants from the Canadian Institutes for Health Research. JFB holds the Canadian Research Chair in Intestinal Physiopathology and is a member of the FRSQ-funded Centre de Recherche Clinique Etienne-LeBel of the CHUS.

6. References

Abraham C, Medzhitov R (2011). Interactions between the host innate immune system and microbes in inflammatory bowel disease. *Gastroenterology,* Vol.140, No.6, (May), pp. 1729-1737, 1528-0012 (Electronic) 0016-5085 (Linking)

Andoh A, Bamba S, Fujiyama Y, Brittan M, Wright NA (2005). Colonic subepithelial myofibroblasts in mucosal inflammation and repair: contribution of bone marrow-derived stem cells to the gut regenerative response. *J Gastroenterol,* Vol.40, No.12, (Dec), pp. 1089-1099, 0944-1174 (Print) 0944-1174 (Linking)

Aufderheide E, Ekblom P (1988). Tenascin during gut development: appearance in the mesenchyme, shift in molecular forms, and dependence on epithelial-mesenchymal interactions. *J Cell Biol,* Vol.107, No.6 Pt 1, (Dec), pp. 2341-2349,

Babyatsky MW, Rossiter G, Podolsky DK (1996). Expression of transforming growth factors alpha and beta in colonic mucosa in inflammatory bowel disease. *Gastroenterology,* Vol.110, No.4, (pp. 975-984,

Beaulieu JF, Vachon PH, Chartrand S (1991). Immunolocalization of extracellular matrix components during organogenesis in the human small intestine. *Anat Embryol (Berl),* Vol.183, No.4, (pp. 363-369,

Beaulieu JF (1992). Differential expression of the VLA family of integrins along the crypt-villus axis in the human small intestine. *J Cell Sci,* Vol.102 (Pt 3), Jul), pp. 427-436,

Beaulieu JF, Vachon PH (1994). Reciprocal expression of laminin A-chain isoforms along the crypt-villus axis in the human small intestine. *Gastroenterology,* Vol.106, No.4, (Apr), pp. 829-839,

Beaulieu JF, Vachon PH, Herring-Gillam FE, Simoneau A, Perreault N, Asselin C *et al* (1994). Expression of the alpha-5(IV) collagen chain in the fetal human small intestine. *Gastroenterology,* Vol.107, No.4, (Oct), pp. 957-967,

Beaulieu JF (1997a). Extracellular matrix components and integrins in relationship to human intestinal epithelial cell differentiation. *Prog Histochem Cytochem,* Vol.31, No.4, (pp. 1-78,

Beaulieu JF (1997b). Recent work with migration/patterns of expression: cell-matrix interactions in human intestinal cell differentiation, In: *The Gut as a Model in Cell and Molecular Biology,* F. Halter, Winton D., Wright N.A., (Eds), 165-179,7923-8726, Kluwer Academic Publisher, Dordrecht.

Beaulieu JF (2001). Role of extracellular matrix proteins on human intestinal cell function: Laminin-epithelial cell interactions, In: *Gastrointestinal Functions,* E.E. Delvin, Lentze M.J., (Eds), 59-75,1093-4715, Vevey/Lippincott Williams & Wilkins, Philadelphia.

Begue B, Wajant H, Bambou JC, Dubuquoy L, Siegmund D, Beaulieu JF *et al* (2006). Implication of TNF-related apoptosis-inducing ligand in inflammatory intestinal epithelial lesions. *Gastroenterology,* Vol.130, No.7, (Jun), pp. 1962-1974, 0016-5085 (Print)

Belanger I, Beaulieu JF (2000). Tenascin in the developing and adult human intestine. *Histol Histopathol,* Vol.15, No.2, (Apr), pp. 577-585,

Benoit YD, Pare F, Francoeur C, Jean D, Tremblay E, Boudreau F *et al* (2010). Cooperation between HNF-1alpha, Cdx2, and GATA-4 in initiating an enterocytic differentiation program in a normal human intestinal epithelial progenitor cell line. *Am J Physiol Gastrointest Liver Physiol,* Vol.298, No.4, (Apr), pp. G504-517, 1522-1547 (Electronic) 0193-1857 (Linking)

Bouatrouss Y, Herring-Gillam FE, Gosselin J, Poisson J, Beaulieu JF (2000). Altered expression of laminins in Crohn's disease small intestinal mucosa. *Am J Pathol,* Vol.156, No.1, (Jan), pp. 45-50,

Bouatrouss YP, J; Beaulieu, JF (1998). Studying the basement membrane, In: *Methods in Disease: investigating the gastrointestinal tract.,* P.V.W. RR, (Ed), 191-200, London Greenwich Medical Media.

Bouma G, Strober W (2003). The immunological and genetic basis of inflammatory bowel disease. *Nat Rev Immunol,* Vol.3, No.7, (Jul), pp. 521-533, 1474-1733 (Print)

Brittan M, Alison MR, Schier S, Wright NA (2007). Bone marrow stem cell-mediated regeneration in IBD: where do we go from here? *Gastroenterology,* Vol.132, No.3, (Mar), pp. 1171-1173, 0016-5085 (Print) 0016-5085 (Linking)

Chadwick VS (1991). Etiology of chronic ulcerative colitis and Crohn's disease, In: *The Large Intestine: Physiology, Pathophysiology, and Disease,* P. S.F., J.H. P., R.G. S., (Eds), 445-463, Raven Press, New York.

Dignass AU, Podolsky DK (1993). Cytokine modulation of intestinal epithelial cell restitution: central role of transforming growth factor beta. *Gastroenterology,* Vol.105, No.5, (pp. 1323-1332,

Dionne S, Ruemmele FM, Seidman EG (1999). Immunopathogenesis of inflammatory bowel disease: role of cytokines and immune cell-enterocyte interactions. *Nestle Nutr Workshop Ser Clin Perform Programme,* Vol.2, pp. 41-57; discussion 58-61.,

Dvorak AM, Dickersin GR (1980). Crohn's disease: transmission electron microscopic studies. I. Barrier function. Possible changes related to alterations of cell coat, mucous coat, epithelial cells, and Paneth cells. *Hum Pathol,* Vol.11, No.5 Suppl, (pp. 561-571,

Fiocchi C (1997a). The immune system in inflammatory bowel disease. *Acta Gastroenterol Belg,* Vol.60, No.2, (Apr-Jun), pp. 156-162,

Fiocchi C (1997b). Intestinal inflammation: a complex interplay of immune and nonimmune cell interactions. *Am J Physiol,* Vol.273, No.4 Pt 1, (pp. G769-G775,

Fiocchi C (2001). TGF-beta/Smad signaling defects in inflammatory bowel disease: mechanisms and possible novel therapies for chronic inflammation. *J Clin Invest,* Vol.108, No.4, (pp. 523-526.,

Francoeur C, Escaffit F, Vachon PH, Beaulieu JF (2004). Proinflammatory cytokines TNF-alpha and IFN-gamma alter laminin expression under an apoptosis-independent mechanism in human intestinal epithelial cells. *Am J Physiol Gastrointest Liver Physiol,* Vol.287, No.3, (Sep), pp. G592-598,

Francoeur C, Bouatrouss Y, Seltana A, Pinchuk IV, Vachon PH, Powell DW *et al* (2009). Degeneration of the pericryptal myofibroblast sheath by proinflammatory cytokines in inflammatory bowel diseases. *Gastroenterology,* Vol.136, No.1, (Jan), pp. 268-277 e263, 1528-0012 (Electronic)

Gabbiani G (2003). The myofibroblast in wound healing and fibrocontractive diseases. *J Pathol,* Vol.200, No.4, (Jul), pp. 500-503,

Goulet O, Kedinger M, Brousse N, Cuenod B, Colomb V, Patey N *et al* (1995). Intractable diarrhea of infancy with epithelial and basement membrane abnormalities. *J Pediatr,* Vol.127, No.2, (pp. 212-219, 0022-3476

Groulx JF, Gagne D, Benoit YD, Martel D, Basora N, Beaulieu JF (2011). Collagen VI is a basement membrane component that regulates epithelial cell-fibronectin interactions. *Matrix Biol,* Vol.30, No.3, (Apr), pp. 195-206, 1569-1802 (Electronic) 0945-053X (Linking)

Hollander D (1993). Permeability in Crohn's disease: altered barrier functions in healthy relatives? *Gastroenterology,* Vol.104, No.6, (pp. 1848-1851,

Korhonen M, Ormio M, Burgeson RE, Virtanen I, Savilahti E (2000). Unaltered distribution of laminins, fibronectin, and tenascin in celiac intestinal mucosa. *J Histochem Cytochem,* Vol.48, No.7, (Jul), pp. 1011-1020,

Kruidenier L, MacDonald TT, Collins JE, Pender SL, Sanderson IR (2006). Myofibroblast matrix metalloproteinases activate the neutrophil chemoattractant CXCL7 from intestinal epithelial cells. *Gastroenterology,* Vol.130, No.1, (Jan), pp. 127-136, 0016-5085 (Print)

Lawrance IC, Maxwell L, Doe W (2001). Altered response of intestinal mucosal fibroblasts to profibrogenic cytokines in inflammatory bowel disease. *Inflamm Bowel Dis,* Vol.7, No.3, (pp. 226-236,

Lohi J (2001). Laminin-5 in the progression of carcinomas. *Int J Cancer,* Vol.94, No.6, (Dec 15), pp. 763-767,

Lussier C, Basora N, Bouatrouss Y, Beaulieu JF (2000). Integrins as mediators of epithelial cell-matrix interactions in the human small intestinal mucosa [In Process Citation]. *MicroscResTech,* Vol.51, No.2, (10/15/2000), pp. 169-178,

Macdonald TT, Monteleone G (2005). Immunity, inflammation, and allergy in the gut. *Science*, Vol.307, No.5717, (Mar 25), pp. 1920-1925, 1095-9203 (Electronic)

MacDonald TT, Monteleone G (2006). Overview of role of the immune system in the pathogenesis of inflammatory bowel disease. *Adv Exp Med Biol*, Vol.579, pp. 98-107, 0065-2598 (Print) 0065-2598 (Linking)

Maki M, Collin P (1997). Coeliac disease. *Lancet*, Vol.349, No.9067, (pp. 1755-1759, 0140-6736

McKaig BC, McWilliams D, Watson SA, Mahida YR (2003). Expression and regulation of tissue inhibitor of metalloproteinase-1 and matrix metalloproteinases by intestinal myofibroblasts in inflammatory bowel disease. *Am J Pathol*, Vol.162, No.4, (Apr), pp. 1355-1360,

McKay DM, Baird AW (1999). Cytokine regulation of epithelial permeability and ion transport. *Gut*, Vol.44, No.2, (pp. 283-289,

Ménard D, Beaulieu JF (1994). Human intestinal brush border membrane hydrolases., In: *Membrane Physiopathology*, G. Bkaily, (Ed), 319-341, Kluweer Academic Publisher, Norwell.

Ménard D, Beaulieu JF, Boudreau F, Perreault N, Rivard N, Vachon PH (2006). Gastrointestinal tract, In: *Cell Siganling and Growth Factors in Development: From molecules to Organogenesis.*, K. Unsicker, Krieglstein K., (Eds), 755-790, Wiley-Vch:, Weinheim.

Otte JM, Rosenberg IM, Podolsky DK (2003). Intestinal myofibroblasts in innate immune responses of the intestine. *Gastroenterology*, Vol.124, No.7, (Jun), pp. 1866-1878, 0016-5085 (Print)

Pageot LP, Perreault N, Basora N, Francoeur C, Magny P, Beaulieu JF (2000). Human cell models to study small intestinal functions: recapitulation of the crypt-villus axis. *Microsc Res Tech*, Vol.49, No.4, (May 15), pp. 394-406,

Perreault N, Herring-Gillam FE, Desloges N, Belanger I, Pageot LP, Beaulieu JF (1998). Epithelial vs mesenchymal contribution to the extracellular matrix in the human intestine. *Biochem Biophys Res Commun*, Vol.248, No.1, (Jul 9), pp. 121-126,

Pinchuk IV, Beswick EJ, Saada JI, Suarez G, Winston J, Mifflin RC *et al* (2007). Monocyte chemoattractant protein-1 production by intestinal myofibroblasts in response to staphylococcal enterotoxin a: relevance to staphylococcal enterotoxigenic disease. *J Immunol*, Vol.178, No.12, (Jun 15), pp. 8097-8106, 0022-1767 (Print)

Podolsky DK (2000). Review article: healing after inflammatory injury--coordination of a regulatory peptide network. *Aliment Pharmacol Ther*, Vol.14 Suppl 1, pp. 87-93,

Powell DW, Mifflin RC, Valentich JD, Crowe SE, Saada JI, West AB (1999). Myofibroblasts. II. Intestinal subepithelial myofibroblasts. *Am J Physiol*, Vol.277, No.2 Pt 1, (pp. C183-C201,

Powell DW, Adegboyega PA, Di Mari JF, Mifflin RC (2005). Epithelial cells and their neighbors I. Role of intestinal myofibroblasts in development, repair, and cancer. *Am J Physiol Gastrointest Liver Physiol*, Vol.289, No.1, (Jul), pp. G2-7, 0193-1857 (Print)

Quaroni A, Beaulieu JF (1997). Cell dynamics and differentiation of conditionally immortalized human intestinal epithelial cells. *Gastroenterology*, Vol.113, No.4, (Oct), pp. 1198-1213, 0016-5085 (Print)

Riedl SE, Faissner A, Schlag P, Von Herbay A, Koretz K, Moller P (1992). Altered content and distribution of tenascin in colitis, colon adenoma, and colorectal carcinoma. *Gastroenterology,* Vol.103, No.2, (Aug), pp. 400-406,

Ruemmele FM, Russo P, Beaulieu J, Dionne S, Levy E, Lentze MJ *et al* (1999). Susceptibility to FAS-induced apoptosis in human nontumoral enterocytes: role of costimulatory factors. *J Cell Physiol,* Vol.181, No.1, (Oct), pp. 45-54,

Saada JI, Pinchuk IV, Barrera CA, Adegboyega PA, Suarez G, Mifflin RC *et al* (2006). Subepithelial myofibroblasts are novel nonprofessional APCs in the human colonic mucosa. *J Immunol,* Vol.177, No.9, (Nov 1), pp. 5968-5979, 0022-1767 (Print)

Sartor RB (2006). Mechanisms of disease: pathogenesis of Crohn's disease and ulcerative colitis. *Nat Clin Pract Gastroenterol Hepatol,* Vol.3, No.7, (Jul), pp. 390-407, 1743-4378 (Print) 1743-4378 (Linking)

Schmehl K, Florian S, Jacobasch G, Salomon A, Korber J (2000). Deficiency of epithelial basement membrane laminin in ulcerative colitis affected human colonic mucosa., Vol.15, No.1, (pp. 39-48, 0179-1958

Simmons JG, Pucilowska JB, Keku TO, Lund PK (2002). IGF-I and TGF-beta1 have distinct effects on phenotype and proliferation of intestinal fibroblasts. *Am J Physiol Gastrointest Liver Physiol,* Vol.283, No.3, (Sep), pp. G809-818,

Simon-Assmann P, Bouziges F, Freund JN, Perrin-Schmitt F, Kedinger M (1990a). Type IV collagen mRNA accumulates in the mesenchymal compartment at early stages of murine developing intestine. *J Cell Biol,* Vol.110, No.3, (Mar), pp. 849-857,

Simon-Assmann P, Simo P, Bouziges F, Haffen K, Kedinger M (1990b). Synthesis of basement membrane proteins in the small intestine. *Digestion,* Vol.46 Suppl 2, pp. 12-21,

Simoneau A, Herring-Gillam FE, Vachon PH, Perreault N, Basora N, Bouatrouss Y *et al* (1998). Identification, distribution, and tissular origin of the alpha5(IV) and alpha6(IV) collagen chains in the developing human intestine. *Dev Dyn,* Vol.212, No.3, (Jul), pp. 437-447,

Teller IC, Beaulieu JF (2001). Interactions between laminin and epithelial cells in intestinal health and disease. *Expert Rev Mol Med,* Vol.3, No.24, (Sep), pp. 1-18, 1462-3994 (Electronic)

Teller IC, Auclair J, Herring E, Gauthier R, Menard D, Beaulieu JF (2007). Laminins in the developing and adult human small intestine: relation with the functional absorptive unit. *Dev Dyn,* Vol.236, No.7, (Jul), pp. 1980-1990, 1058-8388 (Print) 1058-8388 (Linking)

Vachon PH, Durand J, Beaulieu JF (1993). Basement membrane formation and re-distribution of the beta 1 integrins in a human intestinal co-culture system. *Anat Rec,* Vol.235, No.4, (Apr), pp. 567-576,

Vallance BA, Gunawan MI, Hewlett B, Bercik P, Van Kampen C, Galeazzi F *et al* (2005). TGF-beta1 gene transfer to the mouse colon leads to intestinal fibrosis. *Am J Physiol Gastrointest Liver Physiol,* Vol.289, No.1, (Jul), pp. G116-128, 0193-1857 (Print)

Verrecchia F, Mauviel A (2002). Transforming growth factor-beta signaling through the Smad pathway: role in extracellular matrix gene expression and regulation. *J Invest Dermatol,* Vol.118, No.2, (pp. 211-215,

Wang F, Schwarz BT, Graham WV, Wang Y, Su L, Clayburgh DR *et al* (2006). IFN-gamma-induced TNFR2 expression is required for TNF-dependent intestinal epithelial barrier dysfunction. *Gastroenterology,* Vol.131, No.4, (pp. 1153-1163. ,

Warhurst AC, Hopkins SJ, Warhurst G (1998). Interferon gamma induces differential upregulation of alpha and beta chemokine secretion in colonic epithelial cell lines. *Gut,* Vol.42, No.2, (pp. 208-213,

2

Manning the Barricades: Role of the Gut Epithelium in Crohn's Disease

Erik P. Lillehoj[1] and Erik P.H. De Leeuw[2]
[1]Department of Pediatrics and
[2]Institute of Human Virology and Department of Biochemistry & Molecular Biology of the University of Maryland Baltimore School of Medicine, USA

1. Introduction

Crohn's disease is a chronic inflammation of the gut that affects an estimated 800,000 people in North-America alone. Crohn's disease most commonly affects the ileum, and to a lesser extent, the colon, however can be found throughout the entire gastro-intestinal tract (Shanahan, 2002). The cause of this disease is as yet largely unknown, despite tremendous progress in research efforts over the last decade. It is increasingly clear that inflammation and disease progression involves a complex interplay between the environment, host genes and microbes (Baumgart and Carding, 2007). Increasingly, and predominantly based on genomic analyses, involvement of components of the innate immune system have been recognized in inflammatory bowel disease (Baumgart and Sandborn, 2007). The first major susceptibilty locus that was identified for Crohn's disease was the IBD1 locus, encoding nucleotide oligomerization domain 2 or NOD2 (Hugot et al., 2001; Ogura et al., 2001). Various variations in genotypes and single nucleotide polymorphisms have been identifed in NOD2 that are strongly associated with Crohn's disease development (Economou et al., 2004; Lesage et al., 2002). In a recent genome-wide study, a total of 71 loci were identified to be associated with Crohn's disease, with the potential involvement of more genes (Franke et al., 2010). Among the genes identified were the autophagy-related 16-1 or *ATG16L1* gene and the interleukin-23 (IL-23) receptor gene. Autophagy is a mechanism that regulates protein degradation and is essential for immune balance. Disturbance of this mechanism may lead to inflammation or disease and therapeutic applications of manipulating this mechanism are under investigation (Fleming et al., 2011). The IL-23 receptor is a key feature of the Th17 subset of T helper cells which are a critical component of the antibacterial defense (Abraham and Cho, 2009). Both IL-17 and the IL-23 receptor ligand are currently targeted for therapy (De Nitto et al., 2010).
The epithelium of the gut is an important component of innate immunity. Epithelial cells perform an essential, yet selective barrier function, physically separating the gut lumen from underlying cells and tissues (Peyrin-Biroulet et al., 2008). This physical barrier limits the exposure of microbes and infectious agents to the underlying mucosal immune system, while at the same time allowing exchange and uptake of fluids and nutrients. More than a physical barrier, the gut epithelium actively participates in host defense. Epithelial cells

form a critical link between mucosal immunity and the microbial intestinal flora via germ-line encoded receptors and specific signaling pathways (Abreu, 2010; Koch and Nusrat, 2009; Wells et al., 2010). For example, epithelial cells from distinct lineages express NOD2 or ATG16L1, critical for recognition and clearance of intracellular microbes and linked to Crohn's disease as mentioned (Bevins, 2004, 2005; Kaser and Blumberg, 2011). Barrier functions of the gastro-intestinal tract is regulated by chemokines and cytokines released in underlying compartments as well (Zimmerman et al., 2008). The exact sites and mechanisms of how cytokines affect epithelial permeability is not known, however it involves mainly the Th1 cytokines tumor necrosis factor-α (TNF-α) and interferon-γ (IFN-γ). Therapy directed against these cytokines is currently widely applied in the clinic (Ford et al., 2011). Additionally, specialized epithelial cells have evolved in the gut that are critical in three areas: **1**) Goblet cells secrete mucins and are a source of trefoil peptides, important for mucosal repair (McGuckin et al., 2011); **2**) Paneth cells secrete antimicrobial peptides (Bevins, 2006; Ouellette, 2011); and **3**) M cells transport antigen and micro-organisms, thus sampling the gut lumen (Miller et al., 2007). In this chapter, we will discuss in detail the active barrier function of the indivdual cellular components of the intestinal epithelium in context of immune homeostasis and Crohn's disease.

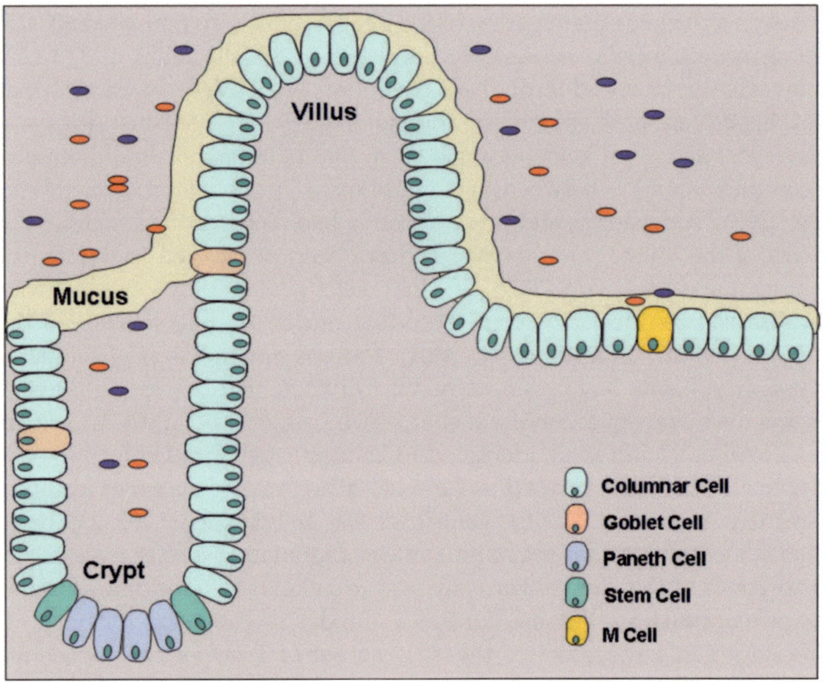

Fig. 1. Epithelial cells of the ileum.

The ileum is predominantly populated by columnar enterocytes or columnar cells which provide essential barrier function to the gut, separating the lumen from underlying tissue. Specialized goblet cells produce mucus, the first line of defence against microorganisms, but also microhabitat for bacteria. Paneth cells produce a host of antimicrobial factors resulting in a relatively sterile environment in the crypt base. Poliplurent stem cells continually self-replicate and differentiate to ensure high turnover rate of epithelial cells. M cells are optimized for antigen sampling and transport and are in close proximity with underlying components of adaptive immunity.

2. Goblet cells

Goblet cells are glandular simple columnar epithelial cells that are found scattered among the epithelia of the intestinal and respiratory tracts, as well as the urogenital, visual, and auditory systems. The primary function of goblet cells is to secrete mucin into the lumen of the gut and airways. The majority of the cytoplasm of goblet cells is occupied by secretory granules containing a variety of proteins that form the mucus layer upon granule exocytosis. Rough endoplasmic reticulum, mitochondria, nucleus, and other organelles are located in the basal portion of the cell. The apical plasma membrane of goblet cells contains microvilli to increase the surface area for secretion.

2.1 Mucus

Mucus comprises a visoelastic layer of fluid that plays an important defensive role against foreign environmental substances. Mucus covers all exposed epithelia of mammals, as well as the epidermis of amphibians and the gills of fish. In addition to trapping and removing foreign substances, mucus serves to lubricate the some epithelial surfaces, principally those of the gastro-intestinal tract. A layer of mucus along the inner walls of the stomach is vital to protect gastric epithelial cells from the highly acidic environment. The average human body produces about one liter of mucus per day (Thorton, 2008). Mucus consists of water, salts and various macromolecules, including mucins, proteinases, proteinase inhibitors, proteoglycans, and defensive proteins. In the latter category are proteins such as lysozyme, lactoferrin, and immunoglobulins. Proper concentrations of these components are required for the optimum function of mucus, and an alteration in the quality or quantity of the individual constituents of mucus may lead to pathological conditions.

2.2 Mucins

Mucins are the primary protein constituents of mucus (Lillehoj and Kim, 2002). These high molecular weight glycoproteins contain variable numbers of tandem repeats (VNTRs) in which serine, threonine, and/or proline residues are highly enriched. Serines and threonines are responsible for extensive mucin glycosylation that contributes to size and charge heterogeneity of the molecules. Glycosylation within the VNTR takes place between the serine/threonine moieties of the peptide backbone and N-acetylgalactosamine of the oligosaccharides, characteristic of O-linked glycoproteins. In addition, a limited amount of N-linked glycosylation between asparagines residues of the protein backbone and N-acetylglucosamine of the oligosaccharides also are present. Mucins can be broadly classified as either gel-forming/secreted mucins or membrane mucins. Gel-forming mucins are produced by goblet cells and account for the visoelastic property of the mucus layer as a result of protein cross-linking between mucin monomers. Cross-linking occurs following disulfide bonding between cysteine-rich D domains in the NH_2- and COOH-termini of the proteins. Membrane mucins are expressed in a polarized fashion on the apical surface of all epithelial cells. Eighteen mucin (MUC) genes have been cloned and the particular distribution of mucin gene expression varies by epithelial type. In the gastro-intestinal tract, 15 mucin glycoproteins are present (McGuckin et al., 2011). These include both gel-forming

(MUC2, MUC5AC, MUC5B, MUC7, and MUC19) and membrane (MUC1, MUC3, MUC4, MUC12, MUC13, MUC15, MUC16, and MUC17) mucins.

2.2.1 MUC2, the major gel-forming mucin of the intestinal tract

MUC2 is the major component of the secreted mucus barrier in the small and large intestines (Figure 2). MUC2 knockout mice spontaneously develop colitis, indicating that MUC2 is critical for colonic protection (Van der Sluis et al., 2006). The MUC2 gene product is a very large, greater than 5,100 amino acids in length, and contains two VNTRs with different amino acid sequences (Gum et al., 1994). The VNTR domain contains 50 -100 threonine/proline-rich 23 amino acid continuous repeats, while the second is composed of a 347 residue irregular and discontinuous serine/threonine/proline-rich repeat. MUC2 contains four cysteine-rich D domains, three located at the NH_2-terminus and the fourth at the COOH-terminus of the protein. This D domain organization is similar to that seen in von Willebrand factor, a glycoprotein involved in hemostasis. The MUC2 D domains contain a characteristic -cysteine-X-X-cysteine- sequence (where X is any amino acid) that mediates mucin oligomerization through disulfide bonding. The glycan moieties of MUC2 contain an equal fraction of neutral (40%) and sialylated (40%) residues with the remainder being sulphated (Karlsson et al., 1996). Mass spectrometry identified the sulfate group attached to C-6 of the N-acetylglucosamine moiety.

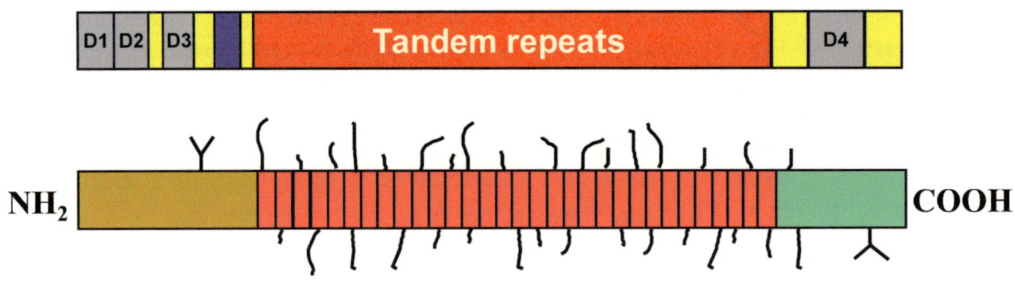

Upper, MUC2 cDNA. D1, D2, D3 = dimerization domains; yellow = cysteine-rich regions; blue = cysteine knot. Lower, MUC2 protein. Tan = non-repeat NH_2–terminal region; red = VNTRs; green = non-repeat COOH-terminal region.

Fig. 2. Schematic structure of MUC2.

2.2.2 MUC3, the major membrane mucin of the intestinal tract

MUC3 is the most abundantly expressed membrane mucin in the small intestine (Kim and Ho). Here, MUC3 expression on epithelial cells shows a maturational gradient with increasing expression from the crypt to villus. The MUC3 protein consists of two subunits, an extracellular region containing heavily O-glycosylated VNTR domains and two epidermal growth factor (EGF)-like domains. The EGF-like regions are separated by a SEA (sperm protein, enterokinase, and agrin) module, containing a proteolytic cleavage site during biosynthesis. A membrane-spanning, hydrophilic region that is responsible for incorporation of MUC3 into the lipid bilayer and an intracellular cytoplasmic tail (CT) with potential phosphorylation sites involved in signalling, lie distal to the SEA domain. The MUC3 ectodomain may be shed from the cell surface by the activation of membrane-associated metalloproteinases, by the separation of two subunits in the SEA domain, or by alternative splicing of its mRNA. Despite the mechanism involved, shed MUC3 contributes to the mucus gel overlying the intestinal epithelium. In mice, the cysteine-rich EGF-like domains inhibit apoptosis and stimulate cell migration, implying a regulatory role in maintaining the structure and function of the intestinal epithelial layer.

2.2.3 MUC1, a membrane mucin with signaling potential

MUC1 was the first mucin gene to be cloned (Gendler et al., 1990; Lan et al., 1990). Several studies have provided evidence that MUC1 plays a critical role in the intestinal tract. First, mice deficient in MUC1 expression have reduced amounts of intestinal mucus (Parmley and Gendler, 1998). Second, lack of intestinal MUC1 mucin in knockout mice impairs cholesterol uptake and absorption (Wang et al., 2004). Similar to MUC3, MUC1 consists of a large extracellular domain which is heavily glycosylated through N-acetylgalactosamine O-linkages, a single-pass transmembrane region, and a cytoplasmic CT (Figure 3). The MUC1 ectodomain serves as a binding site for pathogenic microorganisms, including *Pseudomonas aeruginosa* (Kato et al.; Lillehoj et al., 2001), *Helicobacter pyori* (Linden et al., 2004; Linden et al., 2009), *Campylobacter jejuni* (McAuley et al., 2007), *Escherichia coli* (Parker et al., 2010; Sando et al., 2009), and *Salmonella enterica* (Parker et al., 2010). During intracellular biosynthesis, the MUC1 ectodomain is autoproteolytically cleaved in its SEA domain to yield two noncovalently associated protein chains. The 72-amino acid CT domain of MUC1 contains 7 evolutionally conserved tyrosine residues. Many of these tyrosines are phosphorylated, leading to MUC1 interaction with receptor and cytosolic kinases as well as various adapter

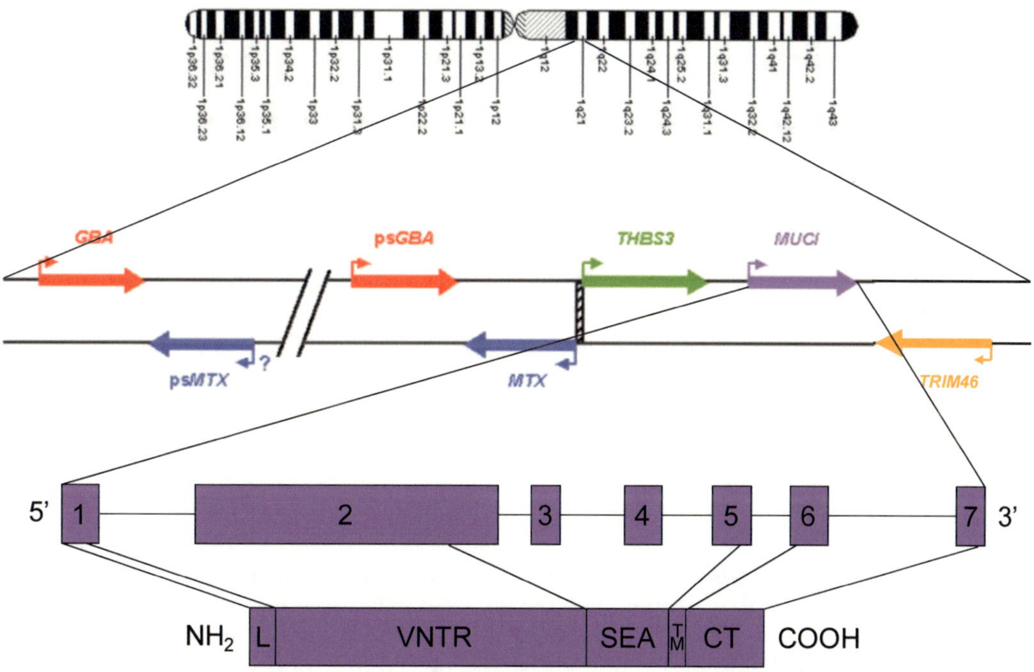

Upper, the MUC1 gene is located on chromosome 1q21 between the genes for thrombospondin 3 (THBS3) and tripartite motif containing 46 (TRIM46). Lower, the seven exon structure of the MUC1 gene and corresponding protein regions. L, leader peptide; VNTR, variable number of tandem repeats; SEA, sperm protein, enterokinase, and agrin; TM, transmembrane; CT, cytoplasmic tail.

Fig. 3. Genomic organization of MUC1.

proteins, including phosphoinositide 3-kinase (PI3K), Shc, phospholipase C-γ (PLC-γ), c-Src, and Grb-2 (Hattrup and Gendler, 2008; Theodoropoulos and Carraway, 2007). Binding of PI3K, c-Src, and Grb-2 to the CT have been experimentally verified, while Shc and PLC-γ are only inferred based upon the presence of the predicted amino acid sequence motifs. Other proteins bind to non-tyrosine sites, including glycogen synthase kinase 3β (GSK3β), protein kinase C-δ (PKC-δ), and β-catenin. Consensus sequences resembling an ITAM (immunoreceptor tyrosine-based activation motif) and ITIM (immunoreceptor tyrosine-based inhibitory motif) are also present in the MUC1 CT region. Estrogen receptor α (ERα), p53, p120ctn, ErbB1-4, adenomatous polyposis coli (APC), heat shock protein 70 (Hsp70), and Hsp90 also have been reported as binding partners of the CT, but specific amino acid residues have not been identified. Analysis of downstream signaling events indicated that the MUC1 CT activated a Ras → MEK1/2 → ERK1/2 pathway, but the mechanism is unclear.

2.3 Mucus proteoglycans

Proteoglycans are large molecular weight glycoconjugates characterized by variable numbers of glycan repeats (Meisenberg, 2006). The basic proteoglycan unit consists of a core protein with one or more covalently attached glycosaminoglycan chain(s) to a serine residue. The serine residue is generally in the sequence -serine-glycine-X-glycine-, although not every protein with this sequence has an attached glycan moiety. The chains are long, linear carbohydrate polymers that are negatively charged under physiological conditions, due to the occurrence of sulfate and uronic acid groups. As a result of the later modifications, proteoglycans are highly acidic in physiologic conditions allowing them to bind to cations, such as Na^+, K^+, and Ca^{2+}. Three types of proteoglycans were shown to be secreted into mucus by epithelial cells cultured *in vitro*, hyaluronic acid containing proteoglycans, chondroitin sulfate containing proteoglycans and heparan sulfate containing proteoglycans (Kim, 1985; Paul et al., 1988; Wu et al., 1985). While the physiologic roles of proteoglycans in mucus remain largely unknown, suggested functions include epithelial development, remodeling, inflammation, and host defense (Forteza et al., 2001; Huang et al., 1999; Ohkawara et al., 2000; Zhao et al., 1999).

2.4 Mucus proteinases and proteinase inhibitors

A number of proteinases are present in mucus, all of which known to be associated with inflammation and derived from inflammatory cells. Among these are elastase and various cathepsins from neutrophils and chymase and tryptase from mast cells. Neutrophil elastase has been shown to cause destruction of elastin (Snider et al., 1984), stimulate mucin release from goblet cells (Kim et al., 1987), and induce chemotaxis via production of IL-8 by the underlying epithelial cells ((Nakamura et al., 1992). Excess elastase released from neutrophils during injury and inflammation is balanced by several proteinase inhibitors, including α1-anti-trypsin, soluble leukocyte protease inhibitor (sLPI), and elafin ((Perlmutter and Pierce, 1989; Sallenave et al., 1993; Thompson and Ohlsson, 1986). Attenuated induction of sLPI and elafin has been reported in Crohn's disease (Schmid et al., 2007). Chymase and trypase are proteinases produced by mast cells, the former being responsible for disruption of the epithelial cell barrier allowing antigens and inflammatory mediators to enter the intestinal mucosa, while the latter is responsible for stimulating mucus secretion as well as TGF-β release from the extracellular matrix (Sommerhoff et al., 1990; Taipale et al., 1995).

2.5 Trefoil peptides

Trefoil peptides, or trefoil factors (TFFs), are a group of molecules that are characterized by having at least one copy of the trefoil motif, a 40-amino acid domain that contains three conserved disulfide bonds (Wong et al., 1999). Trefiol peptides are stable secretory proteins expressed in the gastro-intestinal tract. Their functions are not well defined, but they may protect the mucosa from insults, stabilize the mucus layer, and regulate healing of the epithelium. The close physical association between trefoil peptides and mucins supports these possible roles. The trefoil domain is found in a variety of extracellular eukaryotic proteins, including TFF1 (or protein pS), a protein secreted by the stomach mucosa, TFF2 (or spasmolytic polypeptide), a protein of about 115 residues that inhibits gastro-intestinal motility, and TFF3 (or intestinal trefoil factor, ITF). Other proteins with trefoil domains are *Xenopus laevis* stomach proteins xP1 and xP4, *Xenopus* integumentary mucins A.1 and C.1, *Xenopus* skin protein xp2, zona pellucida sperm-binding protein B (ZP-B), and intestinal sucrase-isomaltase. TFF1 and TFF3 contain one trefoil domain, TFF2 contains two domains, and the *Xenopus* proteins contain multiple copies. All three human proteins are clustered on chromosome 21q22.3. Overexpression of human TFF1 in mice was reported to reduce their susceptibility to dextran sodium sulfate (DSS)-induced colitis and TFF-deficient mice exhibited increased disease susceptibility (Mashimo et al., 1996; Playford et al., 1996). Unfortunately, however, these animal studies have not been translated into an effective clinical therapy (Mahmood et al., 2005).

3. Paneth cell

Paneth cells are specialized intestinal epithelial cells located at the base of ileal crypts in healthy individuals (Bevins, 2004; Ouellette, 2011). These cells are pivotal in maintaining the balance between the host and the microbiome. These cells act as sentinels for the detection of microbial molecules which are recognized by Toll-like receptors (TLRs), germ-line encoded receptors specific for bacterial and viral antigens. Genetic polymorphisms in these receptors and their signaling pathways affect Paneth cell function and have been associated with Crohn's disease (Inohara et al., 2005; Kobayashi et al., 2005). Paneth cell function is regulated by two additional mechanisms, the so-called unfolded protein response or UPR and autophagy, a process involved in clearance of intracellular microbes. The process of autophagy is induced by stress in the endoplasmatic reticulum (ER), which in turn is activated by UPR. Genetic mutations in proteins involved in both of these mechanisms have been linked to Crohn's disease as well. Variations in the autophagy protein ATG16L1 were identified in genome-wide studies and found to be associated with increased risk of disease development (Hampe et al., 2007; Rioux et al., 2007). Alterations in the gene encoding the UPR transcription factor protein Xbox-binding protein 1 or XBP-1 are signifiantly associated with inflammatory bowel disease in humans (Kaser et al., 2008). Further, loss of XBP-1 decreases the number of Paneth cells and thus the antimicrobial capacity of the intestine and leads to spontaneous enteritis in mice (Kaser and Blumberg, 2009; Kaser et al., 2008). Paneth cells are equipped with a vast arsenal of antimicrobial agents which are deployed following the recognition of potential microbial threats. These include enzymes, such as lysozyme , trypsin, phospholipase A2 and matrix metalloproteases, cytokines such as TNF-α and IL-17, as well as the bactericidal defensin peptides (Figure 4). In the following sections, we will discuss in detail the role of defensins as effectors of the innate immune system and their involvement in epithelial mucosal barrier function.

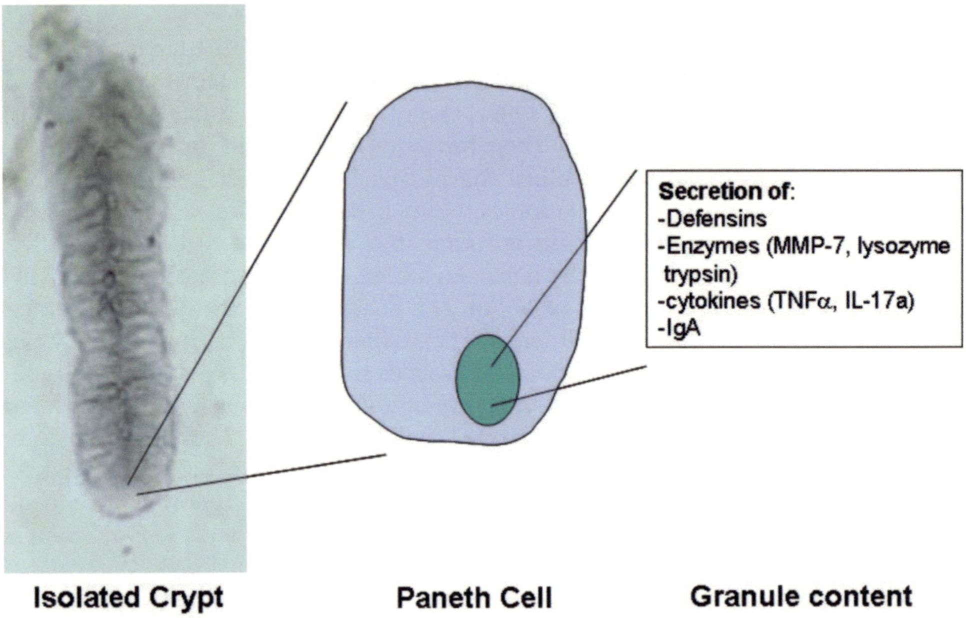

(Left) Light microscope image of isolated human ileal crypt. Paneth cells are localized at the base of the crypt as indicated. The box on the right lists confirmed compounds localized in dense secretory granules.

Fig. 4. Localization and cellular contents of Paneth cells.

3.1 Defensins

Defensins constitute a major family of antimicrobial peptides that play a protective role against microbial invasion of various epithelial surfaces, including the skin, respiratory tract and gastro-intestinal tract. Primarily, these small cationic peptides act as effectors of the innate immune system with the ability to kill a variety of microbial pathogens, including bacteria, fungi and viruses (Ganz, 2003; Zasloff, 2002). Based on a difference in disulfide connectivity of six conserved cysteine residues, defensins have been divided in two families, termed α and β. Both families are believed to have evolved from a common ancestral β-defensin gene (Patil et al., 2004; Schutte et al., 2002), and share similar tertiary structures despite low amino acid sequence identity (Hill et al., 1991; Pazgiera et al., 2006; Szyk et al., 2006). In humans, β-defensins are widely expressed in epithelial cells. Defensins of the α-family are expressed predominantly in neutrophils (termed human neutrophil peptides, or HNPs) or in ileal Paneth cells in the case of Human Defensin 5 and 6 (HD-5 and HD-6) (Porter et al., 2002; Selsted and Ouellette, 2005).

In addition to their antimicrobial activities, increasing evidence suggests that defensins play a significant role in innate and adaptive immunity. Such functions include chemoattraction and immune cell activation and promotion of cell proliferation, often involving interactions with cellular receptors (Aarbiou et al., 2002; Biragyn et al., 2002; Grigat et al., 2007; Yang et al., 1999). The capacity to chemoattractant monocytes was first described for HNPs (Territo et al., 1989). Subsequently, HNPs were shown to chemoattract different subsets of T lymphocytes and immature dendritic cells (Chertov et al., 1997; Yang et al., 2000). Similar functions were reported for β-defensins, which were shown to selectively chemoattract immature dendritic cells and memory T lymphocytes (Yang et al., 1999; Yang et al., 2001). More recently, β-defensins were shown to act as endogenous ligands for TLRs on immature dendritic cells directly. This interaction mediated signaling for dendritic cell maturation and triggered a polarized immune response *in vivo* (Biragyn et al., 2002). In the case of human β-defensin-2 (HBD-2), the observed chemotaxis of immature dendritic cells and memory T cells was shown to result from directly binding the chemokine receptor CCR6 (Yang et al., 1999). Subsequently, a murine β-defensin was shown to recruit tumor-infiltrating dendritic cell precursors through CCR6 also (Conejo-Garcia et al., 2004). In contrast to these earlier studies, it was reported recently that β-defensins chemoattract mast cells and macrophages but not dendritic cells and lymphocytes and that CCR6 was not involved (Soruri et al., 2007). Specific receptors for the chemotactic activity of α-defensins have not been identified. Several studies however have shown that also for α-defensins this activity is blocked by pertussis toxin, indicating the involvement of $G_{i□}$-coupled receptors (Chertov et al., 1996; Yang et al., 2000).

3.1.1 Alpha-Defensins and gastro-intestinal inflammation

There is increasing evidence that aberrant defensin expression is correlated to inflammation of the gastro-intestinal tract. A specific deficiency of the enteric α-defensin HD-5 was observed in patients suffering from ileal Crohn's disease (Wehkamp et al., 2005b). Interestingly, the HD-5 deficiency was more pronounced in patients carrying loss-of-function mutations in the cellular receptor NOD2, an intracellular receptor for the bacterial peptidoglycan component muramyl dipeptide (Inohara et al., 2005). NOD2 is predominantly expressed in the distal part of the ileum in a number of cell types including Paneth cells, which are the sole source of HD-5 (Bevins, 2006; Porter et al., 2002). In addition to recognition of bacterial ligands, NOD2 monitors the expression of enteric α-defensins. Genetic polymorphisms in the *NOD2/CARD15* gene have been identified to be tightly linked with susceptibility to Crohn's disease (Hugot et al., 2001; Ogura et al., 2001) and with decreased defensin expression.

A number of recent animal model studies have underscored the importance of NOD2 and defensin expression in relation to infection. Compared with wild-type mice, NOD2 deficient mice showed reduced expression of certain α-defensins, resulting in increased susceptibility to oral infection by *Listeria monocytogenes* (Kobayashi et al., 2005). Similarly, mice that lack mature cryptdins (the murine orthologue for α-defensins) are more susceptible to ileal colonization by non-invasive *Escherichia coli* (Wilson et al., 1999). Paneth cell expression of HD-5 rendered mice markedly resistant to oral, but not peritoneal, challenge with a virulent strain of *Salmonella typhymurium* (Salzman et al., 2003). Interestingly, HD-5 transgenic mice showed a striking loss of segmented filamentous bacteria and had fewer IL-17-producing lamina propria T cells (Salzman et al., 2010). These findings are in support of the notion that defensin deficiency may alter the microbiome, which in turn affects the adaptive immune response of the host. IL-17-producing T cells, however, were also observed in wild-type mice with functional defensins, in the specific absence of this class of bacteria. Additionally, HD-5 was shown to slightly improve mortality in lethal DSS-induced colitis in mice by intraperitoneal injection; however no effect on disease was noted when the defensin was administered orally (Ishikawa et al., 2009). This may suggest that HD-5 directly affects components of adaptive immunity in addition to affecting the microbiome.

A number of recent studies report on the role of ileal defensins in mucosal immunity and inflammation in humans. Single nucleotide polymorphisms in the gene encoding HD-5 have also been described recently in a New Zealand Caucasian population that may confer susceptibility to inflammatory bowel disease (Ferguson et al., 2008). Luminal processing of pro-HD-5 to its mature form was found to be impaired in Crohn's patients specifically (Elphick et al., 2008). As in mice, human enteric defensins HD-5 and HD-6 are synthesized as pro-peptides in Paneth cells and processed after secretion by trypsin in humans (Ghosh et al., 2002). In the majority of Crohn's disease patients, HD-5 appeared in a complex with its processing enzyme trypsin or chymotrypsin, thus rendering the peptide inactive (Elphick et al., 2008). Additionally, expression of HD-5 was markedly decreased in transplanted human small intestinal allografts (Fishbein et al., 2008). Rejection of allografts resembles Crohn's disease clinically and pathologically (Podolsky, 2002; Shanahan, 2002). Notably, decrease in the expression of HD-5 preceded visible damage to the intestinal epithelium. Finally, expression of both HD-5 and HD-6 was reported to be non-significantly decreased in active ileal Crohn's disease and decreased expression correlated positively with decreased *Vil1* expression, a marker for epithelial integrity (Arijs et al., 2009).

3.1.2 Beta-Defensins and gastro-intestinal inflammation

Impaired induction of β-defensins in the mucosal epithelium has been predominantly linked to colonic Crohn's disease (Fellermann and Stange, 2001; Wehkamp et al., 2002; Wehkamp et al., 2005a; Wehkamp et al., 2005c). The most widely studied β-defensin in the context of gut inflammation is human β-defensin-2 or HBD-2. Genetic polymorphisms (Fellermann et al., 2006), and especially gene copy number of HBD-2 (Fellermann et al., 2006; Hollox, 2008; Hollox et al., 2003), have been identified as risk factors in colonic Crohn's. More recently, expression of HBD-2 at both RNA and protein levels was found to be dysregulated in biopsies from colonic Crohn's patients (Aldhous et al., 2009). Interestingly, in this study, HBD-2 expression correlated with IL-10 production, irrespective of variations in HBD-2 gene copy number or variations in the HBD-2 promoter region. Additional studies on other members of the human β-defensin family emphasize their involvement in mucosal defense. Expression of HBD-1 was found to be protective in colonic Crohn's disease (Peyrin-Biroulet et al., 2010). Protective expression of HBD-1 occured via activation of the peroxisome proliferator-activated receptor (PPAR)-γ with rosiglitazone (Peyrin-Biroulet et al., 2010) or independently via a single nucleotide polymorphism in the HBD-1 gene promoter region (Kocsis et al., 2008). Two studies have reported on colonic Crohn's association of gene copy number of the gene encoding HBD-2, however with contrasting results (Bentley et al., 2010; Fellermann et al., 2006).

4. M cells

M cells, or microfold cells, are specialized epithelial cells of the ileum that have evolved to sample the gut lumen and relay this information to the underlying tissues. They are located in a region of the epithelium that is commonly referred to as the follicle-associated epithelium, or FAE, comprising the Peyer's patches and underlying lymphoid follicles (Figure 5). M cells exhibit microfolds, but not microvilli, and display a thin glycocalyx compare with absorptive enterocytes, making them more accessible to microbes (Gebert, 1996; Kyd and Cripps, 2008). Sensing and transport of microbes by M cells is facilitated by the expression of TLRs, integrins and microbial adhesion molecules such as galectin-9 (Kyd and Cripps, 2008; Pielage et al., 2007).

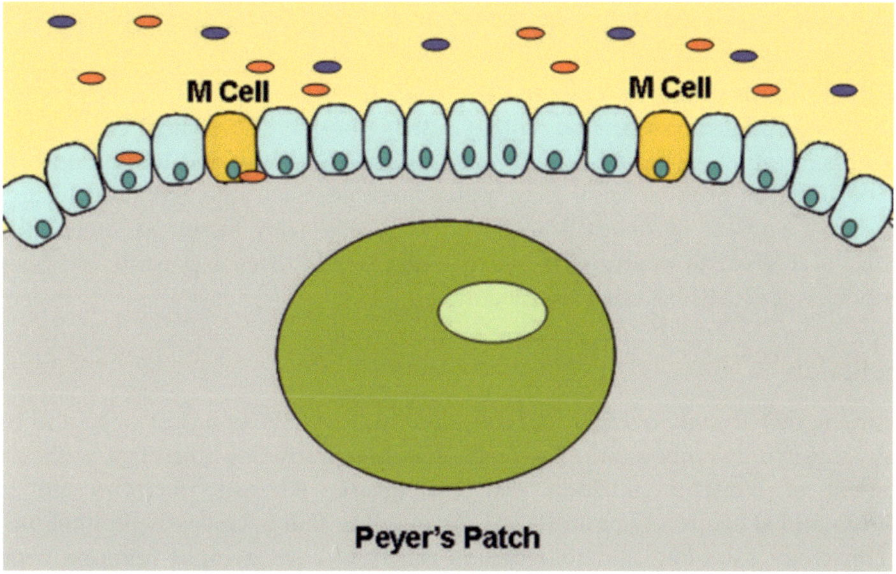

Microfold (M) cells specialize in antigen sampling of the gut lumen and act as a selective conduit to underlying components of adaptive immunity without compromising epithelial barrier function.

Fig. 5. Structure of the follicle-associated epithelium.

M cells do not harbor many lysosomes and do not express major histocompatibility (MHC) class II molecules, suggesting that most antigens that are transported are not degraded (Owen et al., 1986; Pickard and Chervonsky, 2010). Because of their relatively weak defenses compared with other sites of the ileal mucosa, M cells are exploited by pathogens as a potential entry site for infection. Such pathogens include EHEC and EPEC strains of *Escherichia coli* (Fitzhenry et al., 2002; Phillips et al., 2000), as well as *Shigella flexneri* and *Salmonella typhymurium* (Jensen et al., 1998). Viruses may also use M cells as a point of entry and specific receptors for HIV (Fotopoulos et al., 2002) and reovirus (Helander et al., 2003) on M cells have been identified.

4.1 M cells and gastro-intestinal inflammation

It is technically challenging to study human M cells *in vitro*, mainly because of the absence of clear cellular markers. Differentiation of enterocytes into M cells likely requires epithelial cell-T lymphocyte cross-talk as indicated by a co-culture model of these two types of cells (Kerneis et al., 1997). Most of our current knowledge on M cells and their role in gastro-intestinal disease comes from animal studies. Various models of chemically induced intestinal inflammation have been used to study M cells, the FAE and interplay with the underlying Peyer's patches. In an indomethacin-induced enteritis model in rats, M cell numbers increased initially and showed increased apoptosis in inflamed tissue only (Kucharzik et al., 2000; Lugering et al., 2004). In the DSS-induced model of colitis in mice, increased severity of disease was associated with lack of both Peyer's patches and lymph nodes, but not with mice lacking Peyer's patches only (Spahn et al., 2002). Three further studies emphasize the role of epithelial cross-talk with the underlying mucosal tissue at the FAE. The SAMP1/Yit mouse strain develops spontaneous ileal inflammation (Matsumoto et al., 1998). In this model, as well as in a water avoidance stress-induced rat model, early inflammatory lesions were observed in the FAE (Kosiewicz et al., 2001; Velin et al., 2004). Very recently, the FAE and M cells were shown to be targeted specifically by adhesive-invasive *E. coli* bacteria associated with Crohn's disease (Chassaing et al., 2011). The interaction between these bacteria and Peyer's patches of mouse and human was shown to depend on bacterial production of long, polar fimbriae. Such interactions may trigger the recruitment of subsets of dendritic cells or Th1 cells with increased potential for the production of TNF-α, as observed in mucosa of Crohn's disease patients (de Baey et al., 2003; Koboziev et al., 2010; Kudo et al., 2004).

5. Conclusion

It is becoming increasingly evident that intestinal health requires a controlled and balanced interplay between microbes and the host. The host provides microbes with a unique environment of constant nutrition and temperture, whereas microbes aid in food degradation and shape host immunity. In maintaining this balance, the epithelium stands guard, constantly sampling and relaying messages to elicit a rapid immune response if neccesary. At the same time, epithelial cells are continually self-renewing and differentiating to cope with the dynamics of this balance and have evolved into specialized, recognizable subsets. Together, these subsets form a selective barrier consisting of physical, chemical and biological components. In spite of harboring a tremendous arsenal of defensive agents, this barrier does have weaknesses which can be exploited by potentially harmful organisms. Some of these weaknesses have become apparent in an environment where the host is genetically predisposed. The inability of the host to timely recognize or eliminate microbes provides a window of opportunity for penetration of the epithlium, which may eventually lead to inflammation.

In addition to chemical drug treatment, biological therapy has proven its efficacy in treatment of active Crohn's disease. In particular, treatment to eliminate excess tumor necrosis factor alpha or decrease cell trafficking and adhesion by administration of monoclonal antibodies is clinically used in mild to severe cases. Both excess of tumor necrosis factor alpha as well as increased cell adhesion negatively affect the barrier function of the epithelium. Whether an epithelial imbalance is primarily caused by changes in innate or adaptive immunty is currently unclear and will likely vary between individuals. It is clear that disturbance of this delicate balance by environmental factors, pathogens or underlying genetic predispositions of the host may lead to inflammation. Clinically, an imbalance caused by one of these factors is often indistuinguishable from the other. For these reasons, having an understanding of the patients genetic background may help to determine the preferential clinical therapy. Restoration of epithelial barrier function will be an important goal of any therapy, either by strenthening the antibacterial capacity of the gut or by restoring the underlying inflammatory cascade. Additionally, as more and more is revealed about the "black box" which we refer to as the microbiome in the human intestinal tract, alternative approaches to restoration of immune balance may become apparent.

6. Acknowledgment

This chapter is dedicated to the loving memory of Johanna Cornelia de Leeuw-Snoeren. The authors would like to gratefully acknowledge the support of the Institute of Human Virology & the University of Maryland Baltimore School of Medicine. Research in the laboratories of Drs. Lillehoj and de Leeuw is supported by U.S. Public Health Service grants AI072291, AI083463 (EPL) and AI092033 (EdL). Dr. de Leeuw's work is also supported by an IHV Institutional Grant.

7. References

Aarbiou, J., Ertmann, M., van Wetering, S., van Noort, P., Rook, D., Rabe, K.F., Litvinov, S.V., van Krieken, J.H., de Boer, W.I., and Hiemstra, P.S. (2002). Human neutrophil defensins induce lung epithelial cell proliferation in vitro. J Leukoc Biol *72*, 167-174.

Abraham, C., and Cho, J.H. (2009). IL-23 and autoimmunity: new insights into the pathogenesis of inflammatory bowel disease. Annu Rev Med *60*, 97-110.

Abreu, M.T. (2010). Toll-like receptor signalling in the intestinal epithelium: how bacterial recognition shapes intestinal function. Nat Rev Immunol *10*, 131-144.

Aldhous, M.C., Noble, C.L., and Satsangi, J. (2009). Dysregulation of human beta-defensin-2 protein in inflammatory bowel disease. PLoS One *4*, e6285.

Arijs, I., De Hertogh, G., Lemaire, K., Quintens, R., Van Lommel, L., Van Steen, K., Leemans, P., Cleynen, I., Van Assche, G., Vermeire, S., *et al.* (2009). Mucosal gene expression of antimicrobial peptides in inflammatory bowel disease before and after first infliximab treatment. PLoS One *4*, e7984.

Baumgart, D.C., and Carding, S.R. (2007). Inflammatory bowel disease: cause and immunobiology. Lancet *369*, 1627-1640.

Baumgart, D.C., and Sandborn, W.J. (2007). Inflammatory bowel disease: clinical aspects and established and evolving therapies. Lancet *369*, 1641-1657.

Bentley, R.W., Pearson, J., Gearry, R.B., Barclay, M.L., McKinney, C., Merriman, T.R., and Roberts, R.L. (2010). Association of higher DEFB4 genomic copy number with Crohn's disease. Am J Gastroenterol *105*, 354-359.

Bevins, C.L. (2004). The Paneth cell and the innate immune response. Curr Opin Gastroenterol *20*, 572-580.

Bevins, C.L. (2005). Events at the host-microbial interface of the gastrointestinal tract. V. Paneth cell alpha-defensins in intestinal host defense. Am J Physiol Gastrointest Liver Physiol *289*, G173-176.

Bevins, C.L. (2006). Paneth cell defensins: key effector molecules of innate immunity. Biochem Soc Trans *34*, 263-266.

Biragyn, A., Ruffini, P.A., Leifer, C.A., Klyushnenkova, E., Shakhov, A., Chertov, O., Shirakawa, A.K., Farber, J.M., Segal, D.M., Oppenheim, J.J., *et al.* (2002). Toll-like receptor 4-dependent activation of dendritic cells by beta-defensin 2. Science *298*, 1025-1029.

Chassaing, B., Rolhion, N., de Vallee, A., Salim, S.Y., Prorok-Hamon, M., Neut, C., Campbell, B.J., Soderholm, J.D., Hugot, J.P., Colombel, J.F., *et al.* (2011). Crohn disease--associated adherent-invasive E. coli bacteria target mouse and human Peyer's patches via long polar fimbriae. J Clin Invest *121*, 966-975.

Chertov, O., Michiel, D.F., Xu, L., Wang, J.M., Tani, K., Murphy, W.J., Longo, D.L., Taub, D.D., and Oppenheim, J.J. (1996). Identification of defensin-1, defensin-2, and CAP37/azurocidin as T-cell chemoattractant proteins released from interleukin-8-stimulated neutrophils. J Biol Chem *271*, 2935-2940.

Chertov, O., Ueda, H., Xu, L.L., Tani, K., Murphy, W.J., Wang, J.M., Howard, O.M., Sayers, T.J., and Oppenheim, J.J. (1997). Identification of human neutrophil-derived cathepsin G and azurocidin/CAP37 as chemoattractants for mononuclear cells and neutrophils. J Exp Med *186*, 739-747.

Conejo-Garcia, J.R., Benencia, F., Courreges, M.C., Kang, E., Mohamed-Hadley, A., Buckanovich, R.J., Holtz, D.O., Jenkins, A., Na, H., Zhang, L., *et al.* (2004). Tumor-infiltrating dendritic cell precursors recruited by a beta-defensin contribute to vasculogenesis under the influence of Vegf-A. Nat Med *10*, 950-958.

de Baey, A., Mende, I., Baretton, G., Greiner, A., Hartl, W.H., Baeuerle, P.A., and Diepolder, H.M. (2003). A subset of human dendritic cells in the T cell area of mucosa-associated lymphoid tissue with a high potential to produce TNF-alpha. J Immunol *170*, 5089-5094.

De Nitto, D., Sarra, M., Cupi, M.L., Pallone, F., and Monteleone, G. (2010). Targeting IL-23 and Th17-cytokines in inflammatory bowel diseases. Curr Pharm Des *16*, 3656-3660.

Economou, M., Trikalinos, T.A., Loizou, K.T., Tsianos, E.V., and Ioannidis, J.P. (2004). Differential effects of NOD2 variants on Crohn's disease risk and phenotype in diverse populations: a metaanalysis. Am J Gastroenterol *99*, 2393-2404.

Elphick, D., Liddell, S., and Mahida, Y.R. (2008). Impaired luminal processing of human defensin-5 in Crohn's disease: persistence in a complex with chymotrypsinogen and trypsin. Am J Pathol *172*, 702-713.

Fellermann, K., Stange, D.E., Schaeffeler, E., Schmalzl, H., Wehkamp, J., Bevins, C.L., Reinisch, W., Teml, A., Schwab, M., Lichter, P., *et al.* (2006). A chromosome 8 gene-cluster polymorphism with low human beta-defensin 2 gene copy number predisposes to Crohn disease of the colon. Am J Hum Genet *79*, 439-448.

Fellermann, K., and Stange, E.F. (2001). Defensins -- innate immunity at the epithelial frontier. Eur J Gastroenterol Hepatol *13*, 771-776.

Ferguson, L.R., Browning, B.L., Huebner, C., Petermann, I., Shelling, A.N., Demmers, P., McCulloch, A., Gearry, R.B., Barclay, M.L., and Philpott, M. (2008). Single nucleotide polymorphisms in human Paneth cell defensin A5 may confer susceptibility to inflammatory bowel disease in a New Zealand Caucasian population. Dig Liver Dis. *40*, 723-730.

Fishbein, T., Novitskiy, G., Mishra, L., Matsumoto, C., Kaufman, S., Goyal, S., Shetty, K., Johnson, L., Lu, A., Wang, A., *et al.* (2008). NOD2-expressing bone marrow-derived cells appear to regulate epithelial innate immunity of the transplanted human small intestine. Gut *57*, 323-330.

Fitzhenry, R.J., Reece, S., Trabulsi, L.R., Heuschkel, R., Murch, S., Thomson, M., Frankel, G., and Phillips, A.D. (2002). Tissue tropism of enteropathogenic Escherichia coli strains belonging to the O55 serogroup. Infect Immun *70*, 4362-4368.

Fleming, A., Noda, T., Yoshimori, T., and Rubinsztein, D.C. (2011). Chemical modulators of autophagy as biological probes and potential therapeutics. Nat Chem Biol *7*, 9-17.

Ford, A.C., Sandborn, W.J., Khan, K.J., Hanauer, S.B., Talley, N.J., and Moayyedi, P. (2011). Efficacy of biological therapies in inflammatory bowel disease: systematic review and meta-analysis. Am J Gastroenterol *106*, 644-659, quiz 660.

Forteza, R., Lieb, T., Aoki, T., Savani, R.C., Conner, G.E., and Salathe, M. (2001). Hyaluronan serves a novel role in airway mucosal host defense. FASEB J *15*, 2179-2186.

Fotopoulos, G., Harari, A., Michetti, P., Trono, D., Pantaleo, G., and Kraehenbuhl, J.P. (2002). Transepithelial transport of HIV-1 by M cells is receptor-mediated. Proc Natl Acad Sci U S A *99*, 9410-9414.

Franke, A., Balschun, T., Sina, C., Ellinghaus, D., Hasler, R., Mayr, G., Albrecht, M., Wittig, M., Buchert, E., Nikolaus, S., *et al.* (2010). Genome-wide association study for ulcerative colitis identifies risk loci at 7q22 and 22q13 (IL17REL). Nat Genet *42*, 292-294.

Ganz, T. (2003). Defensins: antimicrobial peptides of innate immunity. Nat Rev Immunol *3*, 710-720.

Gebert, A. (1996). M-cells in the rabbit tonsil exhibit distinctive glycoconjugates in their apical membranes. J Histochem Cytochem *44*, 1033-1042.

Gendler, S.J., Lancaster, C.A., Taylor-Papadimitriou, J., Duhig, T., Peat, N., Burchell, J., Pemberton, L., Lalani, E.N., and Wilson, D. (1990). Molecular cloning and expression of human tumor-associated polymorphic epithelial mucin. J Biol Chem *265*, 15286-15293.

Ghosh, D., Porter, E., Shen, B., Lee, S.K., Wilk, D., Drazba, J., Yadav, S.P., Crabb, J.W., Ganz, T., and Bevins, C.L. (2002). Paneth cell trypsin is the processing enzyme for human defensin-5. Nat Immunol *3*, 583-590.

Grigat, J., Soruri, A., Forssmann, U., Riggert, J., and Zwirner, J. (2007). Chemoattraction of macrophages, T lymphocytes, and mast cells is evolutionarily conserved within the human alpha-defensin family. J Immunol *179*, 3958-3965.

Gum, J.R., Jr., Hicks, J.W., Toribara, N.W., Siddiki, B., and Kim, Y.S. (1994). Molecular cloning of human intestinal mucin (MUC2) cDNA. Identification of the amino terminus and overall sequence similarity to prepro-von Willebrand factor. J Biol Chem *269*, 2440-2446.

Hampe, J., Franke, A., Rosenstiel, P., Till, A., Teuber, M., Huse, K., Albrecht, M., Mayr, G., De La Vega, F.M., Briggs, J., *et al.* (2007). A genome-wide association scan of nonsynonymous SNPs identifies a susceptibility variant for Crohn disease in ATG16L1. Nat Genet *39*, 207-211.

Hattrup, C.L., and Gendler, S.J. (2008). Structure and function of the cell surface (tethered) mucins. Annu Rev Physiol *70*, 431-457.

Helander, A., Silvey, K.J., Mantis, N.J., Hutchings, A.B., Chandran, K., Lucas, W.T., Nibert, M.L., and Neutra, M.R. (2003). The viral sigma1 protein and glycoconjugates containing alpha2-3-linked sialic acid are involved in type 1 reovirus adherence to M cell apical surfaces. J Virol *77*, 7964-7977.

Hill, C.P., Yee, J., Selsted, M.E., and Eisenberg, D. (1991). Crystal structure of defensin HNP-3, an amphiphilic dimer: mechanisms of membrane permeabilization. Science *251*, 1481-1485.

Hollox, E.J. (2008). Copy number variation of beta-defensins and relevance to disease. Cytogenet Genome Res *123*, 148-155.

Hollox, E.J., Armour, J.A., and Barber, J.C. (2003). Extensive normal copy number variation of a beta-defensin antimicrobial-gene cluster. Am J Hum Genet *73*, 591-600.

Huang, J., Olivenstein, R., Taha, R., Hamid, Q., and Ludwig, M. (1999). Enhanced proteoglycan deposition in the airway wall of atopic asthmatics. Am J Respir Crit Care Med *160*, 725-729.

Hugot, J.P., Chamaillard, M., Zouali, H., Lesage, S., Cezard, J.P., Belaiche, J., Almer, S., Tysk, C., O'Morain, C.A., Gassull, M., *et al.* (2001). Association of NOD2 leucine-rich repeat variants with susceptibility to Crohn's disease. Nature *411*, 599-603.

Inohara, Chamaillard, McDonald, C., and Nunez, G. (2005). NOD-LRR proteins: role in host-microbial interactions and inflammatory disease. Annu Rev Biochem *74*, 355-383.

Ishikawa, C., Tanabe, H., Maemoto, A., Ito, T., Watari, J., Kono, T., Fujiya, M., Ashida, T., Ayabe, T., and Kohgo, Y. (2009). Precursor processing of human defensin-5 is essential to the multiple functions in vitro and in vivo. J Innate Immun *2*, 66-76.

Jensen, V.B., Harty, J.T., and Jones, B.D. (1998). Interactions of the invasive pathogens Salmonella typhimurium, Listeria monocytogenes, and Shigella flexneri with M cells and murine Peyer's patches. Infect Immun *66*, 3758-3766.

Karlsson, N.G., Johansson, M.E., Asker, N., Karlsson, H., Gendler, S.J., Carlstedt, I., and Hansson, G.C. (1996). Molecular characterization of the large heavily glycosylated domain glycopeptide from the rat small intestinal Muc2 mucin. Glycoconj J *13*, 823-831.

Kaser, A., and Blumberg, R.S. (2009). Endoplasmic reticulum stress in the intestinal epithelium and inflammatory bowel disease. Semin Immunol *21*, 156-163.

Kaser, A., and Blumberg, R.S. (2011). Autophagy, microbial sensing, endoplasmic reticulum stress, and epithelial function in inflammatory bowel disease. Gastroenterology *140*, 1738-1747.

Kaser, A., Lee, A.H., Franke, A., Glickman, J.N., Zeissig, S., Tilg, H., Nieuwenhuis, E.E., Higgins, D.E., Schreiber, S., Glimcher, L.H., *et al.* (2008). XBP1 links ER stress to intestinal inflammation and confers genetic risk for human inflammatory bowel disease. Cell *134*, 743-756.

Kato, K., Lillehoj, E.P., Kai, H., and Kim, K.C. (2010). MUC1 expression by human airway epithelial cells mediates Pseudomonas aeruginosa adhesion. Front Biosci (Elite Ed) *2*, 68-77.

Kerneis, S., Bogdanova, A., Kraehenbuhl, J.P., and Pringault, E. (1997). Conversion by Peyer's patch lymphocytes of human enterocytes into M cells that transport bacteria. Science *277*, 949-952.

Kim, K.C. (1985). Possible requirement of collagen gel substratum for production of mucin-like glycoproteins by primary rabbit tracheal epithelial cells in culture. In Vitro Cell Dev Biol *21*, 617-621.

Kim, K.C., Wasano, K., Niles, R.M., Schuster, J.E., Stone, P.J., and Brody, J.S. (1987). Human neutrophil elastase releases cell surface mucins from primary cultures of hamster tracheal epithelial cells. Proc Natl Acad Sci U S A *84*, 9304-9308.

Kim, Y.S., and Ho, S.B. (2010). Intestinal goblet cells and mucins in health and disease: recent insights and progress. Curr Gastroenterol Rep *12*, 319-330.

Kobayashi, K.S., Chamaillard, M., Ogura, Y., Henegariu, O., Inohara, N., Nunez, G., and Flavell, R.A. (2005). Nod2-dependent regulation of innate and adaptive immunity in the intestinal tract. Science *307*, 731-734.

Koboziev, I., Karlsson, F., and Grisham, M.B. (2010). Gut-associated lymphoid tissue, T cell trafficking, and chronic intestinal inflammation. Ann N Y Acad Sci *1207 Suppl 1*, E86-93.

Koch, S., and Nusrat, A. (2009). Dynamic regulation of epithelial cell fate and barrier function by intercellular junctions. Ann N Y Acad Sci *1165*, 220-227.

Kocsis, A.K., Lakatos, P.L., Somogyvari, F., Fuszek, P., Papp, J., Fischer, S., Szamosi, T., Lakatos, L., Kovacs, A., Hofner, P., *et al.* (2008). Association of beta-defensin 1 single nucleotide polymorphisms with Crohn's disease. Scand J Gastroenterol *43*, 299-307.

Kosiewicz, M.M., Nast, C.C., Krishnan, A., Rivera-Nieves, J., Moskaluk, C.A., Matsumoto, S., Kozaiwa, K., and Cominelli, F. (2001). Th1-type responses mediate spontaneous ileitis in a novel murine model of Crohn's disease. J Clin Invest *107*, 695-702.

Kucharzik, T., Lugering, N., Rautenberg, K., Lugering, A., Schmidt, M.A., Stoll, R., and Domschke, W. (2000). Role of M cells in intestinal barrier function. Ann N Y Acad Sci *915*, 171-183.

Kudo, T., Nagata, S., Aoyagi, Y., Suzuki, R., Matsuda, H., Ohtsuka, Y., Shimizu, T., Okumura, K., and Yamashiro, Y. (2004). Polarized production of T-helper cell type 1 cells in Peyer's patches in Crohn's disease. Digestion *70*, 214-225.

Kyd, J.M., and Cripps, A.W. (2008). Functional differences between M cells and enterocytes in sampling luminal antigens. Vaccine *26*, 6221-6224.

Lan, M.S., Batra, S.K., Qi, W.N., Metzgar, R.S., and Hollingsworth, M.A. (1990). Cloning and sequencing of a human pancreatic tumor mucin cDNA. J Biol Chem *265*, 15294-15299.

Lesage, S., Zouali, H., Cezard, J.P., Colombel, J.F., Belaiche, J., Almer, S., Tysk, C., O'Morain, C., Gassull, M., Binder, V., *et al.* (2002). CARD15/NOD2 mutational analysis and genotype-phenotype correlation in 612 patients with inflammatory bowel disease. Am J Hum Genet *70*, 845-857.

Lillehoj, E.P., Hyun, S.W., Kim, B.T., Zhang, X.G., Lee, D.I., Rowland, S., and Kim, K.C. (2001). Muc1 mucins on the cell surface are adhesion sites for Pseudomonas aeruginosa. Am J Physiol Lung Cell Mol Physiol *280*, L181-187.

Lillehoj, E.R., and Kim, K.C. (2002). Airway mucus: its components and function. Arch Pharm Res *25*, 770-780.

Linden, S., Mahdavi, J., Hedenbro, J., Boren, T., and Carlstedt, I. (2004). Effects of pH on Helicobacter pylori binding to human gastric mucins: identification of binding to non-MUC5AC mucins. Biochem J *384*, 263-270.

Linden, S.K., Sheng, Y.H., Every, A.L., Miles, K.M., Skoog, E.C., Florin, T.H., Sutton, P., and McGuckin, M.A. (2009). MUC1 limits Helicobacter pylori infection both by steric hindrance and by acting as a releasable decoy. PLoS Pathog *5*, e1000617.

Lugering, A., Floer, M., Lugering, N., Cichon, C., Schmidt, M.A., Domschke, W., and Kucharzik, T. (2004). Characterization of M cell formation and associated mononuclear cells during indomethacin-induced intestinal inflammation. Clin Exp Immunol *136*, 232-238.

Mahmood, A., Melley, L., Fitzgerald, A.J., Ghosh, S., and Playford, R.J. (2005). Trial of trefoil factor 3 enemas, in combination with oral 5-aminosalicylic acid, for the treatment of mild-to-moderate left-sided ulcerative colitis. Aliment Pharmacol Ther *21*, 1357-1364.

Mashimo, H., Wu, D.C., Podolsky, D.K., and Fishman, M.C. (1996). Impaired defense of intestinal mucosa in mice lacking intestinal trefoil factor. Science *274*, 262-265.

Matsumoto, S., Okabe, Y., Setoyama, H., Takayama, K., Ohtsuka, J., Funahashi, H., Imaoka, A., Okada, Y., and Umesaki, Y. (1998). Inflammatory bowel disease-like enteritis and caecitis in a senescence accelerated mouse P1/Yit strain. Gut *43*, 71-78.

McAuley, J.L., Linden, S.K., Png, C.W., King, R.M., Pennington, H.L., Gendler, S.J., Florin, T.H., Hill, G.R., Korolik, V., and McGuckin, M.A. (2007). MUC1 cell surface mucin is a critical element of the mucosal barrier to infection. J Clin Invest *117*, 2313-2324.

McGuckin, M.A., Linden, S.K., Sutton, P., and Florin, T.H. (2011). Mucin dynamics and enteric pathogens. Nat Rev Microbiol *9*, 265-278.

Miller, H., Zhang, J., Kuolee, R., Patel, G.B., and Chen, W. (2007). Intestinal M cells: the fallible sentinels? World J Gastroenterol *13*, 1477-1486.

Nakamura, H., Yoshimura, K., McElvaney, N.G., and Crystal, R.G. (1992). Neutrophil elastase in respiratory epithelial lining fluid of individuals with cystic fibrosis induces interleukin-8 gene expression in a human bronchial epithelial cell line. J Clin Invest *89*, 1478-1484.

Ogura, Y., Bonen, D.K., Inohara, N., Nicolae, D.L., Chen, F.F., Ramos, R., Britton, H., Moran, T., Karaliuskas, R., Duerr, R.H., *et al.* (2001). A frameshift mutation in NOD2 associated with susceptibility to Crohn's disease. Nature *411*, 603-606.

Ohkawara, Y., Tamura, G., Iwasaki, T., Tanaka, A., Kikuchi, T., and Shirato, K. (2000). Activation and transforming growth factor-beta production in eosinophils by hyaluronan. Am J Respir Cell Mol Biol *23*, 444-451.

Ouellette, A.J. (2011). Paneth cell alpha-defensins in enteric innate immunity. Cell Mol Life Sci *68*, 2215-2229.

Owen, R.L., Pierce, N.F., Apple, R.T., and Cray, W.C., Jr. (1986). M cell transport of Vibrio cholerae from the intestinal lumen into Peyer's patches: a mechanism for antigen sampling and for microbial transepithelial migration. J Infect Dis *153*, 1108-1118.

Parker, P., Sando, L., Pearson, R., Kongsuwan, K., Tellam, R.L., and Smith, S. (2010). Bovine Muc1 inhibits binding of enteric bacteria to Caco-2 cells. Glycoconj J *27*, 89-97.

Parmley, R.R., and Gendler, S.J. (1998). Cystic fibrosis mice lacking Muc1 have reduced amounts of intestinal mucus. J Clin Invest *102*, 1798-1806.

Patil, A., Hughes, A.L., and Zhang, G. (2004). Rapid evolution and diversification of mammalian alpha-defensins as revealed by comparative analysis of rodent and primate genes. Physiol Genomics *20*, 1-11.

Paul, A., Picard, J., Mergey, M., Veissiere, D., Finkbeiner, W.E., and Basbaum, C.B. (1988). Glycoconjugates secreted by bovine tracheal serous cells in culture. Arch Biochem Biophys *260*, 75-84.

Pazgiera, M., Hoover, D.M., Yang, D., Lu, W., and Lubkowski, J. (2006). Human beta-defensins. Cell Mol Life Sci *63*, 1294-1313.

Perlmutter, D.H., and Pierce, J.A. (1989). The alpha 1-antitrypsin gene and emphysema. Am J Physiol *257*, L147-162.

Peyrin-Biroulet, L., Beisner, J., Wang, G., Nuding, S., Oommen, S.T., Kelly, D., Parmentier-Decrucq, E., Dessein, R., Merour, E., Chavatte, P., *et al.* (2010). Peroxisome proliferator-activated receptor gamma activation is required for maintenance of innate antimicrobial immunity in the colon. Proc Natl Acad Sci U S A *107*, 8772-8777.

Peyrin-Biroulet, L., Desreumaux, P., Sandborn, W.J., and Colombel, J.F. (2008). Crohn's disease: beyond antagonists of tumour necrosis factor. Lancet *372*, 67-81.

Phillips, A.D., Navabpour, S., Hicks, S., Dougan, G., Wallis, T., and Frankel, G. (2000). Enterohaemorrhagic Escherichia coli O157:H7 target Peyer's patches in humans and cause attaching/effacing lesions in both human and bovine intestine. Gut *47*, 377-381.

Pickard, J.M., and Chervonsky, A.V. (2010). Sampling of the intestinal microbiota by epithelial M cells. Curr Gastroenterol Rep *12*, 331-339.

Pielage, J.F., Cichon, C., Greune, L., Hirashima, M., Kucharzik, T., and Schmidt, M.A. (2007). Reversible differentiation of Caco-2 cells reveals galectin-9 as a surface marker molecule for human follicle-associated epithelia and M cell-like cells. Int J Biochem Cell Biol *39*, 1886-1901.

Playford, R.J., Marchbank, T., Goodlad, R.A., Chinery, R.A., Poulsom, R., and Hanby, A.M. (1996). Transgenic mice that overexpress the human trefoil peptide pS2 have an increased resistance to intestinal damage. Proc Natl Acad Sci U S A *93*, 2137-2142.

Podolsky, D.K. (2002). Inflammatory bowel disease. N Engl J Med *347*, 417-429.

Porter, E.M., Bevins, C.L., Ghosh, D., and Ganz, T. (2002). The multifaceted Paneth cell. Cell Mol Life Sci *59*, 156-170.

Rioux, J.D., Xavier, R.J., Taylor, K.D., Silverberg, M.S., Goyette, P., Huett, A., Green, T., Kuballa, P., Barmada, M.M., Datta, L.W., *et al.* (2007). Genome-wide association study identifies new susceptibility loci for Crohn disease and implicates autophagy in disease pathogenesis. Nat Genet *39*, 596-604.

Sallenave, J.M., Silva, A., Marsden, M.E., and Ryle, A.P. (1993). Secretion of mucus proteinase inhibitor and elafin by Clara cell and type II pneumocyte cell lines. Am J Respir Cell Mol Biol *8*, 126-133.

Salzman, N.H., Chou, M.M., de Jong, H., Liu, L., Porter, E.M., and Paterson, Y. (2003). Enteric salmonella infection inhibits Paneth cell antimicrobial peptide expression. Infect Immun *71*, 1109-1115.

Salzman, N.H., Hung, K., Haribhai, D., Chu, H., Karlsson-Sjoberg, J., Amir, E., Teggatz, P., Barman, M., Hayward, M., Eastwood, D., *et al.* (2010). Enteric defensins are essential regulators of intestinal microbial ecology. Nat Immunol *11*, 76-83.

Sando, L., Pearson, R., Gray, C., Parker, P., Hawken, R., Thomson, P.C., Meadows, J.R., Kongsuwan, K., Smith, S., and Tellam, R.L. (2009). Bovine Muc1 is a highly polymorphic gene encoding an extensively glycosylated mucin that binds bacteria. J Dairy Sci *92*, 5276-5291.

Schmid, M., Fellermann, K., Fritz, P., Wiedow, O., Stange, E.F., and Wehkamp, J. (2007). Attenuated induction of epithelial and leukocyte serine antiproteases elafin and secretory leukocyte protease inhibitor in Crohn's disease. J Leukoc Biol *81*, 907-915.

Schutte, B.C., Mitros, J.P., Bartlett, J.A., Walters, J.D., Jia, H.P., Welsh, M.J., Casavant, T.L., and McCray, P.B., Jr. (2002). Discovery of five conserved beta -defensin gene clusters using a computational search strategy. Proc Natl Acad Sci U S A *99*, 2129-2133.

Selsted, M.E., and Ouellette, A.J. (2005). Mammalian defensins in the antimicrobial immune response. Nat Immunol *6*, 551-557.

Shanahan, F. (2002). Crohn's disease. Lancet *359*, 62-69.

Snider, G.L., Lucey, E.C., Christensen, T.G., Stone, P.J., Calore, J.D., Catanese, A., and Franzblau, C. (1984). Emphysema and bronchial secretory cell metaplasia induced in hamsters by human neutrophil products. Am Rev Respir Dis *129*, 155-160.

Sommerhoff, C.P., Nadel, J.A., Basbaum, C.B., and Caughey, G.H. (1990). Neutrophil elastase and cathepsin G stimulate secretion from cultured bovine airway gland serous cells. J Clin Invest *85*, 682-689.

Soruri, A., Grigat, J., Forssmann, U., Riggert, J., and Zwirner, J. (2007). beta-Defensins chemoattract macrophages and mast cells but not lymphocytes and dendritic cells: CCR6 is not involved. Eur J Immunol *37*, 2474-2486.

Spahn, T.W., Herbst, H., Rennert, P.D., Lugering, N., Maaser, C., Kraft, M., Fontana, A., Weiner, H.L., Domschke, W., and Kucharzik, T. (2002). Induction of colitis in mice deficient of Peyer's patches and mesenteric lymph nodes is associated with increased disease severity and formation of colonic lymphoid patches. Am J Pathol *161*, 2273-2282.

Szyk, A., Wu, Z., Tucker, K., Yang, D., Lu, W., and Lubkowski, J. (2006). Crystal structures of human alpha-defensins HNP4, HD5, and HD6. Protein Sci *15*, 2749-2760.

Taipale, J., Lohi, J., Saarinen, J., Kovanen, P.T., and Keski-Oja, J. (1995). Human mast cell chymase and leukocyte elastase release latent transforming growth factor-beta 1 from the extracellular matrix of cultured human epithelial and endothelial cells. J Biol Chem *270*, 4689-4696.

Territo, M.C., Ganz, T., Selsted, M.E., and Lehrer, R. (1989). Monocyte-chemotactic activity of defensins from human neutrophils. J Clin Invest *84*, 2017-2020.

Theodoropoulos, G., and Carraway, K.L. (2007). Molecular signaling in the regulation of mucins. J Cell Biochem *102*, 1103-1116.

Thompson, R.C., and Ohlsson, K. (1986). Isolation, properties, and complete amino acid sequence of human secretory leukocyte protease inhibitor, a potent inhibitor of leukocyte elastase. Proc Natl Acad Sci U S A *83*, 6692-6696.

Van der Sluis, M., De Koning, B.A., De Bruijn, A.C., Velcich, A., Meijerink, J.P., Van Goudoever, J.B., Buller, H.A., Dekker, J., Van Seuningen, I., Renes, I.B., *et al.* (2006). Muc2-deficient mice spontaneously develop colitis, indicating that MUC2 is critical for colonic protection. Gastroenterology *131*, 117-129.

Velin, A.K., Ericson, A.C., Braaf, Y., Wallon, C., and Soderholm, J.D. (2004). Increased antigen and bacterial uptake in follicle associated epithelium induced by chronic psychological stress in rats. Gut *53*, 494-500.

Wang, H.H., Afdhal, N.H., Gendler, S.J., and Wang, D.Q. (2004). Lack of the intestinal Muc1 mucin impairs cholesterol uptake and absorption but not fatty acid uptake in Muc1-/- mice. Am J Physiol Gastrointest Liver Physiol *287*, G547-554.

Wehkamp, J., Fellermann, K., Herrlinger, K.R., Baxmann, S., Schmidt, K., Schwind, B., Duchrow, M., Wohlschlager, C., Feller, A.C., and Stange, E.F. (2002). Human beta-defensin 2 but not beta-defensin 1 is expressed preferentially in colonic mucosa of inflammatory bowel disease. Eur J Gastroenterol Hepatol *14*, 745-752.

Wehkamp, J., Fellermann, K., Herrlinger, K.R., Bevins, C.L., and Stange, E.F. (2005a). Mechanisms of disease: defensins in gastrointestinal diseases. Nat Clin Pract Gastroenterol Hepatol *2*, 406-415.

Wehkamp, J., Salzman, N.H., Porter, E., Nuding, S., Weichenthal, M., Petras, R.E., Shen, B., Schaeffeler, E., Schwab, M., Linzmeier, R., *et al.* (2005b). Reduced Paneth cell alpha-defensins in ileal Crohn's disease. Proc Natl Acad Sci U S A *102*, 18129-18134.

Wehkamp, J., Schmid, M., Fellermann, K., and Stange, E.F. (2005c). Defensin deficiency, intestinal microbes, and the clinical phenotypes of Crohn's disease. J Leukoc Biol *77*, 460-465.

Wells, J.M., Rossi, O., Meijerink, M., and van Baarlen, P. (2010). Epithelial crosstalk at the microbiota-mucosal interface. Proc Natl Acad Sci U S A *108 Suppl 1*, 4607-4614.

Wilson, C.L., Ouellette, A.J., Satchell, D.P., Ayabe, T., Lopez-Boado, Y.S., Stratman, J.L., Hultgren, S.J., Matrisian, L.M., and Parks, W.C. (1999). Regulation of intestinal alpha-defensin activation by the metalloproteinase matrilysin in innate host defense. Science *286*, 113-117.

Wong, W.M., Poulsom, R., and Wright, N.A. (1999). Trefoil peptides. Gut *44*, 890-895.

Wu, R., Yankaskas, J., Cheng, E., Knowles, M.R., and Boucher, R. (1985). Growth and differentiation of human nasal epithelial cells in culture. Serum-free, hormone-supplemented medium and proteoglycan synthesis. Am Rev Respir Dis *132*, 311-320.

Yang, D., Chen, Q., Chertov, O., and Oppenheim, J.J. (2000). Human neutrophil defensins selectively chemoattract naive T and immature dendritic cells. J Leukoc Biol *68*, 9-14.

Yang, D., Chertov, O., Bykovskaia, S.N., Chen, Q., Buffo, M.J., Shogan, J., Anderson, M., Schroder, J.M., Wang, J.M., Howard, O.M., *et al.* (1999). Beta-defensins: linking innate and adaptive immunity through dendritic and T cell CCR6. Science *286*, 525-528.

Yang, D., Chertov, O., and Oppenheim, J.J. (2001). Participation of mammalian defensins and cathelicidins in anti-microbial immunity: receptors and activities of human defensins and cathelicidin (LL-37). J Leukoc Biol *69*, 691-697.

Zasloff, M. (2002). Antimicrobial peptides of multicellular organisms. Nature *415*, 389-395.
Zhao, J., Sime, P.J., Bringas, P., Jr., Gauldie, J., and Warburton, D. (1999). Adenovirus-mediated decorin gene transfer prevents TGF-beta-induced inhibition of lung morphogenesis. Am J Physiol *277*, L412-422.
Zimmerman, N.P., Vongsa, R.A., Wendt, M.K., and Dwinell, M.B. (2008). Chemokines and chemokine receptors in mucosal homeostasis at the intestinal epithelial barrier in inflammatory bowel disease. Inflamm Bowel Dis *14*, 1000-1011.

3

Genotyping of *CARD15/NOD2*, *ATG16L1* and *IL23R* Genes in Polish Crohn's Disease (CD) Patients – Are They Related to the Localization of the Disease and Extra-Intestinal Symptoms?

Ludwika Jakubowska-Burek et al.*
Department of Gastroenterology, Human Nutrition and Internal Diseases,
Poznan University of Medical Sciences
Poland

1. Introduction

Crohn's Disease (CD), together with ulcerative colitis (UC) belongs to inflammatory bowel diseases (IBD). Among its typical symptoms are inflammation, abdominal pain, melaena, diarrhea, ulcers and even fistulas. So far the etiology of CD remains unclear, but what is certain, is that it is multifactorial. Causing chronic inflammation and starting an immunological response requires both genetic factors, as well as environmental ones. What is more, CD is multigenetic - various genes could be a potential cause of the disease; among them are e.g. CARD15/NOD2, *ATG16L1 and IL23R (*Barrett et al., 2008; Cukovic-Cavka 2006, Cho 2008, Lesage 2002).

2. Aim of the study

The aim of this study was to investigate the polymorphisms in the *CARD15/NOD2* rs2066845 (p.Gly908Arg), *ATG16L1* rs2241879, *ATG16L1* rs2241880, *IL23R* rs7517847 and *IL23R* rs1004819 gene. Firstly, this research project focuses on determining whether there are any differences in the frequency of these polymorphisms among CD (Crohn's disease) patients and in the population group. Secondly, the aim of the study is to determine any

---

* Elzbieta Kaczmarek[2], Justyna Hoppe-Golebiewska[3], Marta Kaczmarek-Rys[3], Szymon Hryhorowicz[4], Marcin A. Kucharski[1], Ryszard Slomski[3,5], Krzysztof Linke[1] and Agnieszka Dobrowolska-Zachwieja[1]
[1] *Department of Gastroenterology, Human Nutrition and Internal Diseases, Poznan University of Medical Sciences, Przybyszewskiego 49, 60-355 Poznan, Poland,*
[2] *Department of Bioinformatics and Computational Biology, Poznan University of Medical Sciences, Dabrowskiego 79, 60-529 Poznan, Poland,*
[3] *Institute for Human Genetics Polish Academy of Sciences, Strzeszynska 32, 60-479 Poznan, Poland,*
[4] *The NanoBioMedical Centre, Adam Mickiewicz University in Poznan, Umultowska 85, 61-614 Poznan, Poland,*
[5] *Department of Biochemistry and Biotechnology, University of Life Sciences in Poznan, Wolynska 35, 60-637 Poznan, Poland*

correlations, or associations between the genotypes and alleles, and the localization of gastrointestinal and extra-intestinal symptoms of the disease.

3. Materials and methods

A total of 289 subjects took part in this study: 139 CD patients (60 women, 79 men) and 150 individuals in a population based control group (73 women, 77 men). All the patients were patients of Poznan University of Medical Sciences, Poland, Department of Gastroenterology, Human Nutrition and Internal Diseases. Moreover, all the subjects participating in this research project were adults, who had agreed to take part in genetic testing. The population group came from the DNA bank of the Institute for Human Genetics at the Polish Academy of Science. Genotyping was performed for all the investigated individuals. If obtaining reliable result was impossible, a given probe was eliminated from further analysis. That is why, the number of individuals in particular analyses may differ. In some cases, obtaining the data pertaining to the localization of the symptoms, as well as other co-existing symptoms was also impossible. Similarly, probes without an complete disease history were not included in further research.

Peripheral blood samples were collected on EDTA in the amount of 5 ml. Next, DNA was isolated from leukocytes, using the GTC (guanidine thiocyanate) and phenol-chlorophorm extraction method (Slomski et al, 2008). The isolates were dissolved in 1xTE buffer to obtain 500ng/µl concentration.

In the investigation of single nucleotide polymorphism (SNP) pyrosequencing was performed. A polymerase chain reaction (PCR) was performed for each probe with a set of primers: two for PCR, including a biothynylated one, and primer for sequencing. The sequences of the primers were designed with the use of computer software software dedicated to pyrosequencing (Table 1).

Primer	Sequence 5'→3'	Amplicon length in bp
ATGrs2241879_Fbiotin	gcttagctgcaggcctagaaa	152
ATGrs2241879_R	tggatactcatcctggttctgg	
ATGrs2241879-SEQ	ccacgcttgatatgg	
ATGrs2241880_F	ttacgaagacacacaaggcagtag	98
ATGrs2241880_Rbiotin	tgtctcttccttcccagtcc	
ATGrs2241880_SEQ	tttaccagaaccaggat	
IL23Rrs7517847_F	cctcttggttttcccatttca	292
IL23Rrs7517847_Rbiotin	tgaatttgaggggcctagga	
IL23Rrs7517847_SEQ	tttcacctattcccaag	
IL23Rrs1004819_F	tagcagcacaagcattctagga	125
IL23Rrs1004819_Rbiotin	actgacctgctttatgctgtga	
IL23Rrs1004819_SEQ	cttatgagaaatgcagatag	
CARD15_908_Fbiotin	gactcttttggccttttcagatt	243
CARD15_908_R	ccaatggtctttttccttactcc	
CARD15_908_SEQ	tcgtcacccactctgt	

Table 1. Primers used for analysis.

SNP	Analyzed sequence
ATGrs2241879	TA/GACAGAGCCTGGCAATTAAAGGGTCC
ATGrs2241880	GAGC/TATCCACATTGTCCTGGGGGACTGGG
IL23Rrs7517847	GCCG/TCAGCTACACCTGTATGTAGGCTAGA
IL23Rrs1004819	CAC/TAGTAAGAATCACAGCATAAAGCAGG
CARD15_908	TGCC/GCCAGAATCTGAAAAGGCCAAAAGAG

Table 2. Analyzed sequences. SNPs are marked.

SNP	Population group		CD patients		p
CARD15_G908R	Amount	%	Amount	%	
CC	139	93,9	136	91,9	ns
CG	9	6,1	11	7,4	ns
GG	0	0,0	1	0,7	ns
ATGrs2241879	Amount	%	Amount	%	
GA	39	55,7	75	48,7	ns
AA	19	27,1	48	31,2	ns
GG	12	17,1	31	20,1	ns
ATG16L1rs2241880	Amount	%	Amount	%	
TC	46	47,9	74	47,4	ns
CC	22	22,9	48	30,8	ns
TT	28	29,2	34	21,8	ns
IL23Rrs 7517847	Amount	%	Amount	%	
GT	51	53,7	75	48,7	ns
TT	33	34,7	62	40,3	ns
GG	11	11,6	17	11,0	ns
IL23Rrs 1004819	Amount	%	Amount	%	
TT	4	4,3	18	15,9	ns
TC	48	51,1	40	35,4	ns
CC	42	44,7	55	48,7	ns

Table 3. Genotype frequencies and statistical significance.

Statistical analysis was performed using the exact Fisher test and the test for differences between two frequencies (odds ratio - OR). A p-value of less than 0.05 was accepted as statistically significant.

Symptoms of CD can be localized in the area of the entire gastrointestinal tract (GIT), starting at the oral cavity and ending with the anus; however, extra-intestinal symptoms are also characteristic of this disease. The GIT symptoms were divided into: symptoms occurring in the oral cavity, esophagus, stomach and duodenum, small intestine, colon, and the presence of perianal fistulas. Extra-intestinal symptoms were divided into: arthralgia, uveitis, iritis, stomatitis aphtosa, erythema nodosum, fatty liver and elevated body temperature.

4. Results

4.1 Genotyping

The first aim of the project was to determine the differences in the genotype and allele frequencies, taking into consideration the two investigated groups of individuals: CD patients and the population group.

A statistical analysis of the genotypes did not reveal any significant differences in genotype frequencies (Table 3), but the allele analysis revealed that the frequency of alleles in ATG_rs2241880 and IL23Rrs7517847 differs significantly between the CD subjects and the population group (Table 4).

SNP	CD patients		Population group		p
CARD15_G908R	Amount	%	Amount	%	
G	12	7,55	9	5,66	ns
C	147	92,45	148	93,08	ns
ATGrs2241879	Amount	%	Amount	%	
G	106	46,29	51	46,29	ns
A	123	53,71	57	53,71	ns
ATG_rs2241880	Amount	%	Amount	%	
T	108	46,96	78	33,91	p=0,0775
C	122	53,04	68	29,57	p=0,0017
IL23Rrs7517847	Amount	%	Amount	%	
T	137	59,83	84	36,68	p=0,0011
G	92	40,17	62	27,07	p=0,0987
IL23Rrs1004819	Amount	%	Amount	%	
T	58	37,91	52	33,99	ns
C	95	62,09	90	58,82	ns

Table 4. Allele frequencies and statistical significance.

4.2 The correlation between genotypes and the localization of GIT symptoms

Symptoms were divided into: symptoms occurring in the oral cavity, esophagus, stomach and duodenum, symptoms displayed by the small intestine, colon, and the presence of fistulas. Genotype analysis and its relation to the localization of GIT symptoms revealed that the only polymorphism that is connected with localization of the disease symptoms in the Polish CD population is *IL23R* rs7517847, and which is related to the symptoms localized in the small intestine.

CARD G908R	oral cavity, esophagus, stomach or duodenum				small intestine				colon				perianal fistulas			
Geno-type	CC	CG	GG	Σ	CC	CG	GG	Σ	CC	CG	GG	Σ	CC	CG	GG	Σ
yes	4	1	0	5	40	3	0	43	50	6	0	56	22	0	0	22
no	73	6	0	79	36	4	0	40	26	1	0	27	55	7	0	62
Total	77	7	0	84	76	7	0	83	76	7	0	83	77	7	0	84
p	ns				ns				ns				ns			
Genotype compa-rison	ns				CC vs GG p<0.0001 CC vs CG p< 0.001				ns				ns			

Table 5. *CARD15/NOD2* G908R genotype analysis and its relation with the localization of GIT symptoms.

Statistical analysis did not indicate any significant discrepancies, but some tendencies were observed. A comparison of the genotypes proved that the CC genotype is statistically more frequent than the GG and CG ones, among patients suffering from enteritis.

ATG rs2241 879	Oral cavity, esophagus, stomach or duodenum				small intestine				colon				perianal fistulas			
Geno-type	GA	AA	GG	Σ	GA	AA	GG	Σ	GA	AA	GG	Σ	GA	AA	GG	Σ
yes	1	1	2	4	22	16	8	46	33	16	10	59	16	3	5	24
no	43	25	16	84	22	9	10	41	11	9	8	28	29	22	13	64
Total	44	26	18	88	44	25	18	87	44	25	18	87	45	25	18	88
p	ns				ns				ns				ns			
Genotype compa-rison	ns				GA vs GG p=0.005				ns				ns			

Table 6. *ATG16L1 rs2241879* genotype analysis and its relation to the localization GIT symptoms.

Genotype comparison revealed certain tendencies, i.e. that in the case of the *ATG* rs2241879 polymorphism, among CD patients with symptoms localized in the small intestine, the GA genotype is significantly more frequent than the GG one.

ATG rs2241 880	Oral cavity, esophagus, stomach or duodenum				small intestine				colon				perianal fistulas			
Geno-type	TC	CC	TT	∑	TC	CC	TT	∑	TC	CC	TT	∑	TC	CC	TT	∑
yes	2	2	1	5	23	15	9	47	35	15	11	61	14	4	6	24
no	44	24	18	86	23	10	10	43	11	10	8	29	33	21	13	67
Total	46	26	19	91	46	25	19	90	46	25	19	90	47	25	19	91
p	ns				ns				ns				ns			
Genotype compa-rison	ns				TCvsTTp=0.005				ns				ns			

Table 7. *ATG16L1 rs2241880* genotype analysis and its relation to the localization of GIT symptoms.

The comparison of genotypes suggests, that among CD patients with symptoms localized in small intestine, as far as the ATG16L1 rs2241880 polymorphism is concerned, the TC genotype is significantly more frequent than the TT one.

IL23R rs1004 819	Oral cavity, esophagus, stomach or duodenum				small intestine				colon				perianal fistulas			
Geno-types	TT	TC	CC	∑	TT	TC	CC	∑	TT	TC	CC	∑	TT	TC	CC	∑
yes	1	1	1	3	3	17	20	40	8	22	25	55	2	9	11	22
no	10	32	35	77	8	15	16	39	3	10	11	24	9	23	25	57
Total	11	33	36	80	11	32	36	79	11	32	36	79	11	32	36	79
p	ns				ns				ns				ns			
Genotype compa-rison	ns				TTvsCCp=0.005				ns				ns			

Table 8. *IL23R rs1004819* genotype analysis and its relation to the localization of GIT symptoms.

Genotype comparison showed that, among CD patients, in the IL23R rs1004819 polymorphism, the TT genotype is significantly more related to the localization of the symptoms in the small intestine than the CC genotype.

IL23Rrs 7517847	Oral cavity, esophagus, stomach or duodenum				small intestine				colon				perianal fistulas			
Geno-types	TT	GT	GG	Σ	TT	GT	GG	Σ	TT	GT	GG	Σ	TT	GT	GG	Σ
yes	1	2	0	3	23	15	7	45	24	28	7	59	11	9	3	23
no	36	37	11	84	14	23	4	41	13	10	4	27	26	30	8	64
Total	37	39	11	87	37	38	11	86	37	38	11	86	37	39	11	87
p	ns				p=0.0364				ns				ns			
Geno-type compa-rison	ns				TTvsGGp<0.0001 GTvsGGp=0.005 GTvsTTp=0.0161				ns				ns			

Table 9. *IL23R rs7517847* genotype analysis and its relation with the localization of GIT symptoms.

Statistical analysis demonstrates that the only polymorphism that can statistically be connected with intestinal localization of CD is rs7517847 in the *IL23R gene (p=0.0364).*
What is more, genotype comparison revealed that the TT genotype is significantly more frequent than the GG one in the case of CD patients, whose symptoms are localized in the small intestine; additionally, the GT genotype prevails over the TT.

	oral cavity, esophagus, stomach or duodenum			small intestine			colon			perianal fistulas		
CARD15 _908	G	C	Σ	G	C	Σ	G	C	Σ	G	C	Σ
yes	1	5	6	3	43	46	6	56	62	0	22	22
no	6	79	85	4	40	44	1	27	28	7	62	69
Total	7	84	91	7	83	90	7	83	90	7	84	91
p	ns			ns			ns			ns		
Genotype compari-son	ns			C vs G p<0.001			C vs G p<0.001			C vs G p<0.001		

Table 10. *CARD15/NOD2 G908R* allele analysis and its relation to the localization of symptoms in the GI track.

4.3 Correlation between alleles frequency and GIT symptoms localization

For each of the investigated polymorphisms, allele distribution analysis was performed, as well as an analysis investigating the correlations between particular alleles and the localization of the symptoms in the GI track. The results are presented in tables 10 – 14. None of the alleles seem to be significantly related with the localization of the GI track symptoms. However, genotype comparison revealed certain tendencies, which are presented in the tables below.

In *CARD15/NOD2 G908R* polymorphism, allele C was more frequent among patients with fistulas and symptoms in the area of the small intestine.

	oral cavity, esophagus, stomach or duodenum			small intestine			colon			perianal fistulas		
ATGrs 2241879	G	A	Σ	G	A	Σ	G	A	Σ	G	A	Σ
yes	3	2	5	30	38	68	43	49	92	21	19	40
no	59	68	127	32	31	63	19	20	39	42	51	93
Total	62	70	132	62	69	131	62	69	131	63	70	133
p	ns			ns			ns			ns		
Genotype comparison	ns			ns			ns			ns		

Table 11. ATG16L1 *rs2241879* alleles analysis and its relation to the localization of symptoms in the GI track.

	oral cavity, esophagus, stomach or duodenum			small intestine			colon			perianal fistulas		
ATGrs 2241880	T	C	Σ	T	C	Σ	T	C	Σ	T	C	Σ
Yes	3	4	7	32	38	70	46	50	96	20	18	38
No	62	68	130	33	33	66	19	21	40	46	54	100
Total	65	72	137	65	71	136	65	71	136	66	72	138
p	ns			ns			ns			ns		
Genotypes comparison	ns			ns			ns			ns		

Table 12. *ATG16L1 rs2241880* allele analysis and its relation to the localization of symptoms in the GI track.

	oral cavity, esophagus, stomach or duodenum			small intestine			colon			perianal fistulas		
IL23Rrs 7517847	T	G	Σ	T	G	Σ	T	G	Σ	T	G	Σ
yes	3	2	5	38	22	60	52	35	87	20	12	32
no	73	48	121	37	27	64	23	14	37	56	38	94
Total	76	50	126	75	49	124	75	49	124	76	50	126
p	ns			ns			ns			ns		
Genotypes compari-son	ns			ns			T vs G p<0.02			ns		

Table 13. *IL23R rs7517847* allele analysis and it's relation to the localization of symptoms in GI track.

In *IL23R* rs7517847 what was observed, was the tendency for the predominant presence of allele T in patients with a colonic manifestation of symptoms.

	oral cavity, esophagus, stomach or duodenum			small intestine			colon			perianal fistulas		
IL23Rrs 1004819	T	C	Σ	T	C	Σ	T	C	Σ	T	C	Σ
yes	2	2	4	20	37	57	30	47	77	11	20	31
no	42	67	109	23	31	54	13	21	34	32	48	80
Total	44	69	113	43	68	111	43	68	111	43	68	111
p	ns			ns			ns			ns		
Genotype compa-rison	ns			ns			C vs T p<0.04			ns		

Table 14. *IL23R rs1004819* alleles analysis and its relation to the localization of symptoms in GI track.

In *IL23R* rs1004819, what was observed, was the tendency for allele C, rather than T to be present more often in patients with a manifestation of the symptoms in the colon.

4.4 The correlation between the frequency of genotypes and the localization of non-GIT symptoms

The second part of this research project was devoted to the analysis of the relations between the genotypes and extra-intestinal symptoms. Extra-intestinal symptoms were divided into: arthralgia, uveitis, iritis, *stomatitis aphtosa,* erythema nodosum, fatty liver or elevated body temperature. The results are presented in tables 15-24.

	Arthralgia				uveitis				iritis				stomatitis aphtosa				erythema nodosum			
CARD G908R	CC	CG	GG	Σ	CC	CG	GG	Σ	CC	CG	GG	Σ	CC	CG	GG	Σ	CC	CG	GG	Σ
Yes	45	5	0	50	10	2	0	12	8	1	0	9	22	2	0	24	15	4	0	19
no	31	2	0	33	65	5	0	70	67	6	0	73	53	5	0	58	60	3	0	63
Total	76	7	0	83	75	7	0	82	75	7	0	82	75	7	0	82	75	7	0	82
p	ns				ns				ns				ns				ns			
Genotype compa-rison	CCvsCG p<0.001 CCvsGG p<0.001				CCvsCG p<0.03				ns				CCvsGG p<0.01 CCvsCGp<p <0.01				CCvsGG p<0.03			

Table 15. Analysis of genotypes and their correlation with the extra-intestinal symptoms.

A comparison of the genotypes revealed the tendency for the CC genotype to be the statistically predominant one in all the investigated cases.

	fatty liver				elevated body temperature			
CARD15 G908R	CC	CG	GG	Σ	CC	CG	GG	Σ
yes	4	1	0	5	35	6	0	41
no	71	6	0	77	40	1	0	41
Total	75	7	0	82	75	7	0	82
p	ns				ns			
Genotype compa-rison	ns				CCvsCG p<0.001 CCvsGG p<0.0001			

Table 16. Analysis of genotypes and their correlation with extra-intestinal symptoms.

Genotype comparison revealed the tendency for the CC genotype to be statistically more frequent than GG and CG ones among patients declaring elevated body temperature. Although, in our opinion, elevated body temperature cannot be treated as a symptom specific to CD (rather as a symptom related to the chronic inflammation), the decision was made to include it into the group of extra-intestinal symptoms, since it was mentioned as a symptom by the patients.

	arthralgia				uveitis				iritis				stomatitis aphtosa				erythema nodosum			
ATG rs2241879	GA	AA	GG	Σ	G A	AA	GG	Σ	GA	AA	GG	Σ	G A	AA	GG	Σ	GA	AA	GG	Σ
Yes	25	15	12	52	9	1	2	12	6	1	3	10	13	5	5	23	11	5	3	19
no	20	10	5	35	35	24	15	74	38	24	14	76	31	20	12	63	33	20	14	67
Total	45	25	17	87	44	25	17	86	44	25	17	86	44	25	17	86	44	25	17	86
p	ns				ns				ns				ns				ns			
Genotype comparison	GAvsAAp <0.01 GAvsGGp <0.01				ns				ns				ns				GAvsGG p<0.02			

Table 17. Analysis of the genotypes, and their correlation with extra-intestinal symptoms.

Genotype comparison showed the tendency for the GA genotype to be the statistically prevailing one among patients declaring joint pain and erythema nodosum.

	fatty liver				elevated body temperature			
ATG rs2241879	GA	AA	GG	Σ	GA	AA	GG	Σ
Yes	3	0	2	5	22	14	6	42
no	41	25	15	81	22	11	11	44
Total	44	25	17	86	44	25	17	86
p	ns				ns			
Genotype comparison					GAvsGG p<0.001			

Table 18. Analysis of the genotypes, and their correlation with extra-intestinal symptoms.

Genotype comparison showed a tendency for the GA genotype to be statistically more frequent than GG genotype in patients declaring an elevated body temperature.

ATG rs2241 880	arthralgia				uveitis				iritis				stomatitis aphtosa				erythema nodosum			
	TC	CC	TT	Σ	TC	CC	TT	Σ	TC	CC	TT	Σ	TC	CC	TT	Σ	TC	CC	TT	Σ
yes	27	15	12	54	8	1	3	12	5	1	4	10	13	6	6	25	12	5	4	21
no	20	10	6	36	38	24	15	77	41	24	14	79	33	19	12	64	34	20	14	68
Total	47	25	18	90	46	25	18	89	46	25	18	89	46	25	18	89	46	25	18	89
p	ns				ns				ns				ns				ns			
Genotype comparison	TCvsTT p<0.01 TCvsCC p<0.01				ns				ns				ns				TCvsTT p<0.04			

Table 19. Analysis of the genotypes, and their correlation with extra-intestinal symptoms.

Genotype comparison showed that in patients complaining of joint pain and erythema nodosum, the TC genotype was statistically the most common one.

ATG rs2241880	fatty liver				elevated body temperature			
	TC	CC	TT	∑	TC	CC	TT	∑
Yes	3	0	2	5	22	14	8	44
no	43	25	16	84	24	11	10	45
Total	46	25	18	89	46	25	18	89
p	ns				ns			
Genotype comparison	ns				TCvsTT p<0.01			

Table 20. Analysis of the genotypes, and their correlation with extra-intestinal symptoms.

The TC genotype was more frequent than the TT one among patients with an elevated body temperature.

	arthralgia				uveitis				iritis				stomatitis aphtosa				erythema nodosum			
IL23R rs7517 847	TT	GT	GG	∑	TT	GT	GG	∑	TT	GT	GG	∑	TT	GT	GG	∑	TT	GT	GG	∑
yes	24	21	8	53	7	3	2	12	4	5	1	10	10	10	4	24	6	8	5	19
no	12	18	3	33	28	36	9	73	31	34	10	75	25	29	7	61	29	31	6	66
Total	36	39	11	86	35	39	11	85	35	39	11	85	35	39	11	85	35	39	11	85
p	ns				ns				ns				ns				ns			
Genotype compa-rison	TTvsGG p<0.01 GTvs GGp<0.01				ns				ns				ns				ns			

Table 21. Analysis of genotypes, and their correlation with extra-intestinal symptoms.

Genotype comparison showed two tendencies: in patients complaining of joint pain, the TT genotype was statistically more frequent than the GG one, but GT was more frequent than GG.

	fatty liver				elevated body temperature			
IL23R rs7517847	TT	GT	GG	∑	TT	GT	GG	∑
yes	2	3	0	5	22	14	5	41
no	33	36	11	80	13	25	6	44
Total	35	39	11	85	35	39	11	85
p	ns				ns			
Genotype comparison	ns				TTvsGG p<0.03 GTvsGG p<0.01			

Table 22. Analysis of the genotypes, and their correlation with extra-intestinal symptoms.

Again, an elevated body temperature was related to the presence of the TT but not the GG genotype, as well as the GT but not GG genotype. However, as it was mentioned above, we do not believe it should be associated with CD specifically.

	arthralgia				uveitis				iritis				stomatitis aphtosa				erythema nodosum			
IL23R rs1004 819	TT	TC	CC	Σ	TT	TC	CC	Σ	TT	TC	CC	Σ	TT	TC	CC	Σ	TT	TC	CC	Σ
Yes	8	19	19	46	3	3	6	12	2	4	3	9	5	7	11	23	2	4	13	19
no	3	13	17	33	8	29	30	67	9	28	33	70	6	25	25	56	9	28	23	60
Total	11	32	36	79	11	32	36	79	11	32	36	79	11	32	36	79	11	32	36	79
p	ns				ns				ns				ns				ns			
Genotype compari-son	ns				ns				ns				ns				TTvsCC p<0.03 TCvsCC p<0.03			

Table 23. Analysis of the genotypes, and their correlation with extra-intestinal symptoms.

Patients with erythema nodosum showed the tendency for statistically prevalent TT and TC genotypes.

	fatty liver				elevated body temperature			
IL23R rs1004819	TT	TC	CC	Σ	TT	TC	CC	Σ
Yes	2	2	1	5	8	11	18	37
no	9	30	35	74	3	21	18	42
Total	11	32	36	79	11	32	36	79
p	ns				P=0.078			
Genotype comparison	ns				CCvsTT p<0.03			

Table 24. Analysis of the genotypes and their correlation with extra-intestinal symptoms.

A comparison of the genotypes revealed the tendency for the CC genotype to be statistically more frequent than the TT one in patients declaring elevated body temperature.

4.5 The correlation between allele frequency and the localization of non-GIT symptoms

The analysis of allele frequency in exact polymorphisms among CD patients was correlated with extra-intestinal symptoms. Although no significant results were obtained, some interesting tendencies have been observed. The results are presented in table 25.

	arthralgia		Uveitis		iritis		stomatitis aphtosa		Erythema nodosum		Fatty liver		Elevated body tempera-ture	
CARD15 G908R	**C**	**G**	**C**	**G**	**C**	**G**	**C**	**G**	**C**	**G**	**C**	**G**	**C**	**G**
no	33	2	70	5	73	6	58	5	63	3	77	6	58	5
yes	50	5	12	0	9	1	24	2	19	4	5	1	24	2
p	ns		ns		ns		ns		ns		ns		ns	
Alleles compa-rison	C vs G p<0.001		ns		ns		ns		ns		ns		C vs G p<0.01	
ATG rs2241879	**A**	**G**	**A**	**G**	**A**	**G**	**A**	**G**	**A**	**G**	**A**	**G**	**A**	**G**
yes	40	37	59	40	62	52	51	43	53	47	66	56	33	33
no	30	25	10	11	7	9	18	18	16	14	3	5	36	28
p	ns		ns		ns		ns		ns		ns		ns	
Alleles compa-rison	ns		ns		ns		ns		ns		ns		ns	
ATG rs2241880	**T**	**C**	**T**	**C**	**T**	**C**	**T**	**C**	**T**	**C**	**T**	**C**	**T**	**C**
yes	39	42	53	62	55	65	55	52	48	54	59	68	34	35
no	26	30	11	9	9	6	19	19	16	17	5	3	30	36
p	ns		ns		ns		ns		ns		ns		ns	
Alleles compa-rison	ns		ns		ns		ns		ns		ns		ns	
IL23R rs7517847	**T**	**G**	**T**	**G**	**T**	**G**	**T**	**G**	**T**	**G**	**T**	**G**	**T**	**G**
yes	45	29	64	45	65	44	54	36	60	37	69	47	38	31
no	40	21	10	5	9	6	20	14	14	13	5	3	36	19
p	ns		ns		ns		ns		ns		ns		ns	
Alleles compa-rison	T vs G p< 0.04		ns		ns		ns		ns		ns		ns	
IL23R rs1004819	**T**	**C**	**T**	**C**	**T**	**C**	**T**	**C**	**T**	**C**	**T**	**C**	**T**	**C**
yes	27	38	37	59	37	61	31	50	37	51	39	65	24	39

no	16	30	6	9	6	7	12	18	6	17	4	3	19	29
p	ns		ns		ns		ns		ns		ns		ns	
Alleles compa-rison	ns		ns		ns		ns		ns		ns		ns	

Table 25. Correlation between allele frequency and the localization of non-GIT symptoms

5. Discussion

Crohn's Disease (CD) has been known to physicians for many decades. In 1904 Antoni Leśniowski, already tried to characterize the disease, and in later years his efforts were undertaken by many other researchers. Unfortunately, up to this day we know very little about CD. There are numerous descriptions of clinical cases presenting different localization of disease symptoms, descriptions of symptoms localized solely in the digestive tract, as well as symptoms accompanying the disease, typical for CD, but not necessarily associated with the digestive tract. Since the second half of XX century it has also been known that CD is conditioned by genetic factors. However, these do not act independently, but instead need to overlap with immunological and environmental factors, resulting in an onset of the disease. All this information sheds much light on the etiology of inflammatory bowel disease (IBD), including CD, but does not entirely solve the puzzle constituted by this complex condition. Genetic research initiated by the discovery of the IBD1 region, and later the CARD15/NOD2 gene lying in its vicinity, appears to have provided answers to the numerous questions and doubts of researchers: What is the cause of CD? What increases the risk of the disease developing and what is the protective factor? Why is its clinical picture so diverse and complex, and what is it determined by? Is it hereditary and if so how? It quickly became clear that what seemed to have provided the answer and cleared all doubts, only opened new perspectives for ascertaining the possible causes of CD, but still did not solve the problem. Today CD is thought to be polygenic, which means that complicated dependencies related to numerous genes lie at its basis. Until recently, it was assumed that a group of 40 genes are involved as possible determinants of the disease, but the most recent findings point to a number twice as large.

While planning this research project, the idea which emerged, was to research the genotype distribution within the human genome, amongst Polish patients diagnosed with Crohn's disease. Although the clinical course might be similar everywhere, research as to the genetic factors underlying CD differs depending on the population which patient stems from. Consequently, we decided to define the span of genotypes and alleles for the Polish population. What is more, having the information about the clinical course of the disease, it seemed interesting to study whether any dependencies exist between a particular genome and the clinical course, as well as localization of the disease symptoms.

Recently, some information surfaced related o the dependency between the localization of the disease symptoms and the particular genotypes. The latest of these studies, (Jurgens et al., 2010), carried out by German researchers on patients with CD, showed that there is a clear dependency between the presence of homozygotic mutations in the CARD15/NOD2 gene and the occurrence of fistulas and simultaneously post-inflammatory intestinal strictures. As part of the research work span of this project, a single change of the SNP type

(G908R) in CARD15/NOD2 gene was studied. However, it did not show a statistically significant change in the frequency of occurrence of particular genotypes and alleles in the patient group, as compared to the healthy population. None the less, certain tendencies were observed, which pointed to a relation between the presence of the CC genotype iand an intestinal localization of the disease (both the small intestine, as well as the colon). Our research also confirmed the association of perianal fistulas with the presence of the CC genotype, in this respect, confirmed the results of the above-mentioned German research project. What is more, our studies also indicated certain tendencies with respect to the occurrence of specific disease symptoms not related to the gastrointestinal tract, such as joint pain, iritis, erythema nodosum, or aphtous ulcerations in the mouth (these symptoms were predominant in patients with the CC genotype). This aspect of the research presented here seems to supplement our current knowledge in an interesting way, as it has not been taken into account in the German study and therefore is in itself innovative and unique.

In this research project two polymorphic changes, located in the IL23R gene (IL23Rrs7517847, as well as IL23Rrs1004819) were analyzed. In the case of the former, statistically significant changes were observed in the frequency of occurrence of the alleles, as compared with the population group (allele T p=0,0011, allele G p=0,0987). This points to the fact that polymorphism IL23Rrs7517847 can be associated with an increased risk of morbidity in significant way. Studies conducted as part of this research project demonstrated the tendency for the development of the disease related changes in the small intestine and colon. Similarly, for IL23Rrs7517847, the TT genotype was significantly more frequent in patients with intestinal changes, while the TG genotype was most frequent in the case of changes within the colon. Although our research does not show any significant association of the IL23R gene with the occurrence of fistulas, it does bear out the results of the German publication cited above.

Another study on the relation between the CARD15/NOD2 gene with the course of the disease is the one conducted on a Croatian group of patients from 2006 (Cukovic-Cavka et al., 2006). They reported that mutations in the CARD15/NOD2 gene were associated with an increased risk of developing CD, and were also responsible for an earlier diagnosis on the disease (the patients were diagnosed at an earlier age) as well as the need for surgical intervention (a more severe disease course). As part of the research conducted on Croatian patients three most common mutations/polymorphisms (Arg702Trp, Gly908Arg, Leu1007fsinsC) occurring in CARD15/NOD2 gene were studied. The research published by Annese i et al. (2005) corroborates the results of the work published above and proves that the existence of even one of the key mutations/polymorphisms is responsible for an aggressive course of the disease. Possibly, because only one analysis, of the mentioned polymorphisms - Gly908Arg –was planned in the project no similar dependence was shown. According to the literature data, the largest impact as far as increasing the risk of developing CD is concerned, as well as a more severe course of the disease is caused by insertional mutation. Although it was not studied as part of this research project as of yet, we do plan to carry out research focussing on this aspect in the future.

Another publication, which confirms the association of the CARD15/NOD2 gene with the clinical symptoms of the disease, is a study by Mendoza et al. from 2003 who scrutinized this dependence in the Spanish population. One aspect makes it particularly interesting; not only does this research point to the influence of the three main SNP changes in the CARD15/NOD2 gene on the occurrence of the intestinal disease symptoms, but also proves that carriers of the G908R mutation show a disease type characterized by intestinal strictures, which additionally requires more frequent surgical interventions, including appendectomy. The results of the study presented here do confirm the Spanish data pertaining to the association of G908R mutation with the intestinal localization of the disease; however, the remaining aspects discussed by Mendoza et. al. are not analyzed in this project, and, therefore, cannot be compared. The need for more frequent surgical intervention associated with the presence of a CARD15/NOD2 gene mutation, was also confirmed in 2010, when pediatric cases of CD were analyzed (Lacher et al., 2010). It was discovered that in the case of children under the age of 17, surgical interventions were more common in those who displayed the presence of the mutation.

A very interesting scientific publications surfaced in 2008, when Barrett et al., performed a GWAS analysis (genome-wide association studies) on a group of 3230 CD patients, as well as a control group of 4829 subjects (GWAP studies include the analysis of a huge number of polymorphisms in the research (patient) group and a subsequent comparison of the same types of changes in the control/ population group; the differences in the occurrence of changes in both of these groups (presented mainly through a very precise and thorough statistical analysis) point to a relation between the potential polymorphisms associations with the disease studied. These studies showed that within the human genome there are at least 32 genes associated with predisposition for CD (11 loci mentioned in earlier publications were confirmed, and 21 new ones were identified). This lends support to the currently held belief that CD may be conditioned by 30-35 different genes.

The reports presented above clearly point to the fact that for a number of years worldwide research has been resorting to multilocus studies. These are not aimed at determining one particular mutation or polymorphism conditioning a given disease, but rather at discovering complex inter-genetic dependencies. Similarly, this research project strives to follow these global trends, at least to an extent. Of course the authors realize that the relatively small patient group (compared to large-scale research projects) is not a match for the reports presented above; nevertheless, we believe it is still an interesting attempt at investigating the described dependencies in the Polish patient population.

Not all of the polymorphisms studied in this doctoral thesis have been analyzed previously in reference to the clinical course of the disease. In Poland this kind of research is quite innovative, although studies of this type have surfaced on the international stage. Most frequently it is the CARD15/NOD2 gene that is subject to analysis as so far, it has seemed to be most closely associated CD. However, recent studies have pointed to other susceptibility genes, for example ATG16L1 or IL23R, which may shed more light on the results obtained so far

In this research project the authors decided to scrutinize those genes which were most frequently linked to CD in publications appearing over the course of last several years. In the planning process of the study presented here we decided to concentrate on the analysis of three chosen genes, as well as the polymorphisms present within them, in order to eventually uncover certain dependencies. We were fortunate to observe certain tendencies in the occurrence of disease symptoms related to a particular genotype; however, we found no relation which might be crucial in explaining the mystery of CD. It is possible that the reason for this is either the absence of such a dependency, or the insufficient size of the research group. Although 160 patients seem to constitute a rather substantial sample, worldwide, these analyses are conducted on groups with numbers going into thousands.

Unfortunately, conducting such large-scale study in Poland is extremely problematic; therefore, a project based on a group of even 160 patients, yet featuring an analysis of 10 polymorphic loci, might be considered a success.
When this research project was still in its infancy, the topic of multilocus analyses of both clinical symptoms and the course of the disease was entirely innovative in Poland; what is more, foreign studies of this type were also extremely scarce. In recent years, the topic has attracted much attention worldwide; nevertheless, in Poland, a genetic multilocus study complemented by an analysis of the clinical symptoms and demonstrating such a wide scope remains a rarity. It is also worth mentioning that despite the fact the relevant genetic dependencies underlying CD remain undiscovered, such a possibility is not unattainable in the future. Global research aimed at unearthing its causes is being carried out as we speak, and it is the authors' firm belief that Polish researchers will also participate in this trend. After all, CD is a complex condition, and the research project presented here does not exhaust all the possible hypotheses pertaining to its etiology.

6. Conclusions

In this research project, 139 patients with Crohn's Disease were analyzed taking into consideration 5 single nucleotide polymorphisms (SNPs):

- CARD15/NOD2 G908R,
- *ATG16L1* rs2241879,
- *ATG16L1* rs2241880,
- *IL23R* rs7517847,
- *IL23R* rs1004819,

The obtained results were compared to an adequate population group.
All SNPs were polymorphic in the Polish population, which has been described in detail in the previous section of this publication. Unfortunately, no statistically significant differences in the distribution of particular genotypes were observed. However, the analysis of alleles showed, that:

- in the *ATG16L1* gene (rs2241880), allele C was statistically significantly more frequent among CD patients than in the population group (p=0.0017, for allele T p=0.0775).
- in the *IL23R* gene (rs7517847), allele T was statistically significantly more frequent among CD patients than in the population group (p=0.0011, for allele G p=0.0987).

Due to these results, it is possible that allele C for *ATG16L1* Thr300Ala (rs2241880) and T for *IL23R* (rs7517847) are connected with a higher risk of developing CD.
The second part of this research project focused on alleles and genotypes; in particular, on their relation to the localization of symptoms. It revealed that there are certain tendencies that can predict some predispositions to exact disease symptoms:

- among the CD patients, in the *CARD15/NOD2* gene G908R, genotype CC and allele C were the most frequent ones, which is connected with the localization of the symptoms in the area of intestines and the presence of perianal fistulas.
- the analysis of the extra-intestinal symptoms also revealed some interesting dependences: patients with joint pain, uveitis, stomatitis aphtosa, erythema nodosum, or elevated body temperature have statistically more frequent alleles C and the CC genotype.

- in the *ATG16L1* gene (rs2241879), patients with symptoms localized in the small intestine more frequently displayed the GA genotype; what is more, the same genotype was observed more often among patients with joint pain and erythema nodosum. Unfortunately, the allele analysis did not reveal statistically significant dependences.
- in the *ATG16L1* gene (rs2241880), the TC genotype was observed more frequently for patients with symptoms localized in the small intestine, arthralgia and erythema nodosum. Allele analysis did not reveal any statistically significant dependences.
- in the *IL23R* gene (rs1004819), the TT genotype was statistically the predominant one in CD patients with the disease symptoms manifested in the small intestine; however, allele analysis revealed that the presence of allele T alone may be crucially connected with the colonic symptoms as well. What is more, the TT and TC genotypes were statistically more frequent among patients declaring the presence of erythema nodosum.
- in the *IL23R* gene (rs7517847) the TT genotype was statistically prevalent among CD patients with symptoms localized in the small intestine. Together with the GT genotype, the TT genotype was statistically more frequent among individuals complaining of joint pain.

Although this research project did not reveal statistically significant differences in the distribution of particular genotypes in CD patients and the population group, some tendencies have been observed. They can be helpful when predicting the development of the disease, but they cannot be treated as a diagnostic parameter; rather, they indicate certain predispositions to the development of the disease. As a result, currently patient history, physical examinations, colonoscopy, histopathology and radiological studies (e.g. USG examination) still remain the main sources of the diagnosis.

It needs to be noted that although spectacular genetic dependencies underlying the causes of CD have not been discovered as of yet, it is still feasible in the future. Indeed, with every next research project - including this one - new advances are made in the field; therefore, it is possible that the genetic background of CD will be determined in the coming years which would constitute a significant advantage for patients.

7. References

Annese V, Lombardi G, Perri F, D'Incà R, Ardizzone S, Riegler G, Giaccari S, Vecchi M, Castiglione F, Gionchetti P, Cocchiara E, Vigneri S, Latiano A, Palmieri O, Andriulli A. Variants of CARD15 are associated with an aggressive clinical course of Crohn's disease--an IG-IBD study. Am J Gastroenterol. 2005 Jan;100(1):84-92

Barrett JC, Hansoul S, Nicolae DL, Cho JH, Duerr RH, Rioux JD, Brant SR, Silverberg MS, Taylor KD, Barmada MM, Bitton A, Dassopoulos T, Datta LW, Green T, Griffiths AM, Kistner EO, Murtha MT, Regueiro MD, Rotter JI, Schumm LP, Steinhart AH, Targan SR, Xavier RJ; NIDDK IBD Genetics Consortium, Libioulle C, Sandor C, Lathrop M, Belaiche J, Dewit O, Gut I, Heath S, Laukens D, Mni M, Rutgeerts P, Van Gossum A, Zelenika D, Franchimont D, Hugot JP, de Vos M, Vermeire S, Louis E; Belgian-French IBD Consortium; Wellcome Trust Case Control Consortium, Cardon LR, Anderson CA, Drummond H, Nimmo E, Ahmad T, Prescott NJ, Onnie CM, Fisher SA, Marchini J, Ghori J, Bumpstead S, Gwilliam R, Tremelling M, Deloukas P, Mansfield J, Jewell D, Satsangi J, Mathew CG, Parkes M, Georges M, &

Daly MJ. Genome-wide association defines more than 30 distinct susceptibility loci for Crohn's disease. Nat Genet. 2008 Aug;40(8):955-62

Cukovic-Cavka S, Vermeire S, Hrstic I, Claessens G, Kolacek S, Jakic- Razumovic J, Krznaric Z, Grubelic K, Radic D, Misak Z, Jadresin O, Rutgeerts P, & Vucelic B. NOD2/CARD15 mutations in Croatian patients with Crohn's disease: prevalence and genotype-phenotype relationship. Eur J Gastroenterol Hepatol 2006 Aug;18(8):895-9.

Cho J. Inflammatory bowel disease: genetic and epidemiologic considerations. World J Gastroenterol 2008 January 21; 14(3):338-347

Jürgens M, Brand S, Laubender RP, Seiderer J, Glas J, Wetzke M, Wagner J, Pfennig S, Tillack C, Beigel F, Weidinger M, Schnitzler F, Kreis ME, Göke B, Lohse P, Herrmann K, Ochsenkühn T. The presence of fistulas and NOD2 homozygosity strongly predict intestinal stenosis in Crohn's disease independent of the IL23R genotype. J Gastroenterol. 2010 Jul;45(7):721-31 Epub 2010 Apr 29

Lacher M, Helmbrecht J, Schroepf S, Koletzko S, Ballauff A, Classen M, Uhlig H, Hubertus J, Hartl D, Lohse P, Schweinitz D, Kappler R. NOD2 mutations predict the risk for surgery in pediatric-onset Crohn's disease Journal of Pediatric Surgery (2010) 45, 1591–1597

Mendoza JL, Murillo LS, Fernández L, Peña AS, Lana R, Urcelay E, Cruz-Santamaría DM, de la Concha EG, Díaz-Rubio M, García-Paredes J. Prevalence of mutations of the NOD2/CARD15 gene and relation to phenotype in Spanish patients with Crohn disease. Scand J Gastroenterol. 2003 Dec;38(12):1235-40

Slomski R. 2008, Wydawnictwo Uniwersytetu Przyrodniczego w Poznaniu 2008, ISBN 978-83-7160-496-6, Poznan

Lesage S, Zouali H, Cézard JP, Colombel JF, Belaiche J, Almer S, Tysk C, O'Morain C, Gassull M, Binder V, Finkel Y, Modigliani R, Gower-Rousseau C, Macry J, Merlin F, Chamaillard M, Jannot AS, Thomas G, Hugot JP; EPWGIBD Group; EPIMAD Group; GETAID Group. CARD15/NOD2 mutational analysis and genotype-phenotype correlation in 612 patients with inflammatory bowel disease. Am J Hum Genet. 2002 Apr;70(4):845-57. Epub 2002 Mar 1

4

Inflammatory Bowel Disease G-Protein Coupled Receptors (GPCRs) Expression Profiling with Microfluidic Cards

Nathalie Taquet[1], Claude Philippe[1],
Jean-Marie Reimund[2,3] and Christian D. Muller [1]
[1]*Laboratoire d'Innovation Thérapeutique UMR CNRS 7200,*
Faculté de Pharmacie, Université de Strasbourg,
[2]*CHU de Caen, Service d'Hépato-Gastro-Entérologie et Nutrition*
[3]*Université de Caen Basse-Normandie, EA 3919, SFR ICORE, UFR de Médecine*
France

1. Introduction

Crohn's disease (CD) and chronic ulcerative colitis (UC) are considered as two distinct forms of inflammatory bowel disease (IBD). In IBDs, the first clinical signs of disease begin typically between adolescence and the third decade of life (Andres & Friedman 1999; Baldassano & Piccoli 1999). CD is a non-specific granulomatous inflammatory disease affecting the lower end of the ileum and often involving the colon and other parts of the intestinal tract (Podolsky 2002). CD was first reported by B. Crohn and his colleagues in 1932 and called Regional Enteritis (Matsuura et al. 1993). CD is diagnosed in four patients per 100 000 in the Northern Europe and the incidence and prevalence is rising (Elson et al. 1995). UC is a chronic disease of unknown etiology characterized by inflammation of the mucosa and sub-mucosa of the rectum (altimes) with a continuous extension to upper parts of the colon without healthy mucosa between inflammatory mucosa, which can be limited to the rectum (proctitis) to the colon below the lefts angle (left colitis), beyond the left angle (extensive colitis) or affect all the colon (pancolitis). UC is mostly characterized by bloody diarrhea. UC may have a prevalence of 100 case per 100 000 population in Northern Europe (Satsangi et al. 1996)

The causes of CD and UC remain to be clarified. However, genetic factors in combination with environmental factors are suspected to be involved in the pathogenesis of Crohn's disease (Baker et al. 1981; Podolsky 2002). Inadequate or prolonged activation of the intestinal immune system plays an important role in the pathophysiology of chronic mucosal inflammation (Elson et al. 1995; Matsuura et al. 1993).

CD and UC are characterized by periods of remission followed by episodes of clinical relapse, characterized by an increase in symptoms usually due to acute intestinal inflammation. Treatment is primarily aimed at reducing inflammation during relapse and secondarily at prolonging the time-spent remission. Conventionally both of these aims are governed by consideration of clinical symptoms rather than objective evidence of inflammatory activity. Gastroenterologists are often faced with the difficulty of differentiating patients with irritable bowel syndrome from those with organic intestinal pathologies, in particular inflammatory bowel disease. Many symptoms are common to both conditions including abdominal pain, bloating, excessive flatus and altered bowel habit while other clinical features such as a predominance of diarrhea and rectal bleeding will increase the likelihood of organic disease. Although symptoms are a surprisingly good guide to a diagnosis, most clinicians proceed to and rely on laboratory tests to aid in the differential diagnosis. The two main forms of IBD are both characterized by an aberrant immune response of intestinal mucosa. The enormous complexity of pathophysiology mandates a systematic approach to identify the molecular events that cause and perpetuate these chronic, relapsing inflammatory disorders. The ability to quantitate the global expression profiles at the level of RNA using oligonucleotide microarrays has recently been applied to investigate transcriptional signatures present in CD peripheral blood and CD gastrointestinal tissue (Lawrance et al. 2001; Warner & Dieckgraefe 2002). These studies identified genes involved in inflammatory response generally up-regulated in IBD and showed that the gastrointestinal tissue transcriptome obtained from UC and CD patients were quite distinct, with gene sets identified that appear to distinguish UC from CD tissue. In contrast to biopsies, peripheral blood is a much more accessible tissue source to distinguish between UC and CD. Circulating peripheral blood mononuclear cells (PBMCs) are responsible for the comprehensive surveillance of the body for signs of infection and disease. PBMCs may therefore serve as a surrogate tissue for evaluation of disease induced gene expression as biomarker of disease status or severity (Rockett et al. 2004).

CD patient PBMC	**Age**	**Gender**
CD1	51	F
CD2	50	F
CD3	18	M
CD4	53	F
Control PBMC	**Age**	**Gender**
C1	30	F
C2	44	M
C3	50	M
C4	24	F
C5	30	M

Biopsies	**Physiological state**	**Age of donor**	**Gender of donor**
CD5	Inflamed	23	F
CD6ni	Non inflamed	24	F
CD6i	Inflamed	24	F
CD7	Inflamed	21	F
CD8	Inflamed	31	F
UC1	Inflamed	45	F
UC2ni	Non inflamed	20	F
UC2i	Inflamed	20	F
IBS 1	Inflamed	28	M
IBS 2	Inflamed	59	F
C6	Non inflamed	55	M

Table 1. Origin of PBMCs and biopsies. CD = Crohn's Disease patient; UC = Ulcerative colitis patient; IBS = Irritable Bowel Syndrome patient, C = Disease free individual.

We here explored expression profiles of PBMCs from four CD patients compared to age and gender matched healthy individuals. We monitored as well the expression profiles of biopsies obtained by endoscopy from five CD patients, three UC, two intestinal disorders functional and one disease free individual (Table 1). To study the transcriptome we used "Taqman Low Density Arrays" microfluidic cards (Applied Biosystems), based on the technology of real-time PCR and Taqman probes. Such strategy is particularly attractive due to the quality of measurements of gene expression, the simplicity of implementation and the 384 wells format thus covering the whole family of G Protein-Coupled Receptor (GPCR) on one plate. In this project, we used cards dedicated to study the GPCR transcriptome and this in two configurations. Card #1 was designed in 2004 by professor J. Haiech (UMR 7200 CNRS, Faculty of Pharmacy, Illkirch). This card contained 355 GPCR, 16 housekeeping genes and 10 genes belonging to various categories. Card #2, used for monitoring biopsies, is produced as it by Applied Biosystems (ref. 4365295). This second card, designed two years later, takes in account updates on GPCR's annotation; it contained 365 GPCR including 4 olfactory GPCR, 14 housekeeping genes and 2 genes of various functions. These two cards have 352 genes in common, including 10 housekeeping genes with 30 genes specific to each card.

2. Materials and methods

2.1 Blood and tissues culture

Healthy donors with no clinical history were selected for PBMCs and tissues studies. Patients blood and tissues were obtained from CD patients at the Gastroentetology units from Strasbourg and Caen Universities hospitals (France). This work was approved by an authorized ethics committee (CPP Nord Ouest 2, Amiens, France), and carried out according to international guidelines. A fragment of each tissue specimen (colon, ileum, small intestine) was used for histopathological studies. The other part was immediately frozen on solution D (Chomczynski and Sacchi 1987) and stored at -70°C. PBMCs from healthy donors were separated as previously described (Boyum 1968).

Peripheral blood diluted in Ca^{2+} and Mg^{2+} free HBSS (CMF-HBSS) containing 100 IU heparin/ml was layered over Histopaque-1077 and centrifuged for 30 min at 400g (20°C). Cells harvested at the interface were washed 3 times in CMF-HBSS and resuspended at a final concentration of 5×10^5 cells/ml in RPMI 1640 supplemented by 10% heat-inactivated fetal bovin serum (FBS). PBMCs were seeded on 24-well culture plates at a final concentration of 5.10^5 cells/ml in RPMI-1640 supplemented with 10% heat-inactivated FBS (v/v) and penicillin-streptomycin (100µg/ml). Control cells and CD patients cells were activated, or not, by LPS (5µg/ml) for 2 hours 30 min at 37°C. PBMCs were centrifuged and the pellets were pooled, frozen in liquid nitrogen and kept at -80°C until testing.

2.2 Flow cytometry

Flow cytometry was performed on a Guava EasyCyte Plus System (Merck/Millipore/ Guava, Hayward, USA) equipped with a 488 nm laser that illuminates each cell then fluorescence is collected at different wavelength (530 ± 15 nm, 575 ± 13 nm and 660 ± 10 nm). The granularity, size, cell number/ml and fluorescence are recorded at a speed of 800 cells per second.

2.3 TNF-α secretion tests

Human PBMCs were incubated in 24 well culture plates in culture medium at $5x10^5$ cells/ml for 24 h at 37°C in a humidified 5% CO_2 / 95% air atmosphere in presence of increasing concentrations of the somatostatin analogues ranging from 10^{-7}M to 10^{-5}M, with or without activation by LPS (5µg/ml). Compounds were dissolved in water. Control samples always contained the same amount of water (without compounds). For ELISA, plates were centrifuged after incubation for 15 min at 200xg (20°C). Supernatants were stored at -80°C until testing. For coating, human TNF-α antibody 0,5mg/ml (BD Pharmingen, Le Pont de Claix, France) was diluted to 1/100 in Binding Solution (Na_2HPO_4 0,1M+NaH_2PO_4 0,1M à pH9) and added in the 96 wells plate (Nunc Maxisorp 96-wells, VWR, Val de Fontenay, France). The plate was sealed to prevent evaporation, and incubated overnight at 4°C. The 96-wells plate was then washed once with PBS 1x/Tween 0,05% then saturated by addition of 200µl PBS/milk 5% during 2 hours at room temperature. After two washes with PBS 1x/Tween 0,05%, PBMC supernatants were added. TNF-α protein standard 1µg/ml (BD Pharmingen, Le Pont de Claix, France) with dilutions (10000, 3333, 1111, 370, 123, 41 and 5pg/ml) was added in corresponding standard wells for the statistic correlation. The detection was done with Human TNF-α biotin 0,5mg/ml (BD Pharmingen, Le Pont de Claix, France) during one hour at room temperature. The plate was washed four times with PBS 1x/Tween 0,05%. Peroxydase/streptavidin 1,25 mg/ml (Zymed, In Vitrogen, Cergy Pontoise, France) was added and the plate incubated for one hour at room temperature. The plate was washed four times in PBS 1x/Tween 0,05%, and OPD (Sigma, Lyon, France) was used to determine the amount of TNF-α detected in each well. The plate was then analysed in a spectrophotometer at 450nm (Molecular Devices, VersaMax Tunable Microplate Reader, Sunnyvale, USA).

2.4 RNA Extraction of tissues and PBMCs

The tissues were defrosted 15 minutes on ice (Chomczynski & Sacchi 1987). The cells were broken with a sterile piston, and put in sodium acetate 2M pH 4, phenol pH 4 saturated and chloriform/isoamylic alcool (49:1). After shaking, the membranes were incubated 15 minutes on ice and centrifuged 20 minutes at 12000g at 4°C. Aqueous phase with the RNA were kept and precipitated with isopropanol one hour at -20°C. The RNA were centrifuged 20 minutes 12000g at 4°C, and washed with 500µl of ethanol 70% stored at -20°C. They were centrifuged 5 minutes 12000g at 4°C and washed again three times. The RNA were dried with Speed Vac, and added with sterile water. RNA was isolated from PBMC cells pellet (5.10^6 cells) with Tri reagent (Molecular Research Center, Inc., Cincinnati, Ohio, USA) according to the manufacturer's instructions.

Total mRNA were checked for integrity and concentration using the RNA 6000 LabChip kit on the Agilent 2100 bio analyzer (ratios of 28S RNA/18S RNA were above 1.6) and for purity by reading the absorbance at 260 and 280 nm (ratios A260/A280 were comprised between 1.8 and 2.0).

2.5 Real-Time RT-PCR and PCR

Five µg of total RNA is reversely transcribed to single-stranded cDNA using the "High-Capacity cDNA AUCive™ Kit" (Applied Biosystems, Foster City, California, USA). RNA is pre-incubated at 25°C for 10 min, followed by 2 hours at 37°C, according to the manufacturer's recommendations (Applied Biosystems, Foster City, California, USA).

Subsequently, cDNA was kept at -20 °C until used. An aliquot of cDNA (850 ng) was mixed carefully in 850µL TaqMan Universal PCR Master Mix (PE Applied Biosystems). On the card keeped at room temperature, 105µL of the sample were loaded into each of 8 ports on the TaqMan Low-Density Array (Applied Biosystems, Foster City, CA). The TaqMan Low-Density Array microfluidic card #1 consists of a preconfigured in a 384-well format to assess the expression of 355 GPCR genes. The card #2 has 365 GPCR genes as well as 4 olfactives GPCR. The cards were then centrifuged twice in custom Buckets (Applied Biosystems, CA USA) in a Heraeus centrifuge (Kendro Scientific, Asheville, NC, USA) for 1 min at 1200 rpm. The cards were immediately sealed with the TaqMan Low-Density Array Sealer (Applied Biosystems, CA USA) to prevent any cross-contamination. Real-time RT-PCR is then performed on an ABI Prism 7900 (Applied Biosystems, Foster City, CA). Thermal cycling, to activate uracil-DNA glycosylase, is carried out for 2 min at 50°C, 10 min at 94.5°C then 40 cycles of 30 s at 97 °C and 60 s at 59.7 °C. Each reaction contained cDNA derived from around 1.5 ng of total RNA.

2.6 Statistics

Real-time RT-PCR data were quantified using the SDS 2.2.1 software package (Applied Biosystems). Results were quantified in a relative comparative study, using an automatic baseline and threshold to record the cycle thresholds (Cts) setting and the 18S rRNA gene expression as a reference for normalization (ΔCts). Student's *t*-test was used with a significance threshold of $P < 0.05$. ELISA data are expressed as a percentage of the basal cytokine secretion level or as means (± SE); 'n' refers to the number of experiments. Results were compared using the non-parametric Mann–Whitney U test. The level of statistical significance was fixed at $P < 0.05$.

3. Results

By monitoring non-orphan RCPGs (*i.e.* 279 among the 382 RCPGs tested) in PBMCs of 10 healthy donors and 10 CD patients we found that the data obtained were highly dependent on RNA integrity. The integrity of RNA molecules is of paramount importance for experiments that try to reflect the snapshot of gene expression at the moment of RNA extraction. The RNA integrity number (RIN) is an important tool regrettably often disregarded, in conducting valid gene expression measurement experiments as real-time PCR or DNA microarray (Schroeder et al. 2006). After RIN determination of our 20 samples, only 4 CD patients and 4 paired healthy donors could be considered reliable due to sample degradation yet with handling and shipping in dry ice from the hospital to the laboratory.

3.1 Standardization

Figure 1 represented a Dot Blot reflecting dispersion of 10 Housekeeping genes (PBMCs and biopsies). Before standardization, values (Ct) of 10 genes presented a distribution around 50% of the median of the samples. However gene *GUSB* had weaker variance and symmetrical distribution compared to median. The distribution of ARNr 18S values is relatively good compared to whole of other Housekeeping genes excepting two samples presenting extreme values. The literature relates that genes of the sugar metabolism were found deregulated in biopsies of IBD patients (Dieckgraefe et al. 2000) this fact encouraged us to choose 18S RNA to standardize our samples. After standardization, genes generally

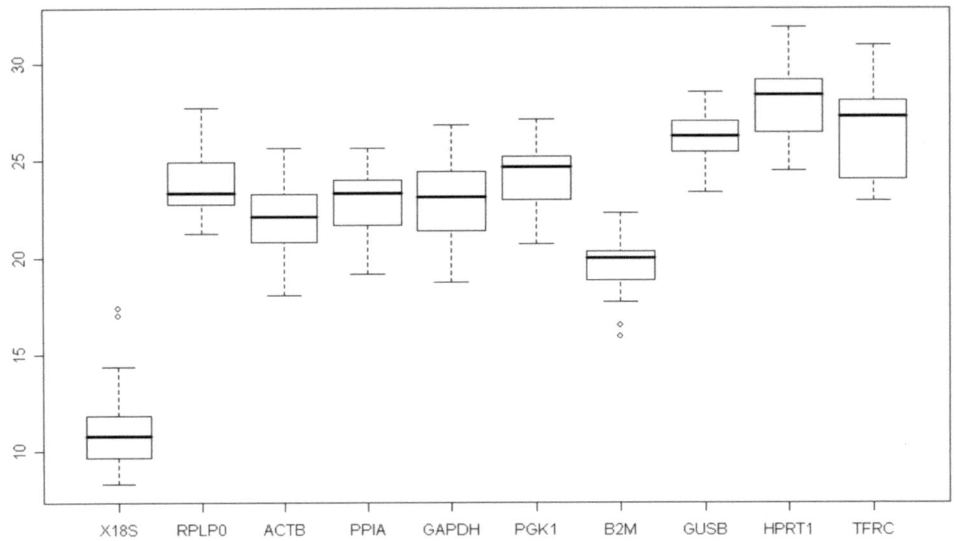

(A)

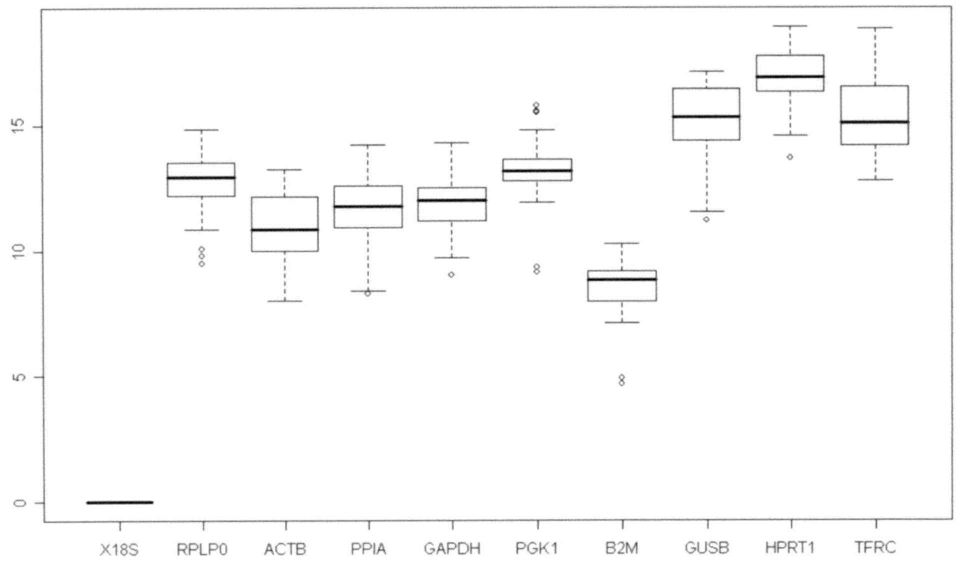

(B)

Fig. 1. Dot blot of 10 Housekeeping genes before (A) and after (B) standardization to 18S RNA.

showed a weaker dispersion, but we noticed that several genes like *PGK1, RPLP0* and *B2M* presented extreme values. The fact that 3 genes out of 10 Housekeeping genes are not standardized the same manner, states clearly that genes are connected to different ways of metabolism which ways are affected by cell deregulation. For example, many reports on ratios show that the level of *GAPDH* messenger does not remain constant. Even if the GAPDH gene was considered for years as a reference in genetic organization, expression and regulation studies, recent evidences demonstrate that mammalian GAPDH displays a number of diverse activities unrelated to its glycolytic function. For example, *GAPDH* messenger variations of enzymatic activity are implied in many mechanisms as varied as replication of DNA, transport of nuclear ARN and organization of cytoskeletal (Sirover 1999) as well as neurodegenerative diseases.(Tatton et al. 2000)

3.2 Gene clustering

Before seeking genes differentially expressed in statistical systems with two classes, we wanted to know if it is possible to group samples in classes that characterize them with profile genes and type of pathology of patient to differentiate CD and UC. We followed a supervised approach which data groups without existing classes. Procedure of clustering consists in classifying a whole of data in several subsets according to their similarities. Data of expression form a matrix whose lines correspond to genes, here genes common to both cards, and columns with 17 samples. First, data were filtered so general average of form of genes is lower than 38 Ct, then standardized compared to ARNr 18S.

The tree diagram or dendrogram illustrates the arrangement of clusters produced by hierarchical clustering. The individuals who resemble the most to each other are gathered in the bottom of the tree. The length of the branches is proportional to their distance among each other. The matrix of expression data is coloured coded according to the relative level of gene expression of genes: colours go from green for level of high expression to red for level of low expression, with black for intermediate level (units expressed in ΔCt).

Figure 2 shows an ascending hierarchical classification by using Pearson's coefficient of correlation to measure the distance between two points. This distance reflects proximity or similarity between two points. Using Euclidean distance, which measures dissimilarity between two points and is more sensitive to amplitude of variations between data, produces regrouping of the data as illustrated into Figure 3.

The data regrouping are obtained in form of two dendrograms, for genes and for individuals for each card. Classification distributes samples in 2 principals groups, PBMCs and biopsies. This first scission marks differences related nature of tissues. Then within each one of these 2 regroupings, we distinguish sub-groups:

- for the PBMC group: the subgroup of healthy individuals differs markedly from that of patients with CD, each of these subgroups appear marginally affected by treatment with LPS.
- for the biopsy group: the formation of sub-groups is less obvious, as is the interpenetration of these sub-groups: healthy subjects, healthy areas of patients with CD, healthy areas of patients with UC and inflammatory areas in patients with CD , inflammatory areas in patients with UC, and finally mucosa of patients with IBS. This behavior is certainly due to an insufficient number of samples representing each class, including healthy people and healthy areas of patients. These ambiguous groupings of biopsies outside their own classes indicate a high level of variation in gene expression in samples.

In addition, dispersion curves (fig. 4 and 5) illustrate the heterogeneity of genes form in samples supposed to represent the same IBS. The correlation curves expression data of biopsies from inflammatory areas of patients with UC show a large dispersion of values in contrast to results obtained with patients CD. Indeed, the correlation coefficient of patients with UC or IBS is much lower (near 0.6) than that obtained with the data on three areas of biopsies from patients with inflammatory CD (around 0.8)

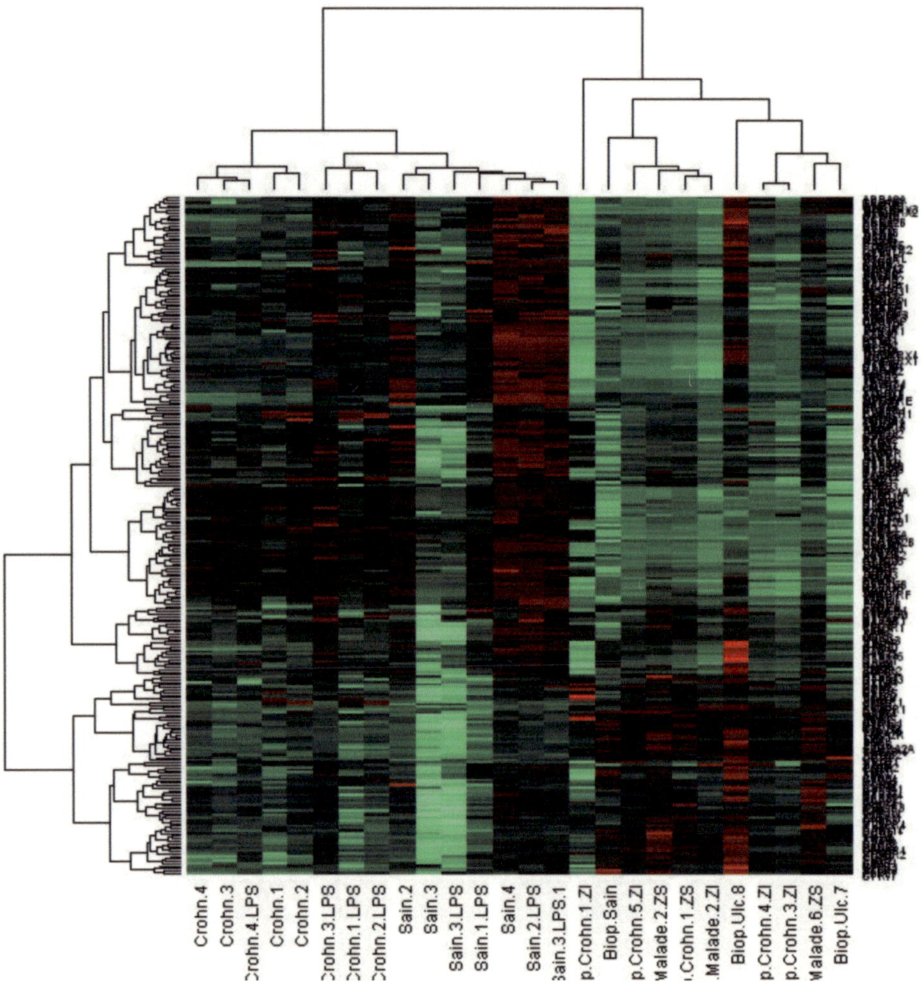

Fig. 2. GPCRs expression profile by ascending hierarchical classification of the samples.

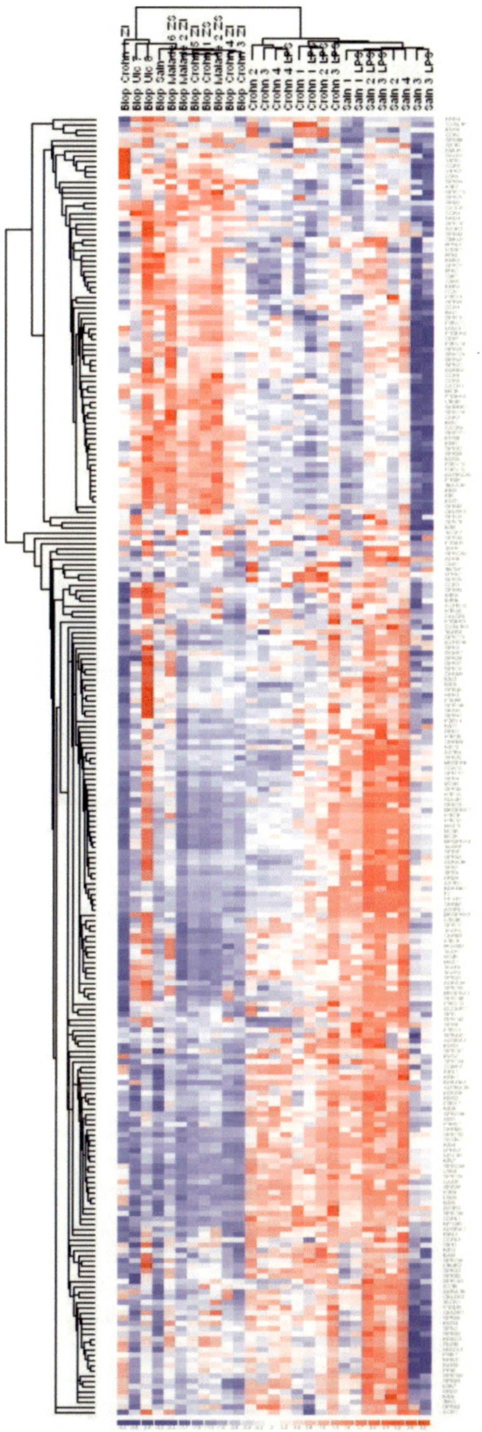

Fig. 3. Ascending hierarchical classification using Euclidean distance to measure dissimilarity and average enters groups for algorithm of aggregation.

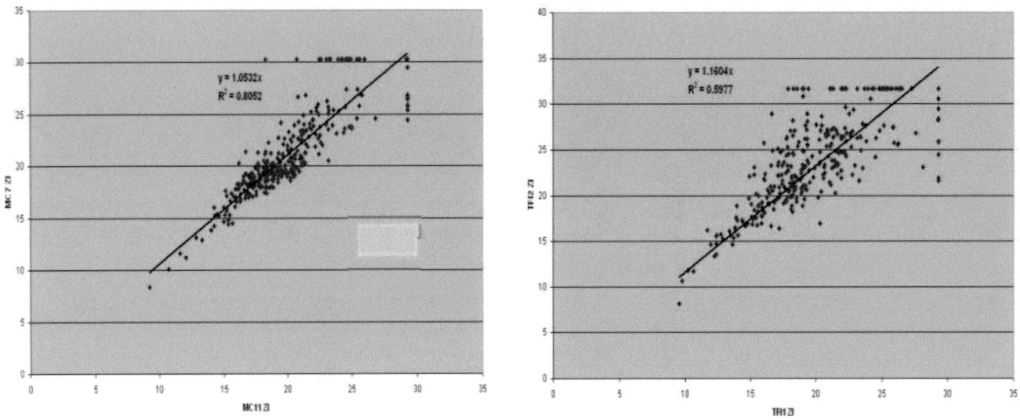

(A) (B)

Fig. 4. Gene dispersion curves for CD (A) and IBS (B) biopsies.

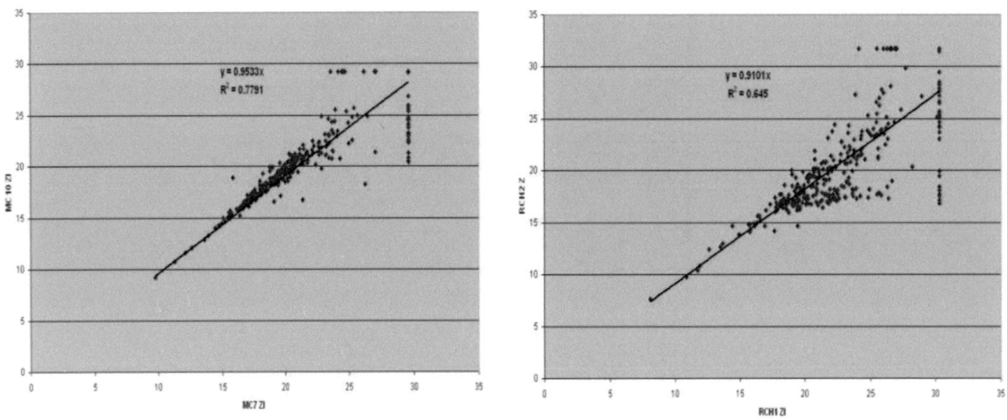

(A) (B)

Fig. 5. Gene dispersion curves for CD (A) and UC (B) biopsies.

The origins of these dispersions are many. First, in a technical point of view, the collection is a delicate operation to achieve in the bowel (colonoscopy) and the removal of the tissue requires expertise to pick the exact target area by damaging the minimum completeness of tissue removed. On the other hand, in a biological point of view, the heterogeneity of individuals (age, sex, treatment, diet, etc..) And the exact position where the taking is in the intestinal tract, are major sources of heterogeneity. The difficulty of our work was to remove background noise genes specifically associated with CD. In addition, changes in profiles of biopsies may represent different levels of evolution and development of the disease. Indeed, there may be a great variability of samples supposed to represent a single disease state or biological replicas considered in the statistical analysis. To achieve this level of interpretation, the data should be obtained on a large number of individuals in a population well characterized.

This grouping study provides assurance that the GPCR expression profiles in PBMCs can distinguish CD from healthy subjects. It shows, however, the existence of heterogeneity of expression profiles of GPCR and a large variance in the expression of genes in the biopsies, this should not be overlooked when analysing the data.

3.3 Normal distribution of data

Parametric statistical tests on the means involve the estimation of parameters such as variance. These tests are generally more powerful than nonparametric tests, but require as a condition for applying the normality of data distribution of the mean. Although the tests called parametric tests are quite robust, *i.e.* are insensitive to a deviation from normality (as long as you estimate the variance) and are often used as the mode of data distribution deviates slightly of normality, it is useful to test the normality of data distribution.

We used the correlation test of Ryan-Joiner, similar to the Shapiro-Wilk test, as proposed in the Minitab software. The test generates a line of Henry and performs a hypothesis test to see if the observations are normally distributed. The assumptions of the test are: H0, the data follow a normal distribution against H1, the data do not follow a normal distribution. Using this test, we submitted the data from 9 housekeeping genes (Table 2) thru the 27 samples for the goodness of fit to a Gaussian distribution.

Gene symbol	Assai ID	Gene Name	NCBI gene reference	Chromo-some
RPLP0	Hs99999902_m1	Ribosomal protein, large, P0	NM_053275	12
PPIA	Hs99999904_m1	Peptidylprolyl isomerase A (cyclophilin A)	NM_203430	7
GAPD	Hs99999905_m1	Glyceraldehyde-3-phosphate dehydrogenase	NM_002046	12
HIST1H1C	Hs00271185_s1	Histone 1, H1c	NM_005319	6
HPRT1	Hs99999909_m1	Hypoxanthine phosphoribosyltransferase 1	NM_000194	X
HSPCA	Hs00743767_sH	Heat shock 90kDa protein, 1 alpha	NM_005348	14
PGK1	Hs99999906_m1	Phosphoglycerate kinase 1	NM_000291	X
K-ALPHA-1	Hs00744842_sH	Tubulin, alpha, ubiquitous	NM_006082	12
RARS	Hs00259879_m1	Arginyl-tRNA synthetase	NM_002887	5
ACTB	Hs99999903_m1	Actin, beta	NM_001101	7
B2M	Hs99999907_m1	Beta-2-microglobulin	NM_004048	15
CYC1	Hs00357717_m1	Cytochrome c-1	NM_001916	8
GUSB	Hs99999908_m1	Glucuronidase, beta	NM_000181	7
TFRC	Hs99999911_m1	Transferrin receptor (p90, CD71)	NM_003234	3
NUP62	Hs00383013_m1	Nucleoporin 62kDa	NM_153719	19
18S		Ribosomal RNA 18S		

Table 2. Housekeeping list presents in the Applied Biosytem microfluidic card.

Of the nine genes tested, 7 of them verify the hypothesis H0, the data follow the normal distribution, the risk of first type α of 0.01 (Figure 6). Only two genes, *PGK1* and *B2M* have p values less than 0.01. These results can be linked with the dispersal rate of expression of these genes, as was noted earlier. The test results are for a normal distribution of data and give us confidence in using the Student test.

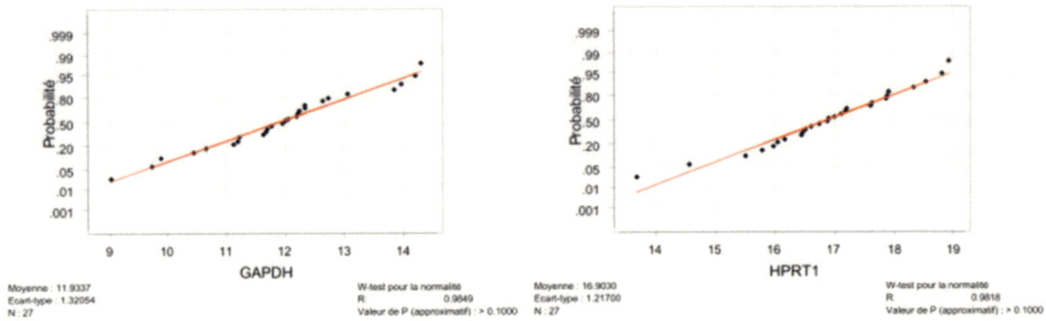

Fig. 6. Test of normality by the Ryan-Joiner test of correlation. The vertical axis represents scale of probabilities and horizontal axis scale of data. A line of least squares is adjusted at raised points and is traced on graph for reference. The line represents an estimate of function of pattern of settlement from where data are extracted. The estimates of parameters average and standard deviations of population are posted under graph.

3.4 Gene expression in PBMCs of CD patients versus control

It is now widely accepted that GPCRs, including cytokine receptors play a critical role in controlling the inflammatory response (Luther & Cyster 2001; Onuffer & Horuk 2002; Thelen 2001). It has been shown that immune cells express many receptors of neuropeptides and neurotransmitters, highlighting the role of mediators in the neuroendocrine modulation of immune response. In addition, there is a bundle of evidence indicating the existence of relationship between GPCR signaling pathways and answers related to antigen receptor of T cells and interleukin-2. Thus, prostaglandins produced by activated macrophages during the immune response can inhibit both cytokine production and proliferation of T cells (Baker et al. 1981). These observations motivated us to work with PBMCs, a more homogeneous cell population much less restrictive than the colon biopsies of patients. In our study on PBMCs taken from four healthy subjects and four patients with CD in remission, the expression profiles of GPCRs were obtained on card #1.

The genes were previously filtered to eliminate those not expressed in any of the samples, so that they are about 85 genes remaining. The were two reason of this operation: i) reduce variance brought by genes not expressed during calculation of ΔCt since these genes have Ct equal to 40; ii) avoid null denominators in calculations in particular standard deviations. This does not mean that all 296 selected genes are expressed. Values are normalized to 18S rRNA in each sample. The differentially expressed genes between the normal subjects and CD patients were obtained from the p-value of the Student test at risk of type α equal to 0.05. The difference in expression between the two classes of individuals was determined from the difference between the average ΔCt healthy subjects and the average ΔCt of CD patients.

$$\Delta\Delta Ct = (\Delta Ct_{healthy} - \Delta Ct_{CD})$$

The data of the 22 differentially expressed genes were subjected to a nonparametric test, more robust and less sensitive to extreme values. The Mann-Whitney test for unpaired data with Minitab software calculates the value p and focuses on the equality of medians of two groups. Figure 7 shows two examples of the report of the results for Minitab for gene *SSTR5* and *ADRA2B* for a threshold of the first kind α of 0.05. The data of the first gene name can reject the hypothesis H0 while those of *ADRA2B* does not allow it.

Assay ID	Gene Symbol	Gene Name	T-TEST	ΔΔCt	Standard Deviation	Mann-Whitney test
Hs00664150_s1	*MRGPRE*	MAS-related GPR, member E	0.007	9.8	2.10	Rejection
Hs00265647_s1	*SSTR5*	somatostatin receptor 5	0.038	9.6	2.50	Rejection
Hs00664166_s1	*GPR142*	G protein-coupled receptor 142	0.011	9.5	2.22	Rejection
Hs00270999_s1	*GPR4*	G protein-coupled receptor 4	0.018	8.4	2.15	Rejection
Hs00266671_s1	*FY*	Duffy blood group	0.020	7.8	2.26	Rejection
Hs00265617_s1	*SSTR1*	somatostatin receptor 1	0.024	7.8	2.10	Rejection
Hs00664089_s1	*GPR148*	G protein-coupled receptor 148	0.023	7.6	2.19	Rejection
Hs00275980_s1	*PPYR1*	pancreatic polypeptide receptor 1	0.022	7.3	2.39	Rejection
Hs00271049_s1	*GPR20*	G protein-coupled receptor 20	0.017	7.2	2.35	Rejection
Hs00265195_s1	*CHRM1*	cholinergic receptor, muscarinic 1	0.035	6.7	2.15	Rejection
Hs00271017_s1	*GPR7*	G protein-coupled receptor 7	0.030	6.3	2.16	Rejection
Hs00271023_s1	*GPR8*	G protein-coupled receptor 8	0.002	6.1	1.52	No rejection
Hs00664201_s1	*BDKRB1*	bradykinin receptor B1	0.049	5.8	2.19	No rejection
Hs00271008_s1	*GPR6*	G protein-coupled receptor 6	0.044	5.5	2.03	No rejection
Hs00706455_s1	*CCR10*	chemokine (C-C motif) receptor 10	0.015	5.3	2.02	No rejection
Hs00268954_s1	*FZD9*	frizzled homolog 9 (Drosophila)	0.016	5.3	1.86	No rejection
Hs00265090_s1	*ADRA2B*	adrenergic, alpha-2B-, receptor	0.047	4.5	1.96	No rejection
Hs00265286_s1	*HTR1B*	5-hydroxytryptamine (serotonin) receptor 1B	0.026	4.1	1.57	No rejection
Hs00184657_m1	*BAI2*	brain-specific angiogenesis inhibitor 2	0.041	-2.4	1.44	No rejection
Hs00222094_m1	*HRH4*	histamine receptor H4	0.050	-2.5	1.57	No rejection
Hs00181231_m1	*ADORA1*	adenosine A1 receptor	0.028	-3.3	1.74	No rejection
Hs00173471_m1	*OPRL1*	opiate receptor-like 1	0.004	-5.1	1.71	Rejection

Table 3. Results of p-values for 22 genes.

The results of the p-values have been reported in Table 3: 14 of 22 genes confirmed the results of the parametric test (*MRGPRE, SSTR5, GPR142, GPR4, FY, SSTR1, GPR148, PPYR1, GPR20, CHRM1, GPR7, FZD9, and HTR1B OPRL1*).

The Mann-Whitney, which addresses to data from samples drawn randomly and independently in two populations of the same variance, is limited here by the low number of individuals tested. Having duplicate data, that is to say to increase the "NR" to 8 instead of 4 and keeping the same values of the medians, produces a p-value less than 0.05. All genes in Table 3 for which the hypothesis H0 could be rejected for NR equal to 4, are regarded significantly different by the mere fact of double samples. This is proven by a ratio of Minitab for *ADRA2B* with NR equal to 8.

Knowing that the signed rank test 2-sample is slightly less powerful than the test samples with 2 grouping of sample variance when the populations are normal, and taking into account the recommendations of Minitab software for populations with different standard deviations, we have privileged a 2-sample t test without pooling the variances for the analysis of differential genes.

Of the 22 genes differentially expressed in PBMC of CD patients compared to normal subjects, 18 were overexpressed, while four are under-expressed. The overexpressed genes are mostly induced in the disease except *ADRA2B* and *GPR8* receptors that are expressed in PBMCs of normal subjects. Among these genes are receptors involved in the inflammatory and immune (*SSTR5, SSTR1, CHRM1, CCR10, FY, BDKRB1, HTR1B*) in other processes (*MRGPRE, PPYR1, FZD9*) and unknown functions (7 orphan receptors: *GPR4, GPR142, GPR148, GPR20, GPR7, GPR8, GPR6*). In a similar approach, Burczynski ME and collaborators research in PBMC gene expression signatures to discriminate CD of UC. They used the Affymetrix microarray platform HG-U133A that allows you to query more than 22 000 genes with a sample of 42 normal individuals and 59 CD patients (Burczynski et al. 2006). Their data were deposited in the database of microarrays GEO "Gene Expression Omnibus" at NCBI and are available to the community in the form of CEL files. CEL files are files that contain Affymetrix raw data. The site also allows to directly visualize the expression profile of a gene selected from across all samples as a histogram. Out of the 22 genes on the TLDA microfluidic cards, 16 are present on the chip. By submitting data at the same t-test that was used at the threshold 0.05, 5 genes appear differentially expressed in CD patients compared to normal individuals (*FZD9, SSTR1, CCR10, HTR1B, OPRL1*) with reports of expression ranging from 1.83 (*FZD9*) and 0.75 (*OPRL1*). The very low expression of these 16 genes on the chip confirms the absence of expression observed in real-time PCR in healthy individuals (*SSTR5, SSTR1, FZD9, CCR10, HTR1B, GPR6, FY, ADORA1, BDKRB1, PPYR1, GPR20, GPR4*). The discrepancy concerning the magnitude of changes in expression levels (less than 2 with the microarray against values higher then 16 in real-time PCR) between the two sets of data can be related to the difference in sensitivity of two technologies, real-time PCR being much more sensitive than the oligonucleotide hybridization technique.

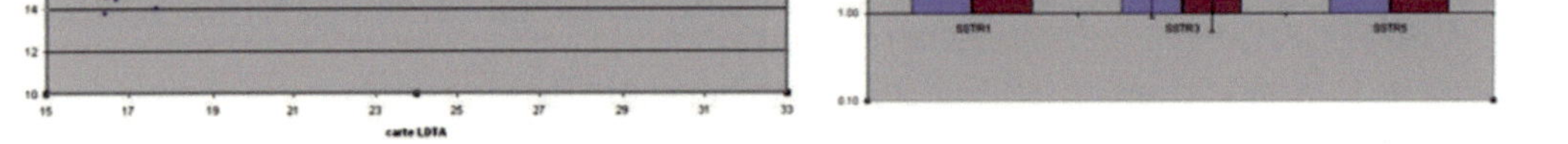

(A) (B)

Fig. 7. Validation of results obtained by real-time PCR in 96 well plates as compared to LDTA card. (A) Correlation curve for SSTR5 data. (B) Ratio of expression rates between CD patient and disease free individuals for 3 somatostatin receptors for data obtained by using microfluidic cards or 96 plates technology..

The presence among this group of receptor genes in the same family, *SSTR1* and *SSTR5*, which in addition show a strong increase of expression in CD patients, is interesting. This prompted us to conduct a new measurement of the expression of these genes by real-time PCR but using 96-well plate format. This makes it possible to assess the performance of the microfluidic card system, i.e. if the differences of expression come from technology, rheology, the depot of the tests in the cards, etc. Complementary DNA has been a resynthesized from total RNA and PCR was conducted under the same conditions of reagents on the ABI Prism 7000 thermocycler. We add to the experience another somatostatin receptor, *SSTR3*, whose expression is unchanged in microfluidic card TLDA. The histogram in Figure 7 confirms the results achieved with the microfluidic card and the curve (Fig.7A) shows good correlation between measurements of two technologies.

3.5 Healthy subjects and CD patients with LPS activation

We tested the ability of PBMC from healthy individuals and CD patients with to induce the production of TNF-α in response to LPS stimulation. After 24 hours incubation with LPS, we measured the release of TNF-α. We observed a production of TNF-α in the two groups of people consolidating us on the effectiveness of PBMC to respond to LPS. PBMCs of CD patients produce TNF-α twice as much as healthy subjects (data not shown).

Concerning gene expression, the data analysis was performed using an approach similar to the one described before. However, we applied here more strict filters by removing genes whose mean Ct was greater than 37. In this area of values measuring variations are significant. They are due on the one hand to the lack of reproducibility of withdrawals that is related to the Gaussian distribution of the sample in a solution containing a small number of copies of cDNA, and secondly, the SDS software that assigns a Ct of 40 to genes for which the amplification curve does not reach a plateau, as they cross the threshold between the 37th and 40th cycle.

Values were first normalized to 18S rRNA then for each individual, the difference of ΔCts, the ΔΔCts between the PBMC stimulated or not by LPS was computed. We also calculated the average values of ΔΔCts obtained from four individuals. The genes whose expression is regulated by the activation of PBMC by LPS in normal subjects were selected on the one hand for an average of ΔΔCts values greater than 1.5 and less than -1.5, and to the other from the p-value of Student's test for paired data at risk of Type α equal to 0.05. We obtained 18 genes (Table 4) whose expression is significantly LPS dependent, of which 4 are overexpressed and 14 repressed. With the exception of *GPRC5A* the three overexpressed genes (*GPR155, SSTR3, H963*) are well expressed in the non-activated PBMC from healthy subjects. Among these genes are many receptors known to be involved in the inflammatory process and immune response (*EDG2, EMR2, EMR3, CCR1, GPR35, FPr1, CCR3, CMKLR1, C5R1, FPRL2, P2RY2, GPBAR1*) with two orphan receptors (*GPR77, GPR162*).

The same experiment conducted with PBMC from CD patients, stimulated or not with LPS, shows a profile of genes regulated by LPS very similar to that obtained in healthy subjects, but with a more important difference between those genes induced and repressed (1 for 19 genes) (Table 5). The appearance of genes such as *CCR5, EDG3, EDNRB* and *IL8RB* strengthens families of genes already controlled by LPS in healthy subjects. We also observe an effect of LPS on the expression of neuropeptide receptors, *BAI1,* and *HTR1A NTSR1.* Conversely, LPS does not seem to affect the expression of *GPRC5A, SSTR3, H963, EMR2 and EMR1* genes in CD patients.

Assay ID	Gene symbol	Gene Name	T-TEST	Average ΔCt
Hs00173681_m1	GPRC5A	retinoic acid induced 3	0.023	4.9
Hs00400624_m1	GPR155	G protein-coupled receptor 155	0.026	2.2
Hs00265633_s1	SSTR3	somatostatin receptor 3	0.005	1.6
Hs00664328_s1	H963	platelet activating receptor homolog	0.027	1.5
Hs00173500_m1	EDG2	endothelial differentiation, lysophosphatidic acid GPCR 2	0.036	-1.7
Hs00203752_m1	EMR2	egf-like module containing, mucin-like, hormone receptor-like 2	0.006	-1.8
Hs00261470_m1	EMR3	egf-like module containing, mucin-like, hormone receptor-like 3	0.028	-2.1
Hs00174298_m1	CCR1	chemokine (C-C motif) receptor 1	0.016	-2.2
Hs00271114_s1	GPR35	G protein-coupled receptor 35	0.005	-2.4
Hs00181830_m1	FPR1	formyl peptide receptor 1	0.002	-2.9
Hs00266213_s1	CCR3	chemokine (C-C motif) receptor 3	0.031	-2.9
Hs00356604_m1	CMKLR1	chemokine-like receptor 1	0.034	-3.0
Hs00356609_g1	C5AR1	complement component 5 receptor 1 (C5a ligand)	0.006	-3.7
Hs00266666_s1	FPRL2	formyl peptide receptor-like 2	0.011	-3.9
Hs00175732_m1	P2RY2	purinergic receptor P2Y, G-protein coupled, 2	0.011	-4.4
Hs00218495_m1	GPR77	G protein-coupled receptor 77	0.038	-4.5
Hs00248078_m1	GPR162	likely ortholog of mouse gene rich cluster, A gene	0.004	-5.0
Hs00544894_m1	GPBAR1	G protein-coupled bile acid receptor 1	0.008	-5.4

Table 4. Genes differentially expressed between PBMCs of control subjects stimulated or not by LPS. Test ID: test Taqman Applied Biosystems identification; T-TEST: value p of the test of Student for paired data; Average of ΔΔCts: average of the difference of ΔΔCt ($\Delta Ct_{healthy}$ - ΔC $Ct_{healthy}$ +LPS) for each individual. The average of ΔΔCts is positive for overexpressed genes and negative for under-expressed genes.

To search for genes regulated by LPS in a different manner in healthy individuals and patients with CD, we used a t test for unpaired data. Table 6 shows the three genes: *P2RY2* gene is repressed by LPS in healthy subjects while remaining unaffected in CD patients, *CCR5* gene is repressed only in CD patients, the gene *GPR4* appears for a regulation in the opposite direction depending on whether LPS acts on PBMC from healthy individuals or CD patients. The difference of expression of *GPR4* between patients and healthy becomes significant. It is interesting to note that the *GPR4* gene was increased in PBMC of CD patients without LPS treatment. To these genes we might add the genes that appear only with the healthy or disease group like *SSTR3, H963, GPRC5A, EMR2* and *EMR3*for the healthy or *NTSR1, EDG3* and *GPRAR* for CD patients, but there is not enough statistical evidence at this level of the study to consider these genes differentially expressed between healthy subjects and patients.

Assay ID	Gene Symbol	Gene Name	T-TEST	Average ΔΔCts
Hs00400624_m1	GPR155	G protein-coupled receptor 155	0.031	1.8
Hs00181777_m1	BAI1	brain-specific angiogenesis inhibitor 1	0.025	-1.7
Hs00173500_m1	EDG2	endothelial differentiation, lysophosphatidic acid GPCR 2	0.039	-1.8
Hs00265014_s1	HTR1A	5-hydroxytryptamine (serotonin) receptor 1A	0.018	-1.8
Hs00152917_m1	CCR5	chemokine (C-C motif) receptor 5	0.003	-1.9
Hs00174304_m1	IL8RB	interleukin 8 receptor, beta	0.004	-2.2
Hs00265090_s1	ADRA2B	adrenergic, alpha-2B-, receptor	0.041	-2.2
Hs00266213_s1	CCR3	chemokine (C-C motif) receptor 3	0.007	-2.3
Hs00356604_m1	CMKLR1	chemokine-like receptor 1	0.021	-2.3
Hs00181830_m1	FPR1	formyl peptide receptor 1	0.034	-2.6
Hs00174298_m1	CCR1	chemokine (C-C motif) receptor 1	0.007	-3.4
Hs00173592_m1	NTSR1	neurotensin receptor 1 (high affinity)	0.008	-3.6
Hs00220561_m1	GPR84	G protein-coupled receptor 84	0.033	-3.7
Hs00266666_s1	FPRL2	formyl peptide receptor-like 2	0.000	-3.8
Hs00356609_g1	C5AR1	complement component 5 receptor 1 (C5a ligand)	0.004	-4.0
Hs00218495_m1	GPR77	G protein-coupled receptor 77	0.003	-4.0
Hs00245464_s1	EDG3	endothelial differentiation, sphingolipid GPCR 3	0.003	-4.1
Hs00240747_m1	EDNRB	endothelin receptor type B	0.010	-4.3
Hs00544894_m1	GPBAR1	G protein-coupled bile acid receptor 1	0.026	-5.2
Hs00248078_m1	GPR162	likely ortholog of mouse gene rich cluster, A gene	0.014	-6.9

Table 5. Genes differentially expressed between PBMC of CD patients stimulated or not by LPS. Test ID: Taqman Applied Biosystems identification test; T-TEST: value p of the test of Student for paired data; Average of ΔΔCts: average of the difference of ΔΔCt (ΔCt_{CD} - $\Delta\Delta C Ct_{CD+LPS}$) for each individual. The average of ΔΔCts is positive for overexpressed genes and negative if under-expressed.

Assai ID	Gene Symbol	Gene Name	T-TEST	Average ΔΔCts
Hs00175732_m1	P2RY2	purinergic receptor P2Y, G-protein coupled, 2	0.049	3.4
Hs00152917_m1	CCR5	chemokine (C-C motif) receptor 5	0.003	-1.5
Hs00270999_s1	GPR4	G protein-coupled receptor 4	0.028	-5.7

Table 6. Genes differentially expressed in PBMCs stimulated by LPS between control and CD patients.

3.6 Expression profiles in biopsies

Biopsies from healthy subjects, CD, UC and IBS patients were analyzed. Data were obtained with the microfluidic card#2 dedicated to GPCR transcriptome. The results presented were obtained from 11 biopsies taken from a sampling of heterogeneous individuals: one biopsy of healthy individuals, four zones of patients with inflammatory CD and a healthy area of a patient with CD, inflammatory zone 2 of patients with UC and a healthy area of a patient with UC, and 2 from patients with IBS. The results presented were obtained from 11 biopsies taken heterogeneous individuals: 1 biopsy of healthy individual only, 4 inflamed zones of CD patients and one healthy zone of CD patients, 2 inflamed zones of UC patients and a healthy zone of UC patient, and 2 inflamed zones of IBS patients.

Due to the heterogeneity and the small number of individuals studied, we tried to present here the most interesting results in spite of all possible combinations. It seemed wise to seek for receptors that expressed specifically in inflamed CD tissue relative to all other samples, biopsy of the healthy individual and those of patients with UC or IBS. This procedure is like comparing the inflammatory tissue of CD with background noise resulting from the combination of all other tissues. To do this, we used the same approach of comparing expression profiles of PBMCs from healthy subjects and patients with a Student test for unpaired data (α equal to 0.05) and the calculation of ΔΔCt averages of two classes ($\Delta\Delta Ct = (\Delta Ct_{non\text{-}CD} - \Delta Ct_{CD})$). The genes were filtered with the criteria of an average of Cts lower than 37 and selected for ΔΔCt higher than 1.5. Thus Table 8 shows 37 genes differentially expressed between biopsies from inflamed zone of CD patients and all the other biopsies (healthy individual, healthy area of CD patient, areas of healthy and inflammatory UC patients and IBS). All 37 genes are overexpressed in CD.

Given the large number of genes revealed, we relied on the David software to highlight the functional categories appropriately represented in an expression profile. David is a Web application of NCBI that uses the NCBI GO terms (Gene Ontology) a vocabulary structured to describe role of genes and their products (The Gene Ontology Consortium, 2001). David interprets terms GO associated with differentially found genes and alternatively compares them with whole of functional categories of genes present on card#2, alternately against the studied genome. Under "immune response", appeared a group of seven genes, including many chemokine receptors (*ADORA1, BLR1, CNR2, CCR6, CCR7, CCR8, IL8RA, IL8RB*). This group corresponds to an ontology enrichment of a factor 2 (8/33 compared to 49/362 in map 2). One can note the strong representation of genes related to neuropeptides, receptor proteins are 17 out of 33 (33 of the 37 gene list have a GO term). However, these receptors do not represent enrichment since they are 162 listed in this category.

We looked for genes characteristic of different types of inflammation of the intestine: IBS, UC and CD. To do this we compare the three groups of tissue two by two and used the criteria previously used to identify "differential" genes. Tables 8 to 11 represent the genes obtained. Table 11 shows a greater number of "differential" genes between inflamed zones between IBS patients and CD patients. All 19 genes are increasing in CD up to several orders of magnitude. These genes are composed in a large majority of neuropeptides receptors. There are also many orphan receptors, like the TAAR family ("Trace Amine Associated Receptor"), for which ligands are likely to have similarities with the metabolites of amino acids as neurotransmitters.

Table 12 shows 4 "differential" genes between UC and IBS: 3 orphan receptors are increased in UC biopsies whereas receptor of chemokine CCBP2 is reduced. Between biopsies of UC and CD (table 10), there are very few genes that are significantly "differently" expressed. Note that among four neuropeptide receptors, two are receptors for peptides from the brain (vasopressin and parathyroid hormone). These hormone receptors may reflect a special relationship of inflammatory bowel area with the central nervous system. Those genes are the significantly different between UC and CD.

Assay ID	Gene Symbol	Gene Name	T-TEST	Average ΔΔCts
Hs00609865_m1	EDNRA	endothelin receptor type A	0.002	6.6
Hs00174146_m1	IL8RA	interleukin 8 receptor, alpha	0.035	6.0
Hs00218495_m1	GPR77	G protein-coupled receptor 77	0.008	5.3
Hs00167241_m1	HTR2A	5-hydroxytryptamine (serotonin) receptor 2A	0.007	4.4
Hs00223340_m1	GPR147	G protein-coupled receptor 147	0.006	4.2
Hs00174304_m1	IL8RB	interleukin 8 receptor, beta	0.044	3.8
Hs00173855_m1	GPR	putative G protein coupled receptor	0.002	3.6
Hs00176122_m1	AVPR1A	arginine vasopressin receptor 1A	0.002	3.4
Hs00200681_m1	ADMR	adrenomedullin receptor	0.049	3.3
Hs00542381_m1	GPR114	G protein-coupled receptor 114	0.015	3.2
Hs00174895_m1	PTHR1	parathyroid hormone receptor 1	0.007	3.1
Hs00171054_m1	CCR7	chemokine (C-C motif) receptor 7	0.001	3.0
Hs00332805_m1	MRGPRF	MAS-related GPR, member F	0.003	3.0
Hs00736776_m1	P2RY8	purinergic receptor P2Y, G-protein coupled, 8	0.002	3.0
Hs00212116_m1	GPRC5B	GPCR, family C, group 5, member B	0.009	3.0
Hs00168765_m1	PTGIR	prostaglandin I2 (prostacyclin) receptor (IP)	0.027	2.9
Hs00174764_m1	CCR8	chemokine (C-C motif) receptor 8	0.016	2.9
Hs00361490_m1	CNR2	cannabinoid receptor 2 (macrophage)	0.028	2.7
Hs00266671_s1	FY	Duffy blood group	0.040	2.7
Hs00391810_m1	GPR116	G protein-coupled receptor 116	0.009	2.6
Hs00237052_m1	CXCR4	chemokine (C-X-C motif) receptor 4	0.006	2.4
Hs00272624_s1	CYSLTR1	cysteinyl leukotriene receptor 1	0.040	2.4
Hs00174910_m1	TSHR	thyroid stimulating hormone receptor	0.030	2.4
Hs00168763_m1	PTGFR	prostaglandin F receptor (FP)	0.028	2.3
Hs00187982_m1	F2RL2	coagulation factor II (thrombin) receptor-like 2	0.047	2.3
Hs00173499_m1	EDG1	endothelial differentiation, sphingolipid GPCR 1	0.010	2.2
Hs00173527_m1	BLR1	Burkitt lymphoma receptor 1, GTP binding protein (chemokine (C-X-C motif) receptor 5)	0.022	2.2
Hs00184657_m1	BAI2	brain-specific angiogenesis inhibitor 2	0.035	2.2
Hs00170665_m1	SMO	smoothened homolog (Drosophila)	0.043	2.1
Hs00262150_m1	GPR124	G protein-coupled receptor 124	0.026	2.1
Hs00274326_s1	P2RY10	purinergic receptor P2Y, G-protein coupled, 10	0.034	2.0
Hs00181231_m1	ADORA1	adenosine A1 receptor	0.042	2.0
Hs00246222_s1	NPY6R	neuropeptide Y receptor Y6 (pseudogene)	0.026	2.0
Hs00168362_m1	HTR2B	5-hydroxytryptamine (serotonin) receptor 2B	0.038	1.9
Hs00173787_m1	CALCRL	calcitonin receptor-like	0.028	1.9
Hs00169258_m1	F2R	coagulation factor II (thrombin) receptor	0.030	1.8
Hs00270873_s1	AGTRL1	angiotensin II receptor-like 1	0.026	1.8
Hs00171121_m1	CCR6	chemokine (C-C motif) receptor 6	0.009	1.8

Table 7. Genes differentially expressed between biopsies of inflamed zone CD patients and biopsies of colon (healthy individual, healthy zone of the CD patient, healthy and inflamed zones of UC patients, inflamed zones of IBS patients).

Assay ID	Gene Symbol	Gene Name	T-TEST	Average ΔΔCts
Hs00174146_m1	IL8RA	interleukin 8 receptor, alpha	0.002	10.8
Hs00218495_m1	GPR77	G protein-coupled receptor 77	0.035	8.4
Hs00220561_m1	GPR84	G protein-coupled receptor 84	0.023	7.9
Hs00174304_m1	IL8RB	interleukin 8 receptor, beta	0.025	6.1
Hs00223340_m1	GPR147	G protein-coupled receptor 147	0.010	5.9
Hs00271072_s1	GPR23	G protein-coupled receptor 23	0.043	5.8
Hs00181830_m1	FPR1	formyl peptide receptor 1	0.035	5.1
Hs00256749_s1	P2RY13	purinergic receptor P2Y, G-protein coupled, 13	0.012	4.0
Hs00266213_s1	CCR3	chemokine (C-C motif) receptor 3	0.034	3.7
Hs00261470_m1	EMR3	egf-like module containing, mucin-like, hormone receptor-like 3	0.040	3.6
Hs00269446_s1	EDG6	endothelial differentiation, G-protein-coupled receptor 6	0.046	3.6
Hs00252658_s1	CYSLTR2	cysteinyl leukotriene receptor 2	0.015	3.1
Hs00171054_m1	CCR7	chemokine (C-C motif) receptor 7	0.012	2.9
Hs00542381_m1	GPR114	G protein-coupled receptor 114	0.031	2.8
Hs00274326_s1	P2RY10	purinergic receptor P2Y, G-protein coupled, 10	0.027	2.4
Hs00252888_s1	VN1R1	vomeronasal 1 receptor 1	0.040	1.7
Hs00176738_m1	MATK	megakaryocyte-associated tyrosine kinase	0.041	-1.3
Hs00191104_m1	GPR37L1	G-protein coupled receptor 37 like 1	0.039	-4.8

Table 8. Genes differentially expressed between biopsies of inflamed zone of CD patients, and biopsies of healthy individual and patients having IBS.

Assay ID	Gene Symbol	Gene Name	T-TEST	Average ΔΔCts
Hs00266671_s1	FY	Duffy blood group	0.040	2.7
Hs00184657_m1	BAI2	brain-specific angiogenesis inhibitor 2	0.035	2.2
Hs00181231_m1	ADORA1	adenosine A1 receptor	0.042	2.0

Table 9. Common genes differentially expressed between biopsies of inflamed zone and PBMCs of CD patients.

Assay ID	Gene Symbol	Gene Name	T-TEST	Average ΔΔCts
Hs00174895_m1	PTHR1	parathyroid hormone receptor 1	0.001	3.9
Hs00176122_m1	AVPR1A	Arginine vasopressin receptor 1A	0.007	2.7
Hs00184657_m1	BAI2	brain-specific angiogenesis inhibitor 2	0.029	2.2
Hs00265081_s1	ADRA2A	adrenergic, alpha-2A-, receptor	0.044	2.1
Hs00174304_m1	IL8RB	interleukin 8 receptor, beta	0.004	-2.2
Hs00266213_s1	CCR3	chemokine (C-C motif) receptor 3	0.007	-2.3
Hs00181830_m1	FPR1	formyl peptide receptor 1	0.034	-2.6
Hs00220561_m1	GPR84	G protein-coupled receptor 84	0.033	-3.7
Hs00218495_m1	GPR77	G protein-coupled receptor 77	0.003	-4.0

Table 10. Genes differentially expressed between biopsies of inflamed zone of CD patients and biopsies of inflamed zone of UC patients.

Assay ID	Gene Symbol	Gene Name	T-TEST	Average ΔΔCts
Hs00601815_s1	TAAR9	trace amine associated receptor 9	0.010	11.7
Hs00365019_s1	MRGPRX2	MAS-related GPR, member X2	0.009	11.4
Hs00265296_s1	HTR1F	5-hydroxytryptamine (serotonin) receptor 1F	0.012	11.2
Hs00609865_m1	EDNRA	endothelin receptor type A	0.026	11.1
Hs00174146_m1	IL8RA	interleukin 8 receptor, alpha	0.006	11.1
Hs00265208_s1	CHRM2	cholinergic receptor, muscarinic 2	0.000	9.9
Hs00220561_m1	GPR84	G protein-coupled receptor 84	0.012	9.4
Hs00269590_s1	TAAR5	trace amine associated receptor 5	0.001	9.3
Hs00754695_s1	MRGPRX3	MAS-related GPR, member X3	0.043	8.8
Hs00265081_s1	ADRA2A	adrenergic, alpha-2A-, receptor	0.036	8.6
Hs00664049_s1	GPR150	G protein-coupled receptor 150	0.017	8.4
Hs00274365_s1	TAAR2	trace amine associated receptor 2	0.002	7.4
Hs00271072_s1	GPR23	G protein-coupled receptor 23	0.002	7.3
Hs00664166_s1	GPR142	G protein-coupled receptor 142	0.044	6.9
Hs00267157_s1	MAS1	MAS1 oncogene	0.003	6.2
Hs00266671_s1	FY	Duffy blood group	0.030	5.8
Hs00271877_s1	CD4R	Melanocortin 4 receptor	0.046	5.1
Hs00269446_s1	EDG6	endothelial differentiation, G-protein-coupled receptor 6	0.029	4.5
Hs00168567_m1	NPY2R	Neuropeptide Y receptor Y2	0.032	3.3

Table 11. Genes differentially expressed between biopsies of inflamed zone of CD patients and IBS patients.

Assay ID	Gene Symbol	Gene Name	T-TEST	Average ΔΔCts
Hs00220561_m1	GPR84	G protein-coupled receptor 84	0.044	8.0
Hs00664166_s1	GPR142	G protein-coupled receptor 142	0.042	7.5
Hs00542396_m1	GPR110	G protein-coupled receptor 110	0.008	4.9
Hs00174299_m1	CCBP2	chemokine binding protein 2	0.039	-2.8

Table 12. Genes differentially expressed between biopsies of inflamed zone of FGD patients and UC patients.

4. Conclusion

Studying the expression of GPCRs in PBMCs has highlighted a number of deregulated genes in CD. In general, among these deregulated genes, the majority is accepted to be involved in mechanisms of inflammation or immune response. After a closer examination of their function, these genes appear to have an opposite contribution in the inflammatory process. Surprisingly, receptor expression is regulated more in favor of a repressor or suppressor effect of a malfunction of inflammatory cells rather than in a pro-inflammatory activity like SSTR5 whose role is to reduce intestinal inflammation.

Expression profiles of PBMC's GPCR distinguish CD patients from healthy donors are represented in Figure 10. The expression of a reduced number of genes makes it even clearly feasible to differentiate PBMCs from healthy individuals and CD patients (Figure 11). These receptors could be a signature for CD, but it remains necessary to test this group of genes with other known genes, for healthy and CD PBMCs, and so to check if clustering classifies correctly these samples. It would be also interesting to compare these profiles with those obtained from PBMCs of patients developing IBS or UC.

Our study activation of PBMCs by LPS shows that PBMCs are able to induce in vitro an immunizing response in answer to exposure to bacterial lipopolysaccharide of production and release in medium of TNF-α, principal mediator of inflammatory answer. This activation of monocytes by LPS was amply described and used in routine way in laboratories to test capacity of monocytes to answer pathogenic microorganisms. Majority of human cells answer molecular signals of microbial invasion of installing locally mechanisms of defense, then by recruiting and activating specialized cells of immune system.

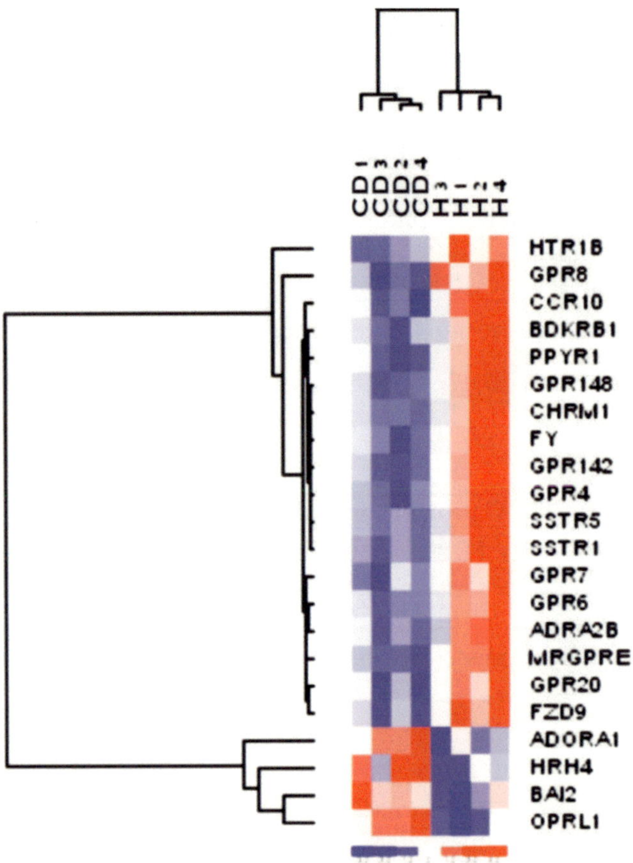

Fig. 10. Signature of GPCR expression in PBMCs from CD patients (CD) versus healthy donors (H). Ascending hierarchic classification was carried out using the software Dchip (Li and Wong 2001) using a correlation matrix of distances and centroid grouping. The matrix of expression data is converted into a thermal colored map according to the relative level of expression of each gene. The colors range from blue to a high level of expression to red for a low level of expression through an intermediate white (values expressed in ΔCt).

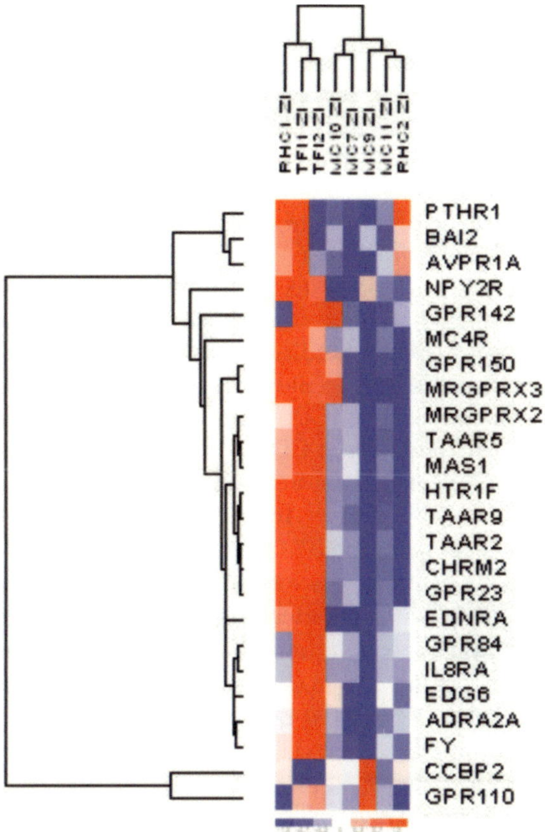

Fig. 11. Signature of expression of GPCRs in biopsies of CD patients (MCxx), UC patients (RHCxx) and IBS patients (TFIxx).

As has been described before, the recognition of TRL4 receptors on the surface of monocytes by a bacterial product such as LPS leads to a cascade of reactions within the cells and release of cytokines TNF-α, but also IL-1, IL-3, I-6, IL-10, and colony stimulating factors (CSFs), chemokines such as IL-8 and macrophage inflammatory proteins (MIFs). The main mechanism underlying the induction of these proteins is at the level of transcription, particularly under the control of the transcription factor NF-κB. We studied here the effect of bacterial stimuli in an original way, first by examining its effect on the expression of almost all GPCRs, second using a macro-arrays technology by real-time PCR. Our results indicate that activation of PBMC by LPS is reflected mainly by a repression of GPCR expression. In a similar approach conducted with larger arrays, the same trend was observed *i.e.* LPS represses 1125 genes out of 1868 differentially expressed genes (Wurfel et al. 2005). Among the overexpressed genes, these authors note the presence of key players in the inflammatory response, primarily cytokines and chemokines. In our hands the only GPCR in the list of 15 genes selected in each category is the chemokine receptor 2 (CCR2) the 2nd most strongly repressed. If we noticed no decrease in CCR2, the experimental condition, origin of LPS, exposure time and concentration of LPS may explain this divergence of results. It is interesting to note that among genes repressed by LPS common to healthy individuals and

CD patients, two families of receptor are represented: chemokine receptors (CCR1, CCR3, CMKLR1, C5AR1) and formylated peptides receptors (FPR1, FPRL2). The receptors involved in chemotaxis and recognition of bacterial peptides (CCR1, CMKLR1, RPF) have been extensively documented for their repression following LPS activation of PBMCs (Boldrick et al. 2002; Nau et al. 2002; Parker et al. 2004). Others observed similar expression profiles in PBMCs (Boldrick et al. 2002). In addition, they noticed that the induction and repression are LPS dose dependent and there are some differences in the profiles along the microorganism and their virulence, suggesting that some pathogens have developed strategies to foil the defense mechanism of host cells. However we observe a suppression of two other chemokine receptors: CCR3, known to have high affinity for eotaxin, a chemokine produced by eosinophil in broncho-alveolar fluid in the animal model of asthma (Jose, Griffiths-Johnson et al. 1994) and C5AR1 studied in neutrophil chemotaxis and linked to many diseases immune complex. Other receptors whose function is less known (EDG2, GPBAR1) and especially 2 orphan receptors (GPR155 one of rare genes activated by LPS and GPR162 repressed by more than 100 times in CD patients) could provide new elements in understanding the signaling pathways that control the inflammatory response.

The decrease in gene expression essential for the defense of an organism, while it is in contact with the invader, may seem paradoxical. One hypothesis is that these mechanisms of repression and induction of certain genes have a regulatory role for antigen-presenting cells (APC). This repression of genes, without which the massive amplification of defense systems quickly destroy infectious agents, allows the APC time to present antigens to T cells, not only at the site of infection but also in secondary lymphoid tissues.

It should be noted that parallel to repression of certain receptors, most of their ligands, cytokines and chemokines, are increased by LPS (Boldrick et al. 2002). This hypothesis reinforces the concept of immune defense mechanism tightly controlled and orchestrated at the transcriptional level as highlighted by studying expression profiles over time. Thus, in monocytes, LPS controls temporally and alternately increase and decrease of expression of different groups of gene (Sharif et al. 2007). In the context of a specific program of control of gene expression, it is not surprising that the time, the origin and the dose of LPS are factors that influence the expression profile. It is interesting to note that in the work of Sharif and coll., 4 receptors of our repertory are among the 72 genes controlled by LPS: after 1 hour of exposure, only ADORA1 is slightly increased but returns to its original level at 4 hours, after four hours, while CCR7 is increased CCR2 and CXR4 are repressed. Our results for these genes obtained after 2 hours 30 of exposure are compatible and consistent with those described before (Sharif et al. 2007). In Table 6 are represented the 3 receptors whose expression varies significantly for CD patients. Why and how genes are regulated in the context of healthy individuals or with the disease and how they are connected to other receptors deregulated in CD patients, are questions difficult to be answered at this level of study. However, the large number of genes controlled by LPS in both healthy subjects and CD patients, compared to three genes differentially controlled, suggests that PBMC from the two populations have the capacity to respond very similarly to LPS activation, suggesting that CD patients PBMCs are only moderately disturbed in response to a bacterial infection. However, we can not exclude that one of the 3 receptors that differentiate two groups of individuals in response to bacterial stimuli, could control a signaling pathway involved, directly or indirectly, in CD. For example, disability and loss of immunological tolerance vis-à-vis certain species of commensal bacteria in the intestine is characteristic of CD patients and are often put forward to explain the chronicity of the inflammatory state (Sartor 2003). The expression profiles of GPCR in inflamed zones of Crohn patients clearly suggest a close relationship between the inflammatory process and the nervous system. Our results have shown unequivocally chemokine receptors (ADORA1, BLR1, CCR6, CCR7, CCR8, IL8RA, IL8RB) many neuropeptide receptors and neurotransmitter in the disease. Neuropeptide receptors and neurotransmitter occupy an essential place in the nervous system to ensure the function of the intestinal wall. The nervous system is complex: the autonomous nervous system consists of a network of nerve fibers connected to the plexus that connect the different layers of the wall and sympathetic and parasympathetic fibers that make synapses in small intramural ganglia. The autonomous nervous system ensures glandular secretion, vasodilation and vasoconstriction, and motility of smooth muscle fibers. The colon wall is also controlled by the vegetative nervous system under the control of the hypothalamic-adrenal-hypophysio-surrenal axis. It is through him that emotions, stress and fatigue affect the functioning of the digestive system (Taylor & Keely 2007).

The presence of chemokine receptors, neuropeptides and neurotransmitters suggests a close relationship and communication between nerve cells, the intestinal lining cells and immune cells in the inflammatory zone. These links are illustrated by the endocrine cells, for example, the colonic epithelium that secrete polypeptide hormones and neurotransmitters such as gastrin, cholecystokinin (CCK), VIP (vasoactive intestinal peptide), substance P, bombesin and somatostatin and serotonin, which also act as neurotransmitters. If the effect of the ligands is relatively well documented in all functions related to the nervous system, transmission potential, secretion, muscle contractility, the role of receptors is more complex. The increase in receptors in the inflammatory tissue of CD is consistent with a general increase in neuronal signaling, described in the literature in terms of neuropeptides and neurotransmitters. At this stage of the study, interpretation of the increase in these receptors and their role in the inflammation is difficult without information on the characteristics of cells in which they are overexpressed.

These increases can be linked to altered activity of nerve cells under the influence of inflammatory mediators or a nervous system response to restore tissue to a normal state. The histology of the intestinal mucosa, as we observed on our CD biopsies, must be accompanied by a remodeling of the enteric system so that it can perform its functions. It is a set of elements that are responsible for these changes: neuronal plasticity, all of these neuronal modulations, changes in morphology, the number and development of new dendrites for connective, but the emergence of new nerve cells (Geboes & Collins 1998). The increase of certain nerve cells may explain the increase in receptors. Enterochromaffin cells contain many neuroactive substances such as serotonin, bradykinin, tachykinin and prostaglandin that are released by multiple stimuli, mechanical, chemical and nervous. The release of serotonin, which has many roles (such as the increase in intestinal motility, vasoconstriction, synaptic transmission), is controlled at the level of enterochromaffin cells by receptors some of which have a stimulatory activity (HTR1, HTR2, MCR3) while others have an inhibitory activity (HTR3, type purinergic receptor P2Y, histamine, neurokinin, somatostatin). In these cells, two receptors HTR2 A and B increased in Crohn's disease, have a role rather amplifier of the disease. It would be the same level of sensory nerves that express a wide range of receptor on their surface. Neuronal activity is controlled mainly by receptor of natural substances such as VIP or substance P, but the activity can be altered by the presence of inflammatory products (serotonin, bradykinin, prostaglandin leukotriene,

ATP) and usually results in hyper excitability. Generally, treatment uses antagonists of these receptors (Hansen 2003).
All nerve cells do not have the same contribution in the development of the disease. For example, in terms of motility disorders, due to alterations in signal transmission at synapses of the enteric nerves, it was shown that motility of the intestine is controlled by the adrenergic sympathetic fibers that decrease while the parasympathetic fibers stimulate the cholinergic (Smith & Smid 2005). Studies show that agents which promote parasympathetic activity also tend to reduce the severity of the disease, and conversely for sympathetic activity (Miceli & Jacobson 2003). It would be interesting to know the repertoire of these receptors in nerve cells and identify those that are deregulated in order to use agonists or antagonists to restore gut motility.
Results reported here are encouraging nevertheless they remain preliminary. It will be necessary to analyze a larger number of samples, identify exactly the biopsy position in the colon and obtain relevant information on individuals before hoping to get molecular signatures of the different types of bowel diseases. In a therapeutic point of view, our results on the transcriptome of GPCRs from Crohn's disease biopsies offer a wide range of potential therapeutic targets, for functions as diverse as those related to the immune response, hormonal regulations, transfers of nervous information nerve, or blood clotting.

5. Acknowledgment

The study was supported by a grant from ACI 2002, MNRT, CNRS-INSERM-CEA, Pathologies-RCPG-Médicaments France. Nathalie Taquet was supported by a grant from FERRING laboratories (Gentilly, France) and Jean-Marie Reimund received a grant from UCB Laboratories, France.

6. References

Andres, P. G. & Friedman, L. S. (1999). Epidemiology and the natural course of inflammatory bowel disease. *Gastroenterol Clin North Am*, Vol.28 N°2 (Jun), pp. 255-281

Baker, P. E., Fahey, J. V. & Munck, A. (1981). Prostaglandin inhibition of T-cell proliferation is mediated at two levels. *Cell Immunol*, Vol.61 N°1 (Jun), pp. 52-61

Baldassano, R. N. & Piccoli, D. A. (1999). Inflammatory bowel disease in pediatric and adolescent patients. *Gastroenterol Clin North Am*, Vol.28 N°2 (Jun), pp. 445-458

Boldrick, J. C., Alizadeh, A. A., Diehn, M., Dudoit, S., Liu, C. L., Belcher, C. E., Botstein, D., Staudt, L. M., Brown, P. O. & Relman, D. A. (2002). Stereotyped and specific gene expression programs in human innate immune responses to bacteria. *Proc Natl Acad Sci U S A*, Vol.99 N°2 (Jan 22), pp. 972-977

Burczynski, M. E., Peterson, R. L., Twine, N. C., Zuberek, K. A., Brodeur, B. J., Casciotti, L., Maganti, V., Reddy, P. S., Strahs, A., Immermann, F., Spinelli, W., Schwertschlag, U., Slager, A. M., Cotreau, M. M. & Dorner, A. J. (2006). Molecular classification of Crohn's disease and ulcerative colitis patients using transcriptional profiles in peripheral blood mononuclear cells. *J Mol Diagn*, Vol.8 N°1 (Feb), pp. 51-61

Chomczynski, P. & Sacchi, N. (1987). Single-step method of RNA isolation by acid guanidinium thiocyanate-phenol-chloroform extraction. *Anal Biochem*, Vol.162 N°1 (Apr), pp. 156-159

Dieckgraefe, B. K., Stenson, W. F., Korzenik, J. R., Swanson, P. E. & Harrington, C. A. (2000). Analysis of mucosal gene expression in inflammatory bowel disease by parallel oligonucleotide arrays. *Physiol Genomics*, Vol.4 N°1 (Nov 9), pp. 1-11

Elson, C. O., Sartor, R. B., Tennyson, G. S. & Riddell, R. H. (1995). Experimental models of inflammatory bowel disease. *Gastroenterology*, Vol.109 N°4 (Oct), pp. 1344-1367

Geboes, K. & Collins, S. (1998). Structural abnormalities of the nervous system in Crohn's disease and ulcerative colitis. *Neurogastroenterol Motil*, Vol.10 N°3 (Jun), pp. 189-202

Hansen, M. B. (2003). The enteric nervous system I: organisation and classification. *Pharmacol Toxicol*, Vol.92 N°3 (Mar), pp. 105-113

Lawrance, I. C., Fiocchi, C. & Chakravarti, S. (2001). Ulcerative colitis and Crohn's disease: distinctive gene expression profiles and novel susceptibility candidate genes. *Hum Mol Genet*, Vol.10 N°5 (Mar 1), pp. 445-456

Luther, S. A. & Cyster, J. G. (2001). Chemokines as regulators of T cell differentiation. *Nat Immunol*, Vol.2 N°2 (Feb), pp. 102-107

Matsuura, T., West, G. A., Youngman, K. R., Klein, J. S. & Fiocchi, C. (1993). Immune activation genes in inflammatory bowel disease. *Gastroenterology*, Vol.104 N°2 (Feb), pp. 448-458

Miceli, P. C. & Jacobson, K. (2003). Cholinergic pathways modulate experimental dinitrobenzene sulfonic acid colitis in rats. *Auton Neurosci*, Vol.105 N°1 (Apr 30), pp. 16-24 1566-0702 (Print)

Nau, G. J., Richmond, J. F., Schlesinger, A., Jennings, E. G., Lander, E. S. & Young, R. A. (2002). Human macrophage activation programs induced by bacterial pathogens. *Proc Natl Acad Sci U S A*, Vol.99 N°3 (Feb 5), pp. 1503-1508

Onuffer, J. J. & Horuk, R. (2002). Chemokines, chemokine receptors and small-molecule antagonists: recent developments. *Trends Pharmacol Sci*, Vol.23 N°10 (Oct), pp. 459-467

Parker, L. C., Whyte, M. K., Vogel, S. N., Dower, S. K. & Sabroe, I. (2004). Toll-like receptor (TLR)2 and TLR4 agonists regulate CCR expression in human monocytic cells. *J Immunol*, Vol.172 N°8 (Apr 15), pp. 4977-4986

Podolsky, D. K. (2002). Inflammatory bowel disease. *N Engl J Med*, Vol.347 N°6 (Aug 8), pp. 417-429

Rockett, J. C., Burczynski, M. E., Fornace, A. J., Herrmann, P. C., Krawetz, S. A. & Dix, D. J. (2004). Surrogate tissue analysis: monitoring toxicant exposure and health status of inaccessible tissues through the analysis of accessible tissues and cells. *Toxicol Appl Pharmacol*, Vol.194 N°2 (Jan 15), pp. 189-199

Sartor, R. B. (2003). Targeting enteric bacteria in treatment of inflammatory bowel diseases: why, how, and when. *Curr Opin Gastroenterol*, Vol.19 N°4 (Jul), pp. 358-365

Satsangi, J., Parkes, M., Louis, E., Hashimoto, L., Kato, N., Welsh, K., Terwilliger, J. D., Lathrop, G. M., Bell, J. I. & Jewell, D. P. (1996). Two stage genome-wide search in inflammatory bowel disease provides evidence for susceptibility loci on chromosomes 3, 7 and 12. *Nat Genet*, Vol.14 N°2 (Oct), pp. 199-202

Schroeder, A., Mueller, O., Stocker, S., Salowsky, R., Leiber, M., Gassmann, M., Lightfoot, S., Menzel, W., Granzow, M. & Ragg, T. (2006). The RIN: an RNA integrity number for assigning integrity values to RNA measurements. *BMC Mol Biol*, Vol.7 pp. 3 1471-2199 (Electronic)

Sharif, O., Bolshakov, V. N., Raines, S., Newham, P. & Perkins, N. D. (2007). Transcriptional profiling of the LPS induced NF-kappaB response in macrophages. *BMC Immunol*, Vol.8 pp. 1

Sirover, M. A. (1999). New insights into an old protein: the functional diversity of mammalian glyceraldehyde-3-phosphate dehydrogenase. *Biochim Biophys Acta*, Vol.1432 N°2 (Jul 13), pp. 159-184

Smith, A. S. & Smid, S. D. (2005). Impaired capsaicin and neurokinin-evoked colonic motility in inflammatory bowel disease. *J Gastroenterol Hepatol*, Vol.20 N°5 (May), pp. 697-704

Tatton, W. G., Chalmers-Redman, R. M., Elstner, M., Leesch, W., Jagodzinski, F. B., Stupak, D. P., Sugrue, M. M. & Tatton, N. A. (2000). Glyceraldehyde-3-phosphate dehydrogenase in neurodegeneration and apoptosis signaling. *J Neural Transm Suppl* N°60 pp. 77-100

Taylor, C. T. & Keely, S. J. (2007). The autonomic nervous system and inflammatory bowel disease. *Auton Neurosci*, Vol.133 N°1 (Apr 30), pp. 104-114

Thelen, M. (2001). Dancing to the tune of chemokines. *Nat Immunol*, Vol.2 N°2 (Feb), pp. 129-134

Warner, E. E. & Dieckgraefe, B. K. (2002). Application of genome-wide gene expression profiling by high-density DNA arrays to the treatment and study of inflammatory bowel disease. *Inflamm Bowel Dis*, Vol.8 N°2 (Mar), pp. 140-157

Wurfel, M. M., Park, W. Y., Radella, F., Ruzinski, J., Sandstrom, A., Strout, J., Bumgarner, R. E. & Martin, T. R. (2005). Identification of high and low responders to lipopolysaccharide in normal subjects: an unbiased approach to identify modulators of innate immunity. *J Immunol*, Vol.175 N°4 (Aug 15), pp. 2570-2578

Part 2

Diagnosis of Crohn's Disease

5

Be or Not to Be a Crohn's Disease: CD and Its Numerous Differential Diagnosis

Amandine Gagneux-Brunon[1], Bernard Faulques[2] and Xavier Roblin[2,*]
[1]*Infectious and Tropical Diseases Department, CHU de Saint-Etienne,*
[2]*Gastroenterology Department, CHU de Saint-Etienne*
France

1. Introduction

Nowadays, there is still no gold standard test for Inflammatory Bowel Disease (IBD). Many etiologies are responsible of an inflammation of the gut. When a patient presents with signs suggestive of IBD (abdominal pain, diarrhea, and sometimes fever), the clinician had to establish whether the patient suffers from an IBD or from one of the numerous alternative diseases. The use of immunosuppressive agents and biotherapies in IBD treatment enforces the necessity to distinguish them from infectious diseases, particularly from tuberculosis. Clinical signs of IBD are not specific. This review will focus on the differential diagnosis of Crohn's Disease (CD) and on the helpful tests for the diagnosis. Histopathological findings are sometimes insufficient to establish the diagnosis, granuloma is not specific and inconstant in CD (only in 15 to 60 % of cases). Serological assays (perinuclear antineutrophil antibodies pANCA and anti-*Saccharomyces cerevisae* antibodies ASCA) are contributing to the diagnosis, but their sensitivity and specificity are too weak for a gold standard. This review will be divided in 2 parts: first, a review of etiologies inducing granulomas in the gut (infections, systemic diseases, drug related disorder…), second, a review of controversies in the distinction between ulcerative colitis (UC) and CD. This review will contribute to provide to clinicians a strategy for differential diagnosis of CD (infection, systemic disease, neoplasm, drug related disorders, non specific inflammation…). Therefore, sensible and specific biomarkers are needed to facilitate the diagnosis of IBD in the future.

Crohn's disease is an Inflammatory Bowel Disease (IBD), able to affect all the gut mucosa. Crohn disease may induce lesion of epithelioid granuloma. However, this type of lesion may be associated with others affections, certain of these affections are infectious diseases, and contra-indicate formally the immunotherapy. Nowadays, there is no gold standard assay to make the etiological diagnosis of granuloma of the gastrointestinal (GI) tract.

2. How differentiate CD from tuberculosis?

The differential diagnosis of CD and tuberculosis of the digestive tract is challenging, as the incidence of CD is dramatically increasing in countries where TB is too prevalent, and as TB epidemic restarts in the developed countries. Since the presence of a caseation necrosis in

* Corresponding Author

endoscopic biopsies confirms TB, this histological findings stay uncommon in the most cases of digestive TB. Surgical biopsies are more efficient to establish the diagnosis of TB (1). A confusion between TB and CD is not Exceptional. In a saoudian study, 21% of the patients treated for a digestive TB, were really affected by CD (2). Clinically, the differential diagnosis is uneasy. Digestive TB is induced by hematogenous spread after the inhalation of the bacillus or by ingestion of *mycobacterium bovis.* In case of an infection by *mycobacterium tuberculosis,* the association with a pulmonary TB is unconsistent. Certain localizations for lesion are more frequent in TB than in CD. Preponderant localizations are presented in table 1. After a comparison between 53 patients with CD and 53 others with digestive TB, *Makharia* et al. establish a clinical, endoscopic et histological score to differentiate TB (3). In this study, chronic diarrhea, blood in the stools, perianal disease and extraintestinal manifestations were significantly more frequent in CD than in TB. On the other side, abdominal pain, constipation, intestinal obstruction, loss of appetite, and weight loss were associated with TB. Sites of CD involvement were more often rectum, sigmoid, ascending and descending colon. The type of lesions in endoscopy was also different in the two groups: skip lesions, friability, aphtous, linear and superficial ulcers, and cobblestoning were more often observed in the CD group. Nodular lesions were more frequent in the TB group. Histological examination found more and larger granulomas per section in TB, and more often lesion of focally enhanced colitis in CD. The developed score is: -2,5*Involvement of sigmoïd colon-2,1* blood in stool+2,3*weight loss-2,1*focally enhanced colitis+7 where each characteristics were given 1 if present and 0 if absent. With a cutt-off of 5,1, this score demonstrated a good sensibility, a good specificity and a good ability to correctly classify the two diseases. The area under the receiver operating curve (AUC-ROC) was 89,2. Endoscopic examination is really helpful to differentiate TB from CD. Considering that anorectal lesions, longitudinal ulcers, aphtous ulcers cobblestone appearance were typical in CD, and that involvement of fewer than four segments, a patulous ileocecal valve, transverse ulcers, and scars of pseudopolypes were typical of intestinal TB, *Lee* et al. hypothesized that CD diagnostic could be made when the number of parameters characteristic of CD was greater than parameters associated with TB (4). With these assumptions, diagnosis was correctly made in 87,5 % of the patients. Histological examination is also useful. However, characteristic lesions of TB as confluent granulomas, more than 10 granulomas per biopsy sites, and caseous necrosis are present in only a limited number of TB cases (50%, 33%, 22% respectively)(5). *Mycobacterium* is found by direct examination of biopsy in only 20 to 50% of intestinal TB cases.

Crohn's Disease	Tuberculosis
Rectum Sigmoid colon Descending colon Jejunum	Ileocecal region Ascending colon Rectum

Table 1. Principal localisations of granuloma in CD and TB

Serological test to differentiate CD and ulcerative colitis (UC) as detection of perinuclear anti-neutrophil antibodies (p-ANCA), and anti-saccharomyces cerevisae antibodies (ASCA) are not useful to differentiate CD from TB. Several studies had shown that IgA and/or IgG level of ASCA was not different between patients with CD and intestinal tuberculosis. P-ANCA was also similar in patients with CD than in patients with intestinal TB. Nowadays, serological test with p-ANCA & ASCA are not helpful to differentiate TB from CD. Intradermoreaction with tuberculin is not enough sensible or enough specific to make the diagnosis of intestinal TB, as it can be positive in the case of infections due to others *Mycobacteriae* and after vaccination and negative in immunocompromised patients. Quantiferon is a blood test of reactivity of lymphocytes T to TB antigens with production of interferon gamma which is not influenced by vaccination. Up today, no study is published on the diagnosis value of quantiferon TB for differentiating between TB and CD. There are only cases reports about positive quantiferon in case of intestinal TB. However, quantiferon is often negative in cases of extrapulmonar TB as osteitis due to *Mycobacteria.*

Cultures of *Mycobacteria* are difficult and long (3 to 8 weeks). Polymerase Chain Reaction (PCR) in intestinal biopsy, or in stools might be a good tool. Yet, the sensibility of the PCR *Mycobacterium tuberculosis* varies from 31 to 60% in biopsies (6). A positive PCR was less frequent than caseation necrosis, and presence of bacillus after Ziehl and Neelsen staining. A PCR positive in stools might help to make the diagnosis of intestinal TB, with a sensibility of 79% and a good specificity, however, this PCR may be positive in case of pulmonary TB without intestinal involvement (7).

3. Non tuberculous *mycobacteria:* Another cause of intestinal granuloma or an agent for CD?

In immuno-compromised patients (particularly HIV-positive subjects and transplanted patients), *Mycobacterium avium paratuberculosis (MAP)* is often incriminated in intestinal granulomatous disorders. However, several authors hypothesized that it might be a causal agent of CD. Long term blood culture from a great number of CD patients are positive for *MAP*, yet a great proportion of healthy controls exhibit positive blood culture. The frequency of *MAP* positive blood culture is greater in the groups of CD patients (8). However, these results are insufficient to conclude that *MAP* is a causal agent for CD. It might be a consequence of a modified commensal microbiota. A defective sensing and killing of bacteria (due to mutation in pattern-recognition receptors) might contribute to the onset of the disease (9). The only temporary efficacy of anti-tuberculous therapy in patients with CD is not in favor of a causal role of *MAP* in CD (10).

4. *Helicobacter pylori* (*HP*): An under-estimated agent of granulomatous gastritis

HP is a potential agent for granulomatous gastritis. Its frequency might be under-estimated. In 18 patients with granulomatous gastritis, HP was found in 14 cases, diagnosis of CD was made in only 1 case (11). For others, infection with HP is only concomitant of CD (12).

5. Gastro-intestinal histoplamosis: A difficult but urgent diagnosis

Histoplasma capsulatum (HC) is a mold which is common in mid-western USA, and south America. The most of patients with a disseminated histoplasmosis exhibits HC in gastrointestinal tract. First, HC is inhaled and disseminated in the all organism. Risk factors for HC are immunodepression: AIDS, CD4 lymphopenia, immunosuppressive agents. Gastrointestinal involvement may occur as a result of the adjacent mediastinal adenitis or fibrosing mediastinitis. Clinical manifestations are dysphagia, upper gastrointestinal bleeding, broncho-oesophageal fistula, abdominal pain, weight loss, lower GI bleeding, intestinal occlusion in the case of an intestinal involvement. However, GI involvement of HC may be asymptomatic. Diagnosis can be made after periodic acid Schiff (PAS) stain, antigen detection in blood and urine, serology and cultures are useful to establish the diagnosis as they are often positive in patients with histoplasmosis (13). This pathology is uncommon, but in the most of cases, no travel in endemic zone is identified. Other manifestations can be seen as hyperferritinemia, macrophagic activation syndrome, pancytopenia. The presence of these extradigestive manifestations in immunocompromised patients may encourage physicians to look for histoplasmosis.

6. *Tropheryma whipplei* (*TW*): A "real" pathogen with frequent asymptomatic carriers

Whipple's disease is unfrequent. Nine percent of the patients with manifestations of Whipple's disease had duodenal biopsies with granulomatous gastritis without caseation necrosis. Clinical manifestations are malabosrption, chronic diarrhea associated with arthritis, arthralgia, neurological disorders: supranuclear ophtalmoplegia, cognitive disorders. PCR for *T. Whipplei* is helpful to make the diagnosis. However, as this PCR is positive in 1 on 174 healthy patients, the diagnosis is definitive when the PAS staining and the PCR are positive, in association with evocating clinical manifestations. Furthermore, this PCR is positive in duodenal biopsies in stools of respectively 5 % and 11% of the patients with gastric disorders. There are many subjects who are asymptomatic carriers of TW (14).

7. GI granuloma: Do not forget Syphilis?

At the secondary and tertiary stage of *Treponema Pallidum* infection, GI involvement is possible with granulomatous lesions (15). Gastric ulcers and upper GI bleeding may be seen. Diagnosis is made with serologies TPHA, VDRL, PCR, and immunofluorescence staining in biopsies. Differential diagnosis are gastric lymphoma and linitis.

8. *Yersinia*: A frequent agent for granulomatous appendicitis

Yersinia enterolitica and *pseudotuberculosis* may cause granulomatous appendicitis, ileitis, mesenteric adenitis and colitis. The cultures are positive in around 25% of granulomatous appendicitis(16). The contamination is due to the ingestion of the bacteria. Some authors hypothesized that the defects in mucosal barrier induced by CD favors infection by *Yersnia* (17).

9. Sarcoïdosis: Rare but not impossible granulomatous involvement of digestive tract

Sarcoïdosis is a systemic granulomatosis, which rarely involves in the gastrointestinal tract (almost 3% of the patients). This is a disease, affecting people from 20 to 40 years old; the incidence is more frequent in blacks and north Europeans. Gastric lesions and extrinsic compression by mediastinal lymphadenopathy are the most frequent (18). Furthermore, any cases were reported of, small bowel polyps and colonic obstruction(19,20). Small bowel involvement may cause a real enteropathy. To confirm the diagnostic, physicians needs to obtain two biopsies from two different sites positive for giant granuloma without caseum, and after having exluded all the other potential diagnosis. Skin biopsies, lymphadenectomy, bronchoscopy with biopsy, 18-fluoro-desoxy-glucose scintigraphy may be useful to confirm the diagnosis. The dosage of the angiotensin converting enzyme (ACE) is not really helpful as every granuloma are secreting (21), as there is a polymorphism for its gene (22), with individuals with low level of ACE, even with sarcoidosis.

10. Other systemic granulomatous disorders: a more frequent GI involvement

Wegener's granulomatosis and Churg-Strauss syndrome affects in 80 % of the cases the GI tract. Clinically, patients exhibit abdominal pains, nausea, diarrhea and digestive hemorrhage (23). Gastroduodenal ulcers may be found. Granuloma is not always found in biopsy. Clinically, asthma is always found in Churg-Strauss syndrome and associated with hypereosinophilia. The dosage of antineutrophil cytoplasmic antibodies is interesting for the diagnosis as the sensibility is almost 70 to 80 % and a similar specificity (23). Anti-PR3 are associated with Wegener's granulomatosis.

11. Other anecdotic etiologies

Gastric lymphoma may represent an alternative diagnosis for a gastric granulomatous lesion (12). It is often T cells lymphoma or, lymphoma of the gut associated lymphoid tissue. Necrosis could be seen in this situation. In Shapiro's study, 2 patients on 42- with a gastric granuloma- were affected by a lymphoma. They also described in this retrospective study, cases of adenocarcinoma of the distal oesophagea. Some toxic agents may cause granuloma; yet, digestive involvement is rare. These agents are beryllium, α-interferon, BCG therapies for bladder cancer, and allopurinol. *Taeniasis* may be associated with granuloma of GI tract. There is a genetic disease, which causes immunodeficiency and systemic granulomatosis. Chronic septic granulomatosis is often linked to X-chromosome. Patients are susceptible to bacterian and fungal infections; it's the consequence of a modified NADPH-oxydase in macrophages. Granulomatous lesions of GI tract are frequent, particularly in colon(24).

12. Which strategy adopting when histopathological examination is not sufficient to make the diagnosis?

First line, second and third line, laboratory assays helpful to make a diagnosis are presented in table 2, 3 and 4. In many cases, the etiological diagnosis is made with all clinical and biological arguments. Finally, when the diagnosis stays difficult, an anti-TB treatment might be started and its efficacy might lead physicians to conclude for a diagnosis of TB.

13. Clinical diagnosis with Crohn's disease among various forms of intestinal inflammation

These diagnosis depend about the anatomic localization of the process

Ileitis:

A variety of conditions may mimic Crohn's iletis. Table 5 report differential diagnosis of ileitis. Some others rare aetiologies can be explain ileitis. Infiltrative diseases (amyloidosis and eosinophilic gastroenteritis), lymphoid nodular hyperplasia and radiation enteritis must be researched also.

Laboratory assays	Diagnostic orientation	Diagnostic value
Hemogram	Lymphopenia : HIV infection, immunodespression Hypereosinophilia : Churg-Strauss syndrome Inflammatory syndrome in all cause of digestive granuloma	No sensibility, No specificity
C-reactive protein	Confirmes inflammation	No sensibility, no specificity
Lactate deshydrogenase	May orientate to lymphoma if increase	No sensibility, no specificity
Creatinine, albumine in urine/creatinine ratio	An associated nephropathy may be observed in Wegener's granulomatosis and Churg-Strauss syndrome	No specificity
Tuberculin test	Tuberculosis, sarcoidosis if asynergy	No specificity (past immunization by BCG), no sensibility in immunocompromised patients
Chest radiography	Tuberculosis	Only 30% patients with TB of GI tract have a pulmonary TB
Testing for HIV by serological assay	Orientate to opportunistic infection : *histoplasmosis* or *non tuberculosis mycobacteria*	Sensible and specific for HIV testing but only give an orientation
Stools cultures Parasitological examination of the stools	*Yersinia,* parasites	Sensible
Helicobacter pylori culture in biopsies, or *Hp* serology	*Hp* infection	Culture may be negative if proton pump inhibitor therapy

Table 2. First line biological examination in patients with evidence of a GI tract granuloma

Laboratory assays	Diagnostic orientation	Diagnostic value
Quantiferon TB gold	Tuberculosis	Not evaluated in digestive tuberculosis
Mycobacterium tuberculosis PCR in stools and biopsies	Tuberculosis	Not enough sensible in biopsies, lack of specificity in stools as it may be positive in pulmonary TB
ANCA detection	Wegener's granulomatosis and Churg-Strauss syndrome Ulcerative colitis	Good sensibility, good specificity for these three etiologies
ASCA detection	Crohn disease	Not specific, may be positive in TB
Angiotensin Converting enzyme	sarcoidosis	Not sensible, not specific and genetic polymorphism
18-FDG scintigraphy	May guide some deep biopsies	Sensible but not specific
Chest and abdominal tomodensitometry	Search other sites of involvement to orientate the diagnosis as infiltrative pneumopathy	Not specific

Table 3. Second line biological or radiological tests

Laboratory assays	Diagnostic orientation	Diagnostic value
Tropheryma Whipplei PCR	Whipple's disease	Good sensibility, but often positive in asymptomatic patients
Urine and blood antigen detection of *histoplasmosis*, serology	Think to histoplasmosis if the patients stayed in endemic area, or in immunocompromised ones	
Angiotensin converting enzyme genotyping	Sarcoidosis to interpret ACE levels	
Yersinia PCR	Yersiniosis	Sensible

Table 4. Third line biological tests

Infection	**Inflammation**	**gynecologic**
Yersinia enterolitica Yersinia pseudotuberculosis Mycobacterium tuberculosis Mycobacterium avium–intracellulare Typhlitis Histoplasma capsulatum Salmonella Cryptococcosis Anisakiasis Actinomycosis israelii	Appendicitis Appendiceal abscess Cecal diverticulitis	Pelvic inflammatory disease Tuboovarian abscess Ovarian cyst or tumor Endometriosis Ovarian torsion Ectopic pregnancy
Neoplasm	**Drug related**	**Vascular**
Cecal or small bowel (ileal) adenocarcinoma Lymphoma Lymphosarcoma Carcinoid tumor Metastatic cancer	Nonsteroidal antiinflammatory drug-related ulcer or stricture Ischemic: oral contraceptives, ergotamine, digoxin, diuretics, antihypertensives	Ischemia Vasculitides: polyarteritis nodosa, Churg–Strauss syndrome, Takayasu's arteritis, Wegener's granulomatosis, lymphomatoid granulomatosis, giant cell arteritis, rheumatoid arthritis vasculitis, thromboangiitis obliterans Henoch-Scho¨nlein purpura Systemic lupus erythematosus Behçet's syndrome

Table 5. Differential diagnosis of ileitis

Proctitis:

In addition to ulcerative proctitis, proctitis may also occasionally be the presentation of crohn's disease. The other differential diagnosis are breaf (Table 6).

Colitis:

The causes of colitis are legion.

Numerous infectious agents may cause a transient colitis, but the clinical course of most enteric infections is usually complete within 2 weeks of onset. The most important infections are: Cytomegalovirus, Shigella, Campylobacter, Clostridium difficile, Salmonella, Aeromonas pleisioides, Amebiasis, Enterohemorrhagic E. coli (EHEC), Mycobacterium tuberculosis, Yersinia enterocolitica, Schistosomiasis and strongylidosis. Nevertheless, others aetiologies must be evocated in function of associated symptoms and patient: Ischemic colitis, diverticulitis, microscopic colitis, diversion colitic or radation, Behçet disease and sarcoidosis.

Infection	Others
Herpes simplex type II *Neisseria gonorrhoeae* Syphilis (*Treponema pallidum*) Lymphogranuloma venereum *Chlamydia trachomatis* Whipworm infestation	Prolapse Solitary rectal ulcer Trauma Chemical injury

Table 6. Differential diagnosis of Crohn's disease or ulcerative proctitis

Drug related colitis must be researched: NSAIDs, gold, penicillamine) or toxic like cannabis; Some aetiologies are rare and must be evocated after these hypothesis: Chronic granulomatous disease, graft-vs-host disease.

	Ulcerative colitis	Crohn's disease
Distribution	Continuous, symmetric, and diffuse, with granularity or ulceration found in entire involved segments;	Often discontinuous and asymmetric with skipped segments, normal intervening mucosa,
Rectum	Typically involving rectum and distributed proximally	Complete or, more often, relative rectal sparing may be present
Mucosal lesions	Microulcers more common, larger ulcers possible, pseudopolyps more common	Aphthous ulcers common in early disease; late disease notable for ulcers with stellate, "rake," "bear-claw," linear or serpiginous ulcers; cobblestonin
Depth of inflammation	Mucosal, not transmural except in fulminant disease	Submucosal, mucosal, and transmural
Histology	Crypt abscesses and ulcers are the defining lesion Crypt abscesses may be present Ulceration on a background of inflamed mucosa	Crypt abscesses may be present Ulceration on a background of inflamed mucosa Hallmark is focally enhanced inflammation, often on a normal background
Complications	Parianal findings not prominent	Parianal lesions (40%), strictures, fistulas

Table 7. Clinical distinctions between ulcerative colitis and Crohn's disease.

When a causative agent is not identified, the issue of sorting out a first presentation of IBD from an acute self-limited colitis arises. Such a distinction relies strongly on histologic rather than endoscopic findings. Once a diagnosis of IBD has been established, Crohn's disease should be distinguished from ulcerative colitis.

14. Controversies in the distinction between ulcerative colitis and Crohn's disease

Many distinctions—clinical, anatomic, histologic—have been drawn between the 2 major forms of IBD (Table 7). A gold standard of diagnosis has yet to be attained, however.
Some clinical distinctions challenged by careful observation. Theorycally, ileum is not involved, except as "backwash" ileitis in panulcerative colitis. Conversely, ileum is often involved in chron's disease. Backwash ileitis has long been recognized as a feature of pan-ulcerative colitis but may yet throw even the experienced diagnostician off the trail if more than a few centimeters of ileal inflammation are present. When ileitis in the setting of pancolitis is more extensive than this, careful appraisal of the ileocecal valve may be helpful. A patulous valve with extensive backwash is more convincing as a feature of ulcerative colitis than lengthy ileitis behind a constricted, stenotic valve, more suggestive of Crohn's disease.
Complications are very frequent in the natural history of Crohn's disease. The 20-year cumulative rate of all complications is more than a population-based cohort (25); CD evolution relates to disease location. Small bowel involvement might be complicated at diagnosis or during the first years after diagnosis by an abcess or fistula, or by a stricture followed by formation of a fistula, whereas colonic disease can remain uncomplicated or inflammatory for many years. Stricturing and penetrating lesions can coexist in the same individual or even within the same intestinal segment. Conversly, in UC perianal findings are not prominent. If fissure or fistula have been present, they shouhd be uncomplicated. Strictures are rarely present and are suggestive of adenocarcinoma. Moreover, fistulas are not present, except for rare occurrence of rectovaginal fistula. In CD, about 20%-30% of patients present with perianal lesions and 15%-20% have or had a fistula (26). Another diagnostic criterion challenged by careful observation is the classic observation of continuous involvement of colonic mucosa without skip areas in ulcerative colitis. Although this distinction is generally true, care must be taken in interpreting the finding of skip areas. Topical therapies may lead to a false impression of "rectal sparing," whereas oral or systemic therapies may result in patchy healing, depending on the timing of endoscopy or completeness of response (27). Accordingly, the most accurate diagnosis may be made at the earliest evaluation, before anatomy and histology have been confounded by treatment.
Given this limitation, it is not surprising that, in some cases, it will be impossible to distinguish between ulcerative colitis and Crohn's disease, with potential implications for prognosis and treatment. Prospective, population-based studies suggest that approximately 1 in 20 patients with IBD will have a diagnosis of indeterminate colitis (28). Subsequent follow-up leads to a firmly established diagnosis of ulcerative colitis in one third of these cases, whereas 17% are assigned a diagnosis of Crohn's disease (29). The clinical value of pANCA or ASCA testing in patients presenting with non-specific gastrointestinal symptoms is limited because of inadequate sensitivity. Thus tests are infrequently positive in

individuals who do not have IBD. With the addition the latest panel of 7 antibodies has improved the positive and negative values of serologies. Using all of the serologic markers reported for CD, the sensitivity for diagnosing CD is greater than 80% and the positive predictive value is over 90% but only when the prevalence of CD is high, 38% (30). ANCA positivity has been observed in other colitides, such as eosinophilic and collagenous colitis. The specificity of ASCA seems to be higher, but ASCA positivity has been observed in patients with Behçet's disease, primary biliary cirrhosis, autoimmune hepatitis, and celiac disease. The cost effectiveness of serologic tests in the sequential diagnostic testing of IBD in children has been shown to avoid unnecessary and costly evaluations (31), but it has not been confirmed by other studies (32).
Serologic evaluation of ANCAs and ASCAs could be of help in patients with indeterminate colitis (33). In these patients, early knowledge of the exact diagnosis could be of clinical importance with regard to therapeutic decisions and prognosis (34). Patients who are pANCA positive and ASCA negative are 19 times more likely to have UC, whereas patients who are ASCA positive and pANCA negative are 16 times more likely to have CD (35). A remarkable finding is that patients who do not have antibodies, to either ASCAs or ANCAs, are remaining indeterminate colitis after a mean duration of 9.9 years (33). Further refinement of serologic tests and/or the combination of serologic testing with routine laboratory and fecal tests testing and noninvasive imaging may offer efficient cost-effective screening in the future.

15. Conclusion

The increases in incidence and prevalence of IBD over the last 15 years and its emergence in developing countries indicate a role of the environment in pathogenesis. Their diagnosis may be difficult and are clinical, endoscopic and histologic assessment. The issue remains that no gold standard test exists for the diagnosis of IBD. For these reasons, diagnosing crohn's disease and ulcerative colitis continues to be a more than occasional challenge to the practicing gastroenterologists. In the time of biotherapies, a casual diagnosis of IBD may result in critical errors in management in that incorrect diagnosis may result in inappropriate or even contraindicated treatment.

16. References

[1] Rao YG, Pande GK, Sahni P, Chattopadhyay TK. Gastroduodenal tuberculosis management guidelines, based on a large experience and a review of the literature. Can J Surg. 2004 Oct;47(5):364-368.
[2] Isbister WH, Hubler M. Inflammatory bowel disease in Saudi Arabia: presentation and initial management. J. Gastroenterol. Hepatol. 1998 Nov;13(11):1119-1124.
[3] Makharia GK, Srivastava S, Das P, Goswami P, Singh U, Tripathi M, et al. Clinical, endoscopic, and histological differentiations between Crohn's disease and intestinal tuberculosis. Am. J. Gastroenterol. 2010 Mar;105(3):642-651.
[4] Lee YJ, Yang S-K, Byeon J-S, Myung S-J, Chang H-S, Hong S-S, et al. Analysis of colonoscopic findings in the differential diagnosis between intestinal tuberculosis and Crohn's disease. Endoscopy. 2006 Jun;38(6):592-597.

[5] Kirsch R, Pentecost M, Hall P de M, Epstein DP, Watermeyer G, Friederich PW. Role of colonoscopic biopsy in distinguishing between Crohn's disease and intestinal tuberculosis. J. Clin. Pathol. 2006 Aug;59(8):840-844.

[6] Pulimood AB, Peter S, Rook GWA, Donoghue HD. In situ PCR for Mycobacterium tuberculosis in endoscopic mucosal biopsy specimens of intestinal tuberculosis and Crohn disease. Am. J. Clin. Pathol. 2008 Jun;129(6):846-851.

[7] Ramadass B, Chittaranjan S, Subramanian V, Ramakrishna BS. Fecal polymerase chain reaction for Mycobacterium tuberculosis IS6110 to distinguish Crohn's disease from intestinal tuberculosis. Indian J Gastroenterol. 2010 Jul;29(4):152-156.

[8] Bentley RW, Keenan JI, Gearry RB, Kennedy MA, Barclay ML, Roberts RL. Incidence of Mycobacterium avium subspecies paratuberculosis in a population-based cohort of patients with Crohn's disease and control subjects. Am. J. Gastroenterol. 2008 May;103(5):1168-1172.

[9] Man SM, Kaakoush NO, Mitchell HM. The role of bacteria and pattern-recognition receptors in Crohn's disease. Nat Rev Gastroenterol Hepatol. 2011 Mar;8(3):152-168.

[10] Selby W, Pavli P, Crotty B, Florin T, Radford-Smith G, Gibson P, et al. Two-year combination antibiotic therapy with clarithromycin, rifabutin, and clofazimine for Crohn's disease. Gastroenterology. 2007 Jun;132(7):2313-2319.

[11] Maeng L, Lee A, Choi K, Kang CS, Kim K-M. Granulomatous gastritis: a clinicopathologic analysis of 18 biopsy cases. Am. J. Surg. Pathol. 2004 Jul;28(7):941-945.

[12] Shapiro JL, Goldblum JR, Petras RE. A clinicopathologic study of 42 patients with granulomatous gastritis. Is there really an "idiopathic" granulomatous gastritis? Am. J. Surg. Pathol. 1996 Apr;20(4):462-470.

[13] Kahi CJ, Wheat LJ, Allen SD, Sarosi GA. Gastrointestinal histoplasmosis. Am. J. Gastroenterol. 2005 Jan;100(1):220-231.

[14] Fenollar F, Puéchal X, Raoult D. Whipple's disease. N. Engl. J. Med. 2007 Jan 4;356(1):55-66.

[15] Chen C-Y, Chi K-H, George RW, Cox DL, Srivastava A, Rui Silva M, et al. Diagnosis of gastric syphilis by direct immunofluorescence staining and real-time PCR testing. J. Clin. Microbiol. 2006 Sep;44(9):3452-3456.

[16] Lamps LW, Madhusudhan KT, Greenson JK, Pierce RH, Massoll NA, Chiles MC, et al. The role of Yersinia enterocolitica and Yersinia pseudotuberculosis in granulomatous appendicitis: a histologic and molecular study. Am. J. Surg. Pathol. 2001 Apr;25(4):508-515.

[17] Lamps LW, Madhusudhan KT, Havens JM, Greenson JK, Bronner MP, Chiles MC, et al. Pathogenic Yersinia DNA is detected in bowel and mesenteric lymph nodes from patients with Crohn's disease. Am. J. Surg. Pathol. 2003 Feb;27(2):220-227.

[18] Liang DB, Price JC, Ahmed H, Farmer N, Montgomery EA, Giday SA. Gastric sarcoidosis: case report and literature review. J Natl Med Assoc. 2010 Apr;102(4):348-351.

[19] Marie I, Sauvetre G, Levesque H. Small intestinal involvement revealing sarcoidosis. QJM. 2010 Jan 1;103(1):60 -62.

[20] Hilzenrat N, Spanier A, Lamoureux E, Bloom C, Sherker A. Colonic obstruction secondary to sarcoidosis: nonsurgical diagnosis and management. Gastroenterology. 1995 May;108(5):1556-1559.
[21] Kwon C-I, Park PW, Kang H, Kim GI, Cha ST, Kim KS, et al. The usefulness of angiotensin converting enzyme in the differential diagnosis of Crohn's disease and intestinal tuberculosis. Korean J. Intern. Med. 2007 Mar;22(1):1-7.
[22] Papadopoulos KI, Melander O, Orho-Melander M, Groop LC, Carlsson M, Hallengren B. Angiotensin converting enzyme (ACE) gene polymorphism in sarcoidosis in relation to associated autoimmune diseases. J. Intern. Med. 2000 Jan;247(1):71-77.
[23] Pagnoux C, Mahr A, Cohen P, Guillevin L. Presentation and outcome of gastrointestinal involvement in systemic necrotizing vasculitides: analysis of 62 patients with polyarteritis nodosa, microscopic polyangiitis, Wegener granulomatosis, Churg-Strauss syndrome, or rheumatoid arthritis-associated vasculitis. Medicine (Baltimore). 2005 Mar;84(2):115-128.
[24] Marciano BE, Rosenzweig SD, Kleiner DE, Anderson VL, Darnell DN, Anaya-O'Brien S, et al. Gastrointestinal involvement in chronic granulomatous disease. Pediatrics. 2004 Aug;114(2):462-468.
[25] Louis E, Collard A, Oger AF, et al. Behaviour of Crohn's disease according to the Vienna classification: changing pattern over the course of the disease. Gut 2001;49:777–782
[26] Cosnes J. Crohn's disease phenotype, prognosis, and long-term complications: what to expect? Acta Gastroenterol Belg 2008; 71:303–307.
[27] Geboes K, Dalle I. Influence of treatment on morphologicalfeatures of mucosal inflammation. Gut 2002;50(suppl 3):S37–S42.
[28] Roseth AG, Aadland E, Grzyb K. Normalization of faecal calprotectin: a predictor of mucosal healing in patients with inflammatory bowel disease. Scand J Gastroenterol 2004;39:1017-20.
[29] Shine B, Berghouse L, Jones JE, Landon J. C-reactive protein as an aid in the differentiation of functional and inflammatory bowel disorders. Clin Chim Acta 1985;148:105-9.
[30] Vernier G, Sendid B, Poulain D, Colombel JF. Relevance of serologic studies in inflammatory bowel disease. Curr Gastroenterol Rep 2004;6:482-7.
[31] Dubinsky MC, Ofman JJ, Urman M, Targan SR, Seidman EG. Clinical utility of serodiagnostic testing in suspected pediatric inflammatory bowel disease. Am J Gastroenterol 2001;96:758-65.
[32] Khan K, Schwarzenberg SJ, Sharp H, Greenwood D, Weisdorf-Schindele S. Role of serology and routine laboratory tests in childhood inflammatory bowel disease. Inflamm Bowel Dis 2002;8:325-9.
[33] Joossens S, Reinisch W, Vermeire S, Sendid B, Poulain D, Peeters M, et al. The value of serologic markers in indeterminate colitis: a prospective follow-up study. Gastroenterology 2002;122:1242-7.
[34] Bossuyt X. Serologic markers in inflammatory bowel disease. Clin Chem 2006;52:171-81.

[35] Abreu MT. Controversies in IBD. Serologic tests are helpful in managing inflammatory bowel disease. Inflamm Bowel Dis 2002;8:224-6; discussion 3, 30-1

6

Crohn's Disease: From an Anesthetist's Perspective

Beyazit Zencirci
Special DEVAKENT Hospital – Department of Anesthesiology & Reanimation
Turkey

1. Introduction

Human biological diversity involves interindividual variability in morphology, behavior, physiology, development, susceptibility to disease and response to stressful stimuli and drug therapy (*phenotypes*). Although the human DNA sequence is 99.9% identical among individuals, the variations may greatly affect a person's disease susceptibility. Many common diseases, and many individual responses to injury, drugs, and non-pharmacologic therapies are genetically complex, characteristically involving an interplay of many genetic variations in molecular and biochemical pathways (1).

The year 2007 marked the publication of adequately powered and successfully replicated genome-wide association studies that identified significant genetic contributors to the risk of common polygenic disease (*e.g., coronary artery disease, MI, types I and II diabetes, atrial fibrillation, obesity, asthma, common cancers, rheumatoid arthritis,* ***Crohn's disease*** *and others*) (1).

Crohn's disease affects a younger age group, with a peak incidence between 10 and 40 years of age. The reported incidence of disease is reported to be 5 to 10 per 100,000/yr (2). Despite advances in medical treatment, many patients still require surgery. The mainstay of management is medical treatment, usually aminosalicylates and steroids. Other immune-modifying agents are used in severe disease. This chapter is going to focus on the relationship between Crohn's disease (*disease and used drugs*) and anesthetic medicine.

2. What is Crohn's disease?

Crohn's disease causes a chronic, nonspecific, transmural inflammation of the intestine that found throughout the GI tract, from the oropharynx to the anus. Crohn's disease also manifests itself in many extraintestinal symptoms of eyes, skin, and joints. The severity and relapsing nature of these symptoms severely affect a patient's quality of life and require dependence on long-term medical therapy (3).

Crohn's disease is incurable, and the natural course of the disease is different for each patient. Patients will have episodes of disease exacerbation followed by periods of relative or complete remission. In a minority of patients, the disease is unrelenting, depending on the location and severity of the disease. The primary treatment of Crohn's disease is medical. Although the time course may vary, at least 75% of patients will require surgery after 20 years with the disease. Surgery is indicated for those who do not respond adequately to medical therapy and develop complications during the disease process (3).

3. Interaction beetween anti-Crohn's drugs and anesthetic drugs

3.1 Aminosalicylates

Sulfasalazine and mesalamine are the two aminosalicylates used for Crohn's disease. The primary antiinflammatory, antipyretic, and analgesic actions of salicylates such as aspirin are due to blockade of prostaglandin synthesis by inhibition of the cyclooxygenase 1 and 2 enzymes. These are effective in maintaining remission in patients with mild-to-moderate diseases (4). Studies demonstrate that both mesalamine and sulfasalazine are efficacious at inducing and maintaining remission, and are often used as long-term maintenance treatments. The improved side effect profile of mesalamine has enabled the use of doses that are much higher in amount than doses possible with sulfasalazine. However, a number of cases of 5-ASA-induced nephrotoxicity have been reported in patients with inflammatory bowel disease (*IBD*) (5, 6). Several case reports have reported renal impairment in the forms of dose-dependent '*analgesic nephropathy*', inhibition of cyclooxygenases or hypersensitivity leading to reversible interstitial nephritis in humans. The incidence of renal impairment in patients with IBD treated with 5-ASA is estimated to be one in 100 patients, and interstitial nephritis occurs in one in 500 patients (7, 8).

Mahmud et al, were unable to show nephrotoxicity after six months of mesalamine treatment in patients with ulcerative colitis using a low dose of 1.2 g/day (9). Similarly, Van Staa et al, were not able to demonstrate a relationship between the dose or type of 5-ASA and the incidence of renal disease among 19,025 IBD patients on 5-ASA (10). Based on their findings, interstitial nephritis related to 5-ASA use appears to be a rare event. Although interstitial nephritis occurs infrequently, renal function can be compromised over time with the use of 5-ASA. According to a recent report, de Jong et al, did not find a significant change in creatinine clearance (*CrCl*) over an 11-year interval in 200 patients with Crohn's disease (11). However, the mean duration of treatment with 5-ASA was 8.6 years, much shorter than the interval that CrCl was measured. This may reflect why the decline in CrCl was reported to be within the expected physiological decline in renal function associated with aging. Fortunately, the kidneys have the capacity to regain function after an insult; thus, creatinine measurements need to be taken at the onset and end of treatment rather than time points outside of the actual treatment interval. Also, no case of interstitial nephritis was reported by same author (11). In brief, the time of development of renal impairment is variable and may be seen as late as after several years. There is also a risk of developing irreversible renal disease if not recognized early, in which discontinuation of 5-ASA could result in recovery of renal function. Monitoring serum creatinine provides an easy and inexpensive way to prevent a detrimental side effect.

3.2 Corticosteroids

For patients with exacerbations leading to moderate or severe Crohn's disease, steroids are the primary therapy. However, they do not help maintain remission and are detrimental when used for long-term treatment. The synthetic analogs of cortisol have been developed with the primary goal of maximizing glucocorticoid activity while minimizing mineralocorticoid effects and decreasing the adverse effects of high quantities of systemically active glucocorticoid. Effects of glucocorticoids that are well documented include inhibition of the production of proinflammatory cytokines such as tumor necrosis factor alpha (*TNF-a*) and interleukin-l (*IL-l*) and chemokines such as IL-8; repression of the transcription of the genes for certain enzymes such as inducible nitric oxide synthase, phospholipase A2, and cyclooxygenase 2; and blockade of adhesion molecule expression. These molecular actions of glucocorticoids result in a blockade of leukocyte migration and function and inhibit the effects of numerous important peptide and lipid-derived mediators of inflammation (3).

Corticosteroids can induce clinical remission in Crohn's disease (*60% success rate compared to 30% placebo response*). The side effects of corticosteroids are extensive and include osteonecrosis, osteoporosis, cataracts, glaucoma, hyperglycemia, hyperlipidemia, hypertension, psychosis, and skin changes (3).

Corticosteroids and its side effects are important in anesthetic practice. Primarily, anesthetist must be aware of the need for corticosteroid replacement not only in patients who have primary adrenal insufficiency but also in patients who have adrenal insufficiency resulting from long-term corticosteroid therapy. Without adequate knowledge, the anesthetist may fail to prepare the patient to withstand the stress of surgery and may open the way for life-threatening hemodynamic abnormalities that accompany inadequate amounts of corticosteroids (12).

Secondly, its known that a long-term medication with prednisolone resulted in a shorter duration of an atracurium-induced neuromuscular block in patients with ulcerative colitis or Crohn's disease. The underlying chronic IBD itself did not influence the time course of the neuromuscular block. Although the mechanism is not fully understood, several possible sites of interaction of steroids with neuromuscular transmission have been suggested: (i) glucocorticoids have been shown to possess a direct facilitatory effect on the impulse generating end of the motor nerve axon; (ii) corticosteroids act presynaptically stimulating synthesis, spontaneous release, and stimulated release of acetylcholine; (iii) however, at large concentrations, corticosteroids might possess a post-synaptic depressant effect on neuromuscular transmission (13).

On the other hand, medication with prednisolone was associated with a prolonged onset time and attenuated maximum block of rocuronium (14). These data are in contrast to the results of the study mentioned in the previous paragraph. The reasons for the differences between atracurium and rocuronium might be alterations in drug metabolism mediated by the glucocorticoid (14). Alternatively, the presence of chronic IBD itself might influence the effect of the neuromuscular blocking drug: in an experimental model of systemic inflammation, resistance to atracurium was attributed to increased drug binding to a1-acid glycoprotein. Changes in acetylcholine receptor expression in systemic inflammation could was not be observed (15).

A reliable effect of neuromuscular blocking drugs is important to all anaesthesiologists in their clinical routine. A delayed recovery from a neuromuscular block might contribute to severe complications; even increased mortality could be proved previously (16). However, an unexpectedly decreased effect of the drug might also lead to intraoperative complications as a result of coughing or sudden movements. Additionally, it might increase laryngeal morbidity, i.e. injuries of the vocal cords (17).

Thirdly; adolescent or child patients, receiving chronic steroid therapy for IBD underwent major intestinal surgery, can develop vasodilation during anesthesia (*especially induction of anesthesia*). Systemic hypotension can occur in patients and we can treate them by large volumes of intravenous crystalloid solution which cause intraoperative and postoperative water retention with resultant hypertension as well as occasional pulmonary edema and seizures. Intravenous fluid administration in excess of maintenance requirements and calculated fluid losses should be given with caution to children/adolescent receiving high-dose steroids who undergo major intestinal surgery. Perioperative fluid retention under those circumstances may be treated best with early diuretic administration (18).

3.3 Antibiotics

Although antibiotics are not used to treat specific bacterial organisms, they have been found to be effective in the treatment of Crohn's disease, especially for the perianal area. Metronidazole is the most common agent employed, although ciprofloxacin has also been used. By decreasing the amount of bacterial flora in the intestinal lumen, they act to prevent the infectious complications of Crohn's disease, such as abscesses and fistulas (3). Clinical trials have shown their efficacy in inducing remission (19, 20).

Although rare, prolonged and high-dose administration of metronidazole may induce cerebellar lesions. Increased awareness of this phenomenon is important, as these lesions are reversible with discontinuation of this drug (21). Therefore, metronidazole dosages should be reduced in patients with liver dysfunction to prevent the accumulation of metronidazole, which can lead to CNS dysfunction and peripheral neuropathy (22).

Knorr et al reported a case of Q-T interval prolongation in a pediatric patient with no known risk factors (*including hypokalemia, hypomagnesemia, hypocalcemia, bradycardia, starvation etc.*) for the development of a long Q-T syndrome (*LQTS*) (23). After 48 hours of ciprofloxacin administration, the patient became bradycardic. Antimicrobial therapy was changed to ampicillin and ciprofloxacin was discontinued. The patient's bradycardia persisted for three days after the initial detection, and his Q-T prolongation was deemed resolved six days after detection; no other cardiac abnormalities have been reported after this day. The patient's Q-T interval was normalized within seven days of ciprofloxacin discontinuation. The patient did not have any further cardiac anomalies.

The pharmacologic mechanism of drug-induced LQTS is proposed to be via the blockade of delayed rectifier potassium channels of the ventricular myocardium during the repolarization phase. This blockade prolongs the cardiac action potential and allows early afterdepolarization (EAD), which results in the development of a second action potential. The second action potential may create a premature ventricular complex on an ECG, and if this dysrhythmia becomes self-sustaining, the resulting pattern of EADs reveals itself as a "twisting of the points" on the ECG. With the development of dysrhythmia, the patient may be asymptomatic or may present with syncope, palpitations, ventricular tachycardia, or sudden death (24, 25). Fluoroquinolone-induced Q-T prolongation is most commonly associated with gatifloxacin, moxifloxacin, and the withdrawn agents sparifloxacin and grepafloxacin (26). This case demonstrated that the use of ciprofloxacin in patients (*esp. pediatric*) should be restricted to situations in which there is no other safe and effective alternative to treat the infection. It is important for clinicians to familiarize themselves with the drugs that may propagate Q-T prolongation as well as the risk factors that increase the probability of developing drug-induced LQTS (23).

3.4 Immunosuppressive drugs

As the increasing number of of evidence points to an immunological etiology of IBD, efforts have been made to utilize various immunotherapies. The drugs most commonly used are azathioprine and its metabolite, 6-mercaptopurine (6-MP), and antimetabolites that inhibit DNA synthesis (27). After administration of azathioprine or 6-MP, the 6-thioguanine nucleotides accumulate intracellularly and are believed to mediate the biological actions of these drugs (3).

Despite over 50 years of investigation, the precise molecular basis for the therapeutic effects of the purine analogs is not known. However, intracellular accumulation of 6-thioguanine nucleotides causes inhibition of the pathways of purine nucleotide metabolism and DNA synthesis and repair, resulting in inhibition of cell division and proliferation. It is plausible, but not proven, that antiproliferative or functionally inhibitory actions on cells of the immune system, such as lymphocytes, underlie the immunosuppressive actions of azathioprine and 6-MP (3). Their value was established in a study that showed 67% of patients with a clinical response compared to 8% in the placebo group, although the effect was delayed by 3 to 6 months. In addition, 75% of patients were able to discontinue or reduce their steroid doses (27). A metaanalysis of nine trials revealed that azathioprine and 6-MP are effective in patients with an active disease, while the adverse side effects approached 10% (28).

Two categories of adverse effects to azathioprine and 6-MP have been described: allergic, occurring early during treatment; and dose-related, generally occurring later. Allergy to these drugs can manifest as pancreatitis, fever, rash, nausea, diarrhea, and an allergic hepatitis. Approximately 50% of the IBD population beginning treatment with azathioprine or 6-MP will experience an allergic reaction to the drug, which can be confirmed by rechallenge if necessary. Dose-related toxicities of azathioprine or 6-MP include bone marrow depression leading to leukopenia (*10% cumulative risk*), anemia, thrombocytopenia, and hepatic toxicity. If severe, leukopenia can potentially cause profound immune suppression and thus predispose to opportunistic infections or neoplasms. If leukopenia and a serious infection develop in a patient receiving azathioprine or 6-MP, reversal of bone marrow suppression is usually possible with granulocyte colony-stimulating factor. Decreases in the white blood cell (*WBC*) or elevations in liver function tests (*LFTs*) are common and generally respond to small dose reductions if needed, without discontinuation. The most important criteria for the success of azathioprine and 6-MP include adequate dosing and duration of treatment and individual metabolism of these drugs based on detectable thiopurine methyltransferase activity (29). Withdrawal of drug has shown a 70% relapse rate (28).

Methotrexate is a folate analog that inhibits purine and pyrimidine synthesis and has been shown in a number of trials to be effective in treating Crohn's disease (30). The principal biochemical action of methotrexate, and the mechanism that is believed to be responsible for the drug's cytotoxic activity, is inhibition of dihydrofolate reductase. It has alternatively been proposed that the antiinflammatory action of methotrexate may be mediated by inhibition of cytokine release or by increased release of the endogenous antiinflammatory autocoid adenosine. Methotrexate may also have effects on activated T lymphocytes, a critical part of the inflammatory infiltrate in IBD. However, this drug has significant side effects, including hepatotoxicity. and bone marrow suppression, and thus is reserved for patients wIth severe Crohn's that is refractory to other therapies (3).

The latest class of drugs that has resulted in huge advancements in the treatment of Crohn's disease are the anti-tumour necrosis factor alpha (TNF-α) agents. Levels of TNF-α are increased in Crohn's disease, and in a study of its efficacy, it was noted to produce fistula healing (3). Infliximab, a monoclonal antibody against TNF-α, is licensed for the management of severe active Crohn's disease and moderate to severe ulcerative colitis in patients whose condition has not responded adequately to treatment with a corticosteroid and a conventional immunosuppressant or who are intolerant of them (31). It has been associated with acute demyelination of the central nervous system (32-34). Recently, Drummonad at al. reported profound postoperative muscle weakness in a patient who had been treated with infliximab (35). However, reports in literature suggesting interactions between infliximab and any anaesthetic drugs are unavailable. It is possible that the immunosuppressive effect of the hydrocortisone bolus (*given at the induction of anesthesia*) or simply of the surgery itself may have interacted with the infliximab, hastening the onset of symptoms. Therefore every patients recently treated with infliximab should have a neurological examination documented at pre-operative assessment in order to provide a in case should problems occur postoperatively.

On the other hand; it is well known that infliximab can worsen congestive heart failure. The preliminary results of a study assessing the heart function (*by means of electro-and echocardiogram*) during infliximab therapy, in twelve paediatric IBD patients (*9 Crohn's disease, 3 ulcerative colitis*), have been published (36). Seven out of 12 patients showed cardiac disturbances consisting of dilation of the cardiac cavities (*5 cases*) and septal hypertrophy (*2 cases*), with a direct correlation between the length of Q–T interval and the systolic and diastolic diameter of the left ventricle. These findings point to an increased risk of developing arrhythmias in these patients. However, further and more complete studies should be done before recommendations about cardiologic work-up required before surgery.

Vitamin B12 (*cyanocobalamin*) is an integral component of two biochemical reactions in humans: the conversion of L-methylmalonyl coenzyme A into succinyl coenzyme A and the formation of methionine by methylation of homocysteine. The transmethylation reaction is essential to DNA synthesis and to the maintenance of the myelin sheath by the methylation of myelin basic protein. Active vitamin B12 contains cobalt in its reduced form (Co^{+}). Nitrous oxide produces irreversible oxidation to the Co^{++} and Co forms that renders vitamin B12 inactive. The etiologies of vitamin B12 deficiency include many situations such as malabsorption (*because of celiac disease, colitis, etc.*). Patients with vitamin B12 deficiency are exceedingly sensitive to neurologic deterioration following nitrous oxide anesthesia. If unrecognized, the neurologic deterioration becomes irreversible and may result in death (37).

4. Certain circumstances in Crohn's disease which may affect anesthesia

4.1 Anemia

Anemia is the most common systemic complication of IBD (38). Anemia in IBD is a prototype of a combination of iron deficiency and anemia of inflammation (*i.e. anemia of chronic disease*) which is caused by negative effects of an activated immune system at different levels of erythropoiesis. Inflammation affects three major steps essential for normal erythropoiesis and can, therefore, lead to the development of anemia of inflammation. These effects are: (i) an immunity-driven diversion of iron traffic leading to retention of the metal in macrophages and thus to iron-deficient erythropoiesis; (ii) blunting of the biological activity of erythropoietin, the major erythropoiesis-stimulating hormone; and (iii) inhibition of the differentiation and proliferation of erythroid progenitor cells (39).

Anemia in IBD can also be induced by deficiency of vitamins, such as cobalamin and folic acid, a condition which further impairs the proliferation of hematopoietic progenitor cells

(40), or by certain medications, such as thiopurine analogs (*6-mercaptopurine, azathioprine*), sulfasalazine and methotrexate, most of which can inhibit erythropoiesis directly (41).

The severity of anemia in IBD varies considerably (42). The lower hemoglobin levels below which anemia was defined as present were those proposed by the World Health Organization (*non-pregnant women, 12.0 g/dL; men 13.0 g/dL).* Most patients with IBD have mild to moderate anemia (*hemoglobin above 10.0g/dL*), but in the presence of bleeding episodes, the hemoglobin concentration may decrease further (41, 43).

The persistence of anemia is associated with impaired cardiac and renal function, reduced systemic oxygen delivery, decreased physical activity, fatigue, and impaired quality of life or ability to work (41, 43, 44). However, anemia is a comorbid condition which is associated with other diseases (*such as transfusion associated hepatitis* C) or even death (45).

Preoperative anemia is a major risk factor for adverse outcome in major surgery and, it's also one of the most important risk factor for perioperative blood transfusions (46). With various multivariate statistics and propensity score matching in some studies, the authors unanimously found that preoperative anemia and perioperative allogeneic blood transfusions (*ABT*) were both independent risk factors for postoperative mortality, ischemia, and infections (47).

The question of what hemoglobin/hematocrit (*Hb/Hct*) level justifies the risks associated with the administration of blood has been widely discussed. The inviolable "10-30" rule has been abandoned. Experience with several patient subpopulations (*renal failure, military casualties, Jehovah's Witnesses*) and systematic study has revealed that considerable greater degrees of anemia can be well tolerated and that, in many situations, morbidity and mortality rates did not increase until Hb levels fell below 7 g/dL (48, 49). As significant as the identification of a 7 g/dL threshold for increased morbidity was the observation that stable general medical-surgical managed to a target Hb of 10g/dL fared less well than a parallel group managed with a transfusion trigger of 7 g/dL (48). That observation implies an adverse effect of transfusion. Accordingly, the contemporary transfusion trigger for stable general medical-surgical patients is 21%/7.0 g/dL (*Hct/Hb*). However, there is evidence that the threshold for patients with cardiac disease should be higher (48). That evidence includes an investigation supporting a threshold of 30%/10 g/dL (*Hct/Hb*) in patients who have suffered a recent acute myocardial infarction (50), and an observational study suggests better outcomes in patients with several cardiac diagnoses (*cardiac and vascular surgery, ischemic heart disease, dysrhythmias*) above a threshold of 9.5g/dL (51). *The Practice Guidelines for Blood Component Therapy* developed by the American Society of Anesthesiologists (*ASA*) state that "*red blood cell transfusion is rarely indicated when the hemoglobin concentration is greater than 10 g/dL and is almost always indicated when it is less than 6 g/dL. The indications for autologous transfusion may be more liberal than for allogeneic (homologous) transfusion*"(52).

Blood transfusions are widely used as an immediate intervention for rapid correction of severe or life-threatening anemia. However, such transfusions do not correct the underlying pathology and do not have a lasting effect. The decision on whether to administer blood should not, therefore, be based only on the hemoglobin level, but should also take clinical symptoms and co-morbidity into account. Whether blood transfusions affect immune function and whether they are cause-effectively linked to mortality in patients undergoing surgery (46) or being treated in intensive care units remains controversial (53).

The clinician's responsibility is to anticipate, on a patient-by-patient basis, the minimum Hb level (*probably in the range of 7 to 10 g/dL*) that will avoid organ damage due to oxygen deprivation. Determining this individual "*transfusion trigger*" requires reference to the many elements of patient condition that determine demand for the delivery of oxygen and the physiologic reserve (54), including ongoing blood loss and the potential for sudden blood loss. Ultimately, the decision to transfuse red blood cells (*RBCs*) should be made on the basis of the clinical judgment that the oxygen-carrying capacity of the blood must be increased to prevent oxygen consumption from outstripping oxygen delivery. That judgment is based on an understanding of the physiologic mechanisms that compensate for anemia and the limits of those mechanisms.

4.2 Respiratory problems

The pathogenesis of IBD-associated respiratory lesions is unknown. The inflammatory lesions seen beneath the bronchial epithelium are similar to those observed beneath the colonic epithelium in IBD. Both epithelia have columnar structures and mucosal glands, and both sites are challenged constantly by foreign antigens. There are two possible hypotheses: (i) a systemic immunologically-mediated phenomenon originating from the intestinal inflammatory process underlies the bronchial/parenchymal changes in the lungs; or (ii) a defect in the regulation of local immune response which is evident in both gastrointestinal and respiratory tract in response to as yet unknown antigens (55).

While clinically apparent bronchopulmonary disease complicating IBD is rare, the function of the small airways and the diffusion capacity of the lungs has been shown to be affected in IBD patients without any clinical respiratory involvement (56, 57). Heatley et al. Reported reduced diffusion capacity for carbon monoxide in 25%, and spirometric abnormalities in 50%, of 102 patients with IBD (58). Adenis et al., using clearance of 99mTechnitium isotopic DTPA, suggested that patients with Crohn's disease may have increased pulmonary vascular permeability due to latent alveolitis (57).

Respiratory symptoms can occur at any time in the history of IBD. Most interstitial lung diseases associated with IBD start gradually with weeks or months of breathlessness associated with cough. Bronchiolitis can progress unrecognised as there is no distinctive pattern of physical signs (59). Despite exertional dyspnoea, there may be no audible signs on auscultation. Radiological signs are also variable. Chest radiographs may show diffuse or patchy infiltrates but can be normal. Computed tomography scan is more helpful in demonstrating diffuse nodular or ground glass opacities which maybe patchy or uniform (60). Pulmonary function tests usually show a restrictive defect in interstitial lung involvement with reduced gas transfer and resting/exercise hypoxaemia. Broncho-alveolar lavage, useful in ruling out infectious causes, generally shows lymphocytosis. A lung biopsy is usually necessary to confirm the diagnosis and may aid in indicating prognosis (61)

Drug-induced interstitial lung disease has been well-reported in IBD, with clinical features very similar to IBD-associated interstitial lung diseases. Most cases have been attributed to salicylates and mesalazine therapy (62). Salicylates (*sulphasalazine and 5-ASA*) can induce different lung diseases such as bronchiolitis obliterans, bronchiolitis obliterans with organising pneumonia (*BOOP*), and interstitial pneumonitis with the most common being eosinophilic pneumonitis.

Drug-induced lung disease can be confirmed by drug rechallenge and improvement has occurred following drug withdrawal. Generally, prognosis is favourable in the majority of salicylate-induced interstitial lung diseases, but fatal outcomes due to irreversible lung fibrosis and rapidly progressive interstitial lung disease have been described (63). Hypersensitivity pneumonitis may occur with methotrexate. This is a serious complication, occasionally fatal, with a reported prevalence of 3.1 to 11.6% in patients receiving long-term low-dose therapy (64, 65). The clinical features include dyspnoea, fever and cough with diffuse alveolar and interstitial shadowing on chest X-ray. Treatment requires the immediate withdrawal of methotrexate and high dose corticosteroids. A few cases of azathioprine-induced interstitial lung diseases have been reported in non-IBD patients. Opportunistic infections have been described in patients treated with immunosuppressants, particularly cyclosporin, and most recently, infliximab (66, 67).

Most respiratory disease associated with IBD responds well to corticosteroids with the exception of constrictive bronchiolitis obliterans (68). But, in some patients, pathological changes such as bronchiectasis and bronchiolitis obliterans are irreversible. Initial treatment of airways inflammation is with inhaled corticosteroids. Systemic corticosteroids are used to treat parenchymal disease (*BOOP, interstitial pneumonitis and necrotic nodules*). Methotrexate or salicylates should be withdrawn as potential causes of interstitial lung disease. The duration and dosage of corticosteroid treatment should be guided by symptomatic response and pulmonary function tests. In the case of BOOP, the duration of corticosteroid treatment is usually six months and clinical improvement can be seen within days to weeks (69).

4.3 Renal problems

Secondary amyloidosis (*SA*) is a rare but serious complication of IBD, generally seen in Crohn's disease. Indeed SA is frequently described as a major cause of death in patients with Crohn's disease (70). At least 1% of patients with Crohn's disease develop SA. In literature, the time lapse between the onset of Crohn's disease and the diagnosis of SA has been reported to range from one to 21 years. In most patients, protein-uria heralded the onset of renal involvement from amyloid and occurred from three to 15 years after Crohn's disease diagnosis (71). Renal failure is the most common clinical presentation of SA, ranging from nephrotic syndrome and impaired renal function–to renal failure, with a potential for high morbidity (72).

So far no effective treatment for SA has been identified. Multiple therapeutic strategies have been employed with discouraging results, including colchicine and immunosuppressive drugs such as tumor necrosis factor alpha inhibitors The therapeutic approach to these patients should be dual. On the one hand it aims at minimizing the activity of the underlying disease in order to mitigate or prevent serum amyloid A (*SAA*) production, the precursor of plasma amyloid that is deposited in tissues and will be responsible for their malfunction. On the other hand it is aimed at treating the disease once it is established. The treatment of SA has two pillars: a) improvement of renal dysfunction; and b) reduction of inflammation, the constant source of SAA, thus trying to prevent the formation of amyloid, and hence curb the progression of disease (73, 74). Dialysis and renal transplantation are reserved for patients with end-stage renal failure. Survival rates for these patients have improved in recent years with the introduction of these drugs, but there is still no standardized treatment, and prognosis remains dismal (75).

4.4 Pain problems

Pain is a common component of IBD, especially during acute inflammatory episodes. The substances involved in visceral hyperalgesia are present throughout the gastrointestinal tract and their synthesis is increased during acute clinical episodes of IBD (76-79). On the other hand, opioid-binding proteins are involved as acutephase reactants and their concentrations are elevated in IBD (80), and the modulation of pain during this disease is therefore unclear.

However, medical management of IBD remains challenging and cannot always control all aspects of the disease. Even with therapy, patients frequently suffer not only from diarrhea and rectal bleeding but also from abdominal pain, cramps and arthralgia. Although the established disease activity indices only include abdominal pain as one variable, pain occurs throughout the body with pain attacks severely diminishing the patient's health-related quality of life (*HRQOL*) and interfering with their social and occupational habits. Localization of pain is a matter of great interest because of the different treatment options for abdominal pain and arthralgia. While the treatment of arthralgia could be composed of physical therapy, steroids or sulfasalazine, abdominal pain requires a more effective anti-inflammatory therapy. In cases of persistent pain despite remission, IBS-like symptoms, depression or drug-related side effects must also be considered (81).

The use of analgesics and their dosage is difficult to gauge and should be well evaluated. Pain killers have a variety of known effects and side effects. Given the gastrointestinal side effects and the possibility of aggravating mucosal inflammation, non-steroidal anti-inflammatory drugs (*NSAID*) should be avoided in IBD. However, opioids might also worsen pain in IBD patients because long-term use of opioids may also be associated with the development of abnormal sensitivity to pain and a progressive decline in plasma cortisol levels (82). Consequently, Smith and coworkers recently showed that treatment with low-dose naltrexone improved disease course and HRQOL of Crohn's disease (83). An alternative explanation for the discrepancy between use of analgesics and perception of pain might be the high prevalence of functional somatic symptoms (*IBS-like symptoms*) among IBD patients (84).

Previous studies have demonstrated an increase in opioid requirements and a large variability in patients with Crohn's disease or ulcerative colitis compared with controls undergoing abdominal major surgery. Two recent studies have indicated the existence of diffuse hyperalgesia during an intestinal inflammatory process (85, 86). Verne and colleagues confirmed that patients with functional bowel disorder have visceral cutaneous hyperalgesia that are distributed over a considerable rostro-caudal distance but are yet optimally expressed in lumbosacral dermatoma (87). Also, that study demonstrate that the inflammatory status seems to influence opioid requirements during surgery for IBD. Inflammation induces visceral and cutaneous hyperalgesia that may explain the decrease in opioid requirements in patients with quiescent IBD compared with those who have an active IBD. On the other hand, during surgery, pain stimulation was much more related to painful stimuli to the abdominal wall than to direct stimuli to the inflammatory bowel. Hence, we may speculate that increased opioid requirements during abdominal wall stimulation are linked to this somatic hyperalgesia in lumbosacral referred dermatoma. However, the decrease in opioid consumption may also be related to changes in pharmacokinetic factors due to the inflammation (88).

5. Conclusion

We are faced with the Crohn's disease in practice of anesthesia. We usually pay attention to the type of surgery. However, our patients's clinical status (*nutrition, blood protein level, etc.*), interactions between anesthetic drugs and patient used drugs are impotant too. Thus we can help prevent complications, early discern to negative signals and start effective treatments. Nothing is simple, nothing is resolved.

6. References

[1] Podgoreanu MV & Mathew JP (2009). Genomic Basis of Perioperative Medicine. In: *Clinical Anesthesia*. Barash PG, Cullen BF, Stoelting RK, Cahalan MK & Stock MC (Eds), 115-36. Lippincott Williams & Wilkins, ISBN 978-078-1787-63-5, Philadelphia.

[2] Carter MJ, Lobo AJ, Travis SP & IBD Section of the British Society of Gastroenterology (2004). Guidelines for the management of inflammatory bowel disease in adults. *Gut*. Vol.53, No.suppl V, (September 2004), pp. v1–v16, ISSN 0017-5749

[3] Welton ML, Shelton AA, Chang GJ & Varma MG (2008). Colon, Rectum, and Anus. In: *Surgery Basic Science and Clinical Evidence 2nd ed*. Norton JA, Barie PS, Bollinger RR, Chang AE, Lowry SF, Mulvihill SJ, Pass HI & Thompson RW (Eds), 1011-1110. Springer, ISBN 978-038-7308-00-5, New York.

[4] Malchow H, Ewe K, Brandes JW, Goebell H, Ehms H, Sommer H & Jesdinsky H (1984). European Cooperative Crohn's Disease Study (ECCDS): results of drug treatment. *Gastroenterology*. Vol.86, No.2 (February 1984), pp. 249-66, ISSN 0016-5085

[5] Corrigan G & Stevens PE (2000). Review article: interstitial nephritis associated with the use of mesalazine in inflammatory bowel disease. *Alimentary Pharmacology & Therapeutics*. Vol.14, No.1 (January 2000), pp. 1-6, 1SSN 1365-2036

[6] Loftus EV Jr, Kane SV & Bjorkman D. Systematic review: short-term adverse effects of 5-aminosalicylic acid agents in the treatment of ulcerative colitis. *Alimentary Pharmacology & Therapeutics*. Vol.19, No.2, (January,2004), pp. 179-89. 1SSN 1365-2036

[7] World MJ, Stevens PE, Ashton MA & Rainford DJ (1996). Mesalazine-associated interstitial nephritis. *Nephrology Dialysis Transplantation*. Vol.11, No.4, (April 1996), pp. 614-21, ISSN 1460-2385

[8] Thuluvath PJ, Ninkovic M, Calam J & Anderson M (1994). Mesalazine induced interstitial nephritis. *Gut*. Vol.35, No.10, (October 1994), pp. 1493-6, ISSN 0017-5749

[9] Mahmud N, O'Toole D, O'Hare N, Freyne PJ, Weir DG & Kelleher D (2002). Evaluation of renal function following treatment with 5-aminosalicylic acid derivatives in patients with ulcerative colitis. *Alimentary Pharmacology & Therapeutics*. Vol.16, No.2, (February 2002), pp. 207-15, 1SSN 1365-2036

[10] Van Staa TP, Travis S, Leufkens HG & Logan RF (2004). 5-aminosalicylic acids and the risk of renal disease: A large British epidemiologic study. *Gastroenterology*. Vol.126, No.7, (July 2004), pp. 1733-9, ISSN 0016-5085

[11] de Jong DJ, Tielen J, Habraken CM, Wetzels JF & Naber AH (2005). 5-Aminosalicylates and effects on renal function in patients with Crohn's disease. *Inflammatory Bowel Disease*. Vol.11, No.11, (November 2005), pp. 972-6, ISSN 1536-4844

[12] Wakim JH & Sledge KC (2006). Anesthetic implications for patients receiving exogenous corticosteroids. *American Association of Nurse Anesthetists Journal*. Vol.74, No.2, (April 2006), pp. 133-9, ISSN 0094-6354

[13] Soltész S, Mencke T, Mey C, Röhrig S, Diefenbach C & Molter GP (2008). Influence of a continuous prednisolone medication on the time course of neuromuscular block of atracurium in patients with chronic inflammatory bowel disease. *British Journal of Anaesthesia*.Vol.100, No.6, (June 2008), pp. 798-802, ISSN 0007-0912

[14] Soltész S, Mencke T, Stunz M, Diefenbach C, Ziegeler S & Molter GP (2009). Attenuation of a rocuronium-induced neuromuscular block in patients receiving prednisolone. *Acta Anaesthesiologica Scandinavica*. Vol.53, No.4, (April 2009), pp. 443-8, ISSN 0001-5172

[15] Fink H, Luppa P, Mayer B, Rosenbrock H, Metzger J, Martyn JA & Blobner M (2003). Systemic inflammation leads to resistance to atracurium without increasing membrane expression of acetylcholine receptors. *Anesthesiology*. Vol.98, No.1, (January 2003), pp. 82-8, ISSN 0003-3022

[16] Arbous MS, Meursing AE, van Kleef JW, de Lange JJ, Spoormans HH, Touw P, Werner FM & Grobbee DE (2005). Impact of anesthesia management characteristics on severe morbidity and mortality. *Anesthesiology*. Vol.102, No.2, (February 2005), pp. 257-68, ISSN 0003-3022

[17] Mencke T, Echternach M, Plinkert PK, Johann U, Afan N, Rensing H, Noeldge-Schomburg G, Knoll H & Larsen R (2006). Does the timing of tracheal intubation based on neuromuscular monitoring decrease laryngeal injury? A randomized prospective, controlled trial. *Anesthesia and Analgesia*. Vol.102, No.1 (January 2006), pp. 306-12, ISSN 0003-2999

[18] Mulvihill SJ & Fonkalsrud EW (1984). Complications of excessive operative fluid administration in children receiving steroids for inflammatory bowel disease. *Journal of Pediatric Surgery*. Vol.19, No.3, (June 1984), pp. 274-7, ISSN 0022-3468

[19] Sutherland L, Singleton J, Sessions J, Hanauer S, Krawitt E, Rankin G, Summers R, Mekhjian H, Greenberger N, Kelly M, Levine J, Thomson A, Alpert E & Prokipchuk E (1991). Double blind, placebo controlled trial of metronidazole in Crohn's disease. *Gut*. Vol.32, No.9 (September 1991), pp. 1071-5, ISSN 0017-5749

[20] Rutgeerts P, Hiele M, Geboes K, Peeters M, Penninckx F, Aerts R & Kerremans R (1995). Controlled trial of metronidazole treatment for prevention of Crohn's recurrence after ileal resection. *Gastroenterology*. Vol.108, No.6, (June 1995), pp. 1617-21, ISSN 0016-5085

[21] Ito H, Maruyama M, Ogura N, Fujioka T, Iwasaki Y, Aikawa A & Hasegawa A (2004). Reversible cerebellar lesions induced by metronidazole therapy for helicobacter pylori. *Journal of Neuroimaging*. Vol.14, No.4, (October 2004), pp. 369-71, ISSN 1552-6569

[22] Horlen CK, Seifert CF & Malouf CS (2000). Toxic metronidazole-induced MRI changes. *Annals of Pharmacotherapy*. Vol.34, No.11, (November 2000), pp.1273-5, ISSN 1542-6270

[23] Knorr JP, Moshfeghi M & Sokoloski MC (2008). Ciprofloxacin-induced Q-T interval prolongation. *American Journal of Health System Pharmacy*. Vol.65, No.6, (March 2008), pp. 547-51, ISSN 1079-2082

[24] Roden DM (2004). Drug-induced prolongation of the QT interval. *New England Journal of Medicine*. Vol.350, No.10, (March 4, 2004), pp. 1013-22, ISSN 0028-4793

[25] Owens RC Jr (2004). QT prolongation with antimicrobial agents: understanding the significance. *Drugs*. Vol.64, No.10, (2004), pp. 1091-124, ISSN 1179-1950

[26] Makaryus AN, Byrns K, Makaryus MN, Natarajan U, Singer C & Goldner B (2006).. Effect of ciprofloxacin and levofloxacin on the QT interval: is this a significant "clinical" event? *Southern Medical Journal*. Vol.99, No.1 (January 2006), pp. 52-6, ISSN 1541-8243

[27] Present DH, Korelitz BI, Wisch N, Glass JL, Sachar DB & Pasternack BS (1980). Treatment of Crohn's disease with 6-mercaptopurine. A long-term, randomized, double-blind study. *New England Journal of Medicine*. Vol.302, No.18, (May 1, 1980), pp. 981-7, ISSN 0028-4793

[28] Pearson DC, May GR, Fick GH & Sutherland LR (1995). Azathioprine and 6-mercaptopurine in Crohn's disease. A meta-analysis. *Annals of Internal Medicine*. Vol.123, No.2, (July 15, 1995), pp.132-42, ISSN 0003-4819

[29] Katz S (2005). Update in medical therapy of ulcerative colitis: newer concepts and therapies. *Journal of Clinical Gastroenterology*. Vol.39, No.7, (August 2005), pp. 557-69, ISSN 0192-0790

[30] Alfadhli AA, McDonald JW & Feagan BG (2009). Methotrexate for induction of remission in refractory Crohn's disease. In: *Cochrane Database of Systematic Reviews*. (21 July 2004), Avaliable from: <http://onlinelibrary.wiley.com/o/cochrane/clsysrev/articles/CD003459/frame.html>

[31] Ngo B, Farrell CP, Barr M, Wolov K, Bailey R, Mullin JM & Thornton JJ (2010). Tumor necrosis factor blockade for treatment of inflammatory bowel disease: efficacy and safety. *Current Molecular Pharmacology*. Vol.3, No.3, (November 1, 2010), pp. 145-52, ISSN 1874-4672

[32] Singer OC, Otto B, Steinmetz H & Ziemann U (2004). Acute neuropathy with multiple conduction blocks after TNFalpha monoclonal antibody therapy. *Neurology*. Vol.63 No.9, (November 9, 2004), pp. 1754, ISSN 0028-3878 .

[33] Richez C, Blanco P, Lagueny A, Schaeverbeke T & Dehais J. Neuropathy resembling CIDP in patients receiving tumor necrosis factor-alpha blockers. *Neurology*. Vol.64, No.8, (April 26, 2005), pp. 1468-70, ISSN 0028-3878

[34] Cocito D, Bergamasco B, Tavella A, Poglio F, Paolasso I, Costa P, Ciaramitaro P & Isoardo G (2005). Multifocal motorneuropathy during treatment with infliximab. *Journal of the Peripheral Nervous System*. Vol.10, No.4, (December 2005), pp. 386-7, ISSN 1085-9489

[35] Drummond AD, Williamson RM, Silverdale MA & Rothwell MP (2008). Postoperative muscle weakness in a patient recently treated with infliximab. *Anaesthesia*. Vol.63, No.5, (May 2008), pp. 548-50, ISSN 0003-2409

[36] Barbato M, Curione M, Viola F, Versacci P, Parisi F, Amato S & Cucchiara S (2006). Cardiac involvement in children with IBD during infliximab therapy. *Inflammatory Bowel Disease*. Vol.12, No.8, (August 2006), pp. 828-9, ISSN 1536-4844

[37] Flippo TS & Holder WD Jr (1993). Neurologic degeneration associated with nitrous oxide anesthesia in patients with vitamin B12 deficiency. *Archives of Surgery*. Vol.128, No.12, (December 1993), pp. 1391-5, ISSN 0004-0010

[38] Gasche C, Berstad A, Befrits R, Beglinger C, Dignass A, Erichsen K, Gomollon F, Hjortswang H, Koutroubakis I, Kulnigg S, Oldenburg B, Rampton D, Schroeder O, Stein J, Travis S & Van Assche G (2007). Guidelines on the diagnosis and management of iron deficiency and anemia in inflammatory bowel diseases. *Inflammatory Bowel Disease*. Vol.13, No.12, (December 2007), pp.1545-53, ISSN 1536-4844

[39] Weiss G & Gasche C (2010). Pathogenesis and treatment of anemia in inflammatory bowel disease. *Haematologica*. Vol.95, No.2, (February 2010), pp. 175-8, ISSN 0390-6078

[40] Rodriguez RM, Corwin HL, Gettinger A, Corwin MJ, Gubler D & Pearl RG (2001). Nutritional deficiencies and blunted erythropoietin response as causes of the anemia of critical illness. *Journal of Critical Care*. Vol.16, No.1 (March 2001), pp. 36-41, ISSN 0883-9441

[41] Gomollon F & Gisbert JP (2009). Anemia and inflammatory bowel diseases. *World Journal of Gastroenterology*. Vol.15, No.37, (October 7, 2009), pp. 4659-65, ISSN 1007-9327

[42] Kulnigg S & Gasche C (2006). Systematic review: managing anaemia in Crohn's disease. *Alimentary Pharmacology & Therapeutics*. Vol.24, No.11-12, (December 2006), pp. 1507-23, ISSN 0953-0673

[43] Gasche C, Lomer MC, Cavill I & Weiss G (2004). Iron, anaemia, and inflammatory bowel diseases. *Gut*. Vol.53, No.8, (August 2004), pp. 1190-7, ISSN 0017-5749

[44] Wells CW, Lewis S, Barton JR & Corbett S (2006). Effects of changes in hemoglobin level on quality of life and cognitive function in inflammatory bowel disease patients. *Inflammatory Bowel Disease*. Vol.12, No.2, (February 2006), pp. 123-30, ISSN 1536-4844

[45] Cucino C & Sonnenberg A (2001). Cause of death in patients with inflammatory bowel disease. *Inflammatory Bowel Disease*. Vol.7, No.3, (August 2001), pp. 250-5, ISSN 1536-4844

[46] Beattie WS, Karkouti K, Wijeysundera DN & Tait G (2009). Risk associated with preoperative anemia in noncardiac surgery: A single-center cohort study. *Anesthesiology*. Vol.110, No.3, (March 2009), pp. 574–81, ISSN 0003-3022

[47] Spahn DR. Anemia and patient blood management in hip and knee surgery: a systematic review of the literature. Anesthesiology. Vol.113, No.2, (August 2010), pp. 482-95, ISSN 0003-3022

[48] Hebert PC, Wells G, Blajchman MA, Marshall J, Martin C, Pagliarello G, Tweeddale M, Schweitzer I & Yetisir E (1999). A multicenter, randomized, controlled clinical trial of transfusion requirements in critical care. Transfusion Requirements in Critical Care Investigators, Canadian Critical Care Trials Group. *New England Journal of Medicine*. Vol.340, No.6 (February 11, 1999), pp. 409-17, ISSN 0028-4793

[49] Hebert PC, McDonald BJ & Tinmouth A (2004): Overview of transfusion practices in perioperative and critical care. *Vox Sanguinis*. Vol.87, No.Suppl 2, (July 2004), pp. 209-17, ISSN 1423-0410

[50] Wu WC, Rathore SS, Wang Y, Radford MJ & Krumholz HM (2001). Blood transfusion in elderly patients with acute myocardial infarction. *New England Journal of Medicine*. Vol.345, No.17, (October 25, 2001), pp. 1230-6, ISSN 0028-4793

[51] Hebert PC, Wells G, Tweeddale M, Martin C, Marshall J, Pham B, Blajchman M, Schweitzer I & Pagliarello G (1997). Does transfusion practice affect mortality in critically ill patients? Transfusion Requirements in Critical Care (TRICC) Investigators and the Canadian Critical Care Trials Group. *American Journal of Respiratory and Critical Care Medicine*. Vol.155, No.5 (May 1997), pp. 1618-23. ISSN 1535-4970

[52] Practice Guidelines for blood component therapy: A report by the American Society of Anesthesiologists Task Force on Blood Component Therapy. *Anesthesiology*. Vol.84, No.3, (March 1996), pp. 732-47, ISSN 0003-3022

[53] Marik PE & Corwin HL (2008). Efficacy of red blood cell transfusion in the critically ill: a systematic review of the literature. *Critical Care Medicine*. Vol 36, No.9, (September 2008), pp. 2667-74, ISSN 0090-3493

[54] Swerdlow PS. Red cell exchange in sickle cell disease. *Hematology*. Vol.2006, pp. 48-53, ISSN 1520-4383

[55] Ho GT, Innes JA, Shand AG & Satsangi J (2006). Bronchopulmonary manifestations of inflammatory bowel disease: a case report and literature review. *The Journal of the Royal College of Physicians of Edinburgh*. Vol.36, No.4, (November 2006), pp. 299-303, ISSN 2042-8189

[56] Tzanakis N, Samiou M, Bouros D, Mouzas J, Kouroumalis E & Siafakas NM (1998). Small airways function in patients with inflammatory bowel disease. *American Journal of Respiratory and Critical Care Medicine*. Vol.157, No.2, (February 1998), pp. 382-6, ISSN: 1535-4970

[57] Adenis A, Colombel JF, Lecouffe P, Wallaert B, Hecquet B, Marchandise X & Cortot A (1992). Increased pulmonary and intestinal permeability in Crohn's disease. *Gut*. Vol.33, No.5, (May 1992), pp. 678-82, ISSN 0017-5749

[58] Heatley RV, Thomas P, Prokipchuk EJ, Gauldie J, Sieniewicz DJ, Bienenstock J. Pulmonary function abnormalities in patients with inflammatory bowel disease. The Quarterly Journal of Medicine. Vol.51, No.203, (Summer 1982), pp. 241-50, ISSN 1460-2393

[59] King TE Jr (1989). Bronchiolitis obliterans. Lung. Vol.167, No.1, (December 1989), pp. 69-93, ISSN 1432-1750

[60] Essadki O & Grenier P (1999). Bronchiolitis: computed tomographic findings. Journal de Radiologie. Vol.80, No.1, (January 1999), pp. 17-24, ISSN 0221-0363
[61] Camus P & Colby TV (2000). The lung in inflammatory bowel disease. European Respiratory Journal. Vol.15, No.1, (January 2000), pp. 5-10, ISSN 1399-3003.
[62] Foucher P, Biour M, Blayac JP Godard P, Sgro C, Kuhn M, Vergnon JM, Vervloet D, Pfitzenmeyer P, Ollagnier M, Mayaud C & Camus P (1997). Drugs that may injure the respiratory system. *European Respiratory Journal.* Vol.10, No.2, (February 1997), pp. 265-79, ISSN 0903-1936
[63] Camus P, Piard F, Ashcroft T, Gal AA & Colby TV (1993). The lung in inflammatory bowel disease. Medicine (Baltimore).Vol.72, No.3, (May 1993), pp. 151-83, ISSN 1536-5964.
[64] Searles G & McKendry RJ (1987). Methotrexate pneumonitis in rheumatoid arthritis: potential risk factors. Four case reports and a review of the literature. Journal of Rheumatology. Vol.14, No.6, (December 1987), pp. 1164-71, ISSN 1499-2752
[65] Egan LJ & Sandborn WJ (1996). Methotrexate for inflammatory bowel disease: pharmacology and preliminary results. Mayo Clinic Proceedings. Vol.71, No.1, (January 1996), pp. 69-80, ISSN 1942-5546
[66] Stein RB & Hanauer SB (2000). Comparative tolerability of treatments for inflammatory bowel disease. Drug Safety. Vol.23, No.5, (November 2000), pp. 429-48, ISSN 0114-5916
[67] Warris A, Bjorneklett A & Gaustad P (2001). Invasive pulmonary aspergillosis associated with infliximab therapy. *New England Journal of Medicine*. Vol.344, No.14, (April 5, 2001), pp. 1099–100, ISSN 0028-4793
[68] Ezri T, Kunichezky S, Eliraz A, Soroker D, Halperin D & Schattner A (1994). Bronchiolitis obliterans–current concepts. *The Quarterly Journal of Medicine*. Vol.87, No.1 (January 1994), pp. 1-10, ISSN 1460-2393
[69] Epler GR, Colby TV, McLoud TC, Carrington CB & Gaensler EA (1985). Bronchiolitis obliterans organizing pneumonia. *New England Journal of Medicine*. Vol. 312, No.3, (January 17, 1985), pp. 152-8, ISSN 0028-4793
[70] Weterman IT, Biemond I & Peña AS (1990). Mortality and causes of death in Crohn's disease. Review of 50 years' experience in Leiden University Hospital. *Gut*, Vol.31, No.12, (December 1990), pp. 1387-90, ISSN 0017-5749
[71] Basturk T, Ozagari A, Ozturk T, Kusaslan R & Unsal A (2009). Crohn's disease and secondary amyloidosis: early complication? A case report and review of the literature. *Journal of Renal Care*. Vol.35, No.3, (September 2009), pp. 147-50, ISSN 1755-6686
[72] Greenstein AJ, Sachar DB, Panday AK, Dikman SH, Meyers S, Heimann T, Gumaste V, Werther JL & Janowitz HD. Amyloidosis and inflammatory bowel disease. A 50-year experience with 25 patients. *Medicine (Baltimore)*. Vol.71, No.5, (September 1992), pp. 261-70, ISSN 1536-5964
[73] Lovat LB, Madhoo S, Pepys MB & Hawkins PN (1997). Long-term survival in systemic amyloid A amyloidosis complicating Crohn's Disease. *Gastroenterology*. Vol.112, No.4, (April 1997), pp. 1362-5, ISSN 0016-5085

[74] Palma CL, Grünholz D & Osorio G (2005). Clinical features of patients with the pathological diagnosis of amyloidosis. *Revista Medica de Chile.* Vol.133, No.6 (June 2005), pp. 655-61, ISSN 0717-6163

[75] Seijo Ríos S, Barreiro de Acosta M, Vieites Pérez-Quintela B, Iglesias Canle J, Forteza J & Domínguez Muñoz JE (2008). Secondary amyloidosis in Crohn's disease. *Revista Espanola de Enfermedades Digestivas.* Vol.100, No.12, (December 2008), pp. 792-7, ISSN 1130-0108.

[76] Mayer EA & Gebhart GF (1994). Basic and clinical aspect of visceral hyperalgesia. *Gastroenrerology.* Vol.107, No.1, (July 1994), pp. 271-93, ISSN 0016-5085

[77] Schreiber S, Raedler A, Stenson WF & MacDermott RP (1992). The role of the mucosal immune system in inflammatory bowel disease. *Gastroenterology Clinics of North America.* Vol.21, No.2, (June 1992), pp. 451-502, ISSN 0889-8553

[78] Dray A (1995). Inflammatory mediators in pain. *British Journal of Anaesthesia.* Vol.75, No.2, (August 1995), pp. 125-31, ISSN 0007-0912

[79] Gebhart GF (1999). Peripheral contributions to visceral hyperalgesia. *Canadian Journal of Gastroenterology.* Vol.13, No.Suppl A, (March 1999), pp. 37A–41A. ISSN 0835-7900

[80] Weeke B & Jarnum S (1971). Serum concentration of 19 serum proteins in Crohn's disease and ulcerative colitis. *Gut.* Vol.12, No.4, (April 1971), pp. 297-302, ISSN 0017-5749

[81] Schirbel A, Reichert A, Roll S, Baumgart DC, Büning C, Wittig B, Wiedenmann B, Dignass A & Sturm A (2010). Impact of pain on health-related quality of life in patients with inflammatory bowel disease. *World Journal of Gastroenterology.* Vol.16, No.25, (July 7, 2010), pp. 3168-77, ISSN 1007-9327

[82] Ballantyne JC & Mao J (2003). Opioid therapy for chronic pain. *New England Journal of Medicine.* Vol.349, No.20, (November 13, 2003), pp. 1943-53, ISSN 0028-4793

[83] Smith JP, Stock H, Bingaman S, Mauger D, Rogosnitzky M & Zagon IS (2007). Low-dose naltrexone therapy improves active Crohn's disease. *American Journal of Gastroenterology.* Vol.102, No.4, (April 2007), pp. 820-8, ISSN 1572-0241

[84] Grover M, Herfarth H & Drossman DA (2009). The functional-organic dichotomy: postinfectious irritable bowel syndrome and inflammatory bowel disease-irritable bowel syndrome. *Clinical Gastroenterology and Hepatology.* Vol.7, No.1, (January 2009), pp. 48-53, ISSN 1542-3565

[85] Gesink-van der Veer BJ, Burm AG, Vletter AA & Bovill JG (1993). Influence of Crohn's disease on the pharmacokinetics and pharmacodynamics of alfentanil. *British Journal of Anaesthesia.* Vol.71, No.6, (December 1993), pp. 827-34, ISSN 0007-0912

[86] Guidat A, Fleyfel M, Vallet B, Desreumaux P, Levron JC, Gambiez L, Colombel JF & Scherpereel P (2003). Inflammation increases sufentanil requirements during surgery for inflammatory bowel diseases. *European Journal of Anaesthesiology.* Vol.20, No.12, (December 2003), pp. 957-62, ISSN 0265-0215

[87] Verne GN, Robinson ME & Price DD (2001). Hypersensitivity to visceral and cutaneous pain in the irritable bowel syndrome. *Pain.* Vol.93, No.1, (July 2001), pp.7-14, ISSN 0304-3959

[88] Fleyfel M, Dusson C, Ousmane ML, Guidat A, Colombel JF, Gambiez L & Vallet B (2008). Inflammation affects sufentanil consumption in ulcerative colitis. *European Journal of Anaesthesiology*. Vol.25, No.3, (March 2008), pp. 188-92. ISSN 0265-0215

7

Detection of *Mycobacterium avium subsp. paratuberculosis* in Crohn's Disease Patients and Ruminants Intestine by In Situ Hybridization

Lucía C. Favila-Humara* et al.
Laboratorio de Tuberculosis. CENID-Microbiología Animal. INIFAP. México

1. Introduction

Mycobacterium avium subsp. *paratuberculosis* is an acid fast rod, extremely slow growing and mycobactin-dependent for its *in vitro* growth. This mycobacterium is the etiological agent of the chronic enteritis that affects domestic and wild ruminants, well-known as paratuberculosis or Johne's disease. In humans, a possible *M. avium* subsp. *paratuberculosis* infection has been suggested to be involved in the pathogenesis of Crohn's disease [1, 2], sarcoidosis; and recently sarcoidosis-like multisystem autosomal-dominant granulomatous disorder (Blau syndrome) [3, 4].

Crohn's disease encompasses a spectrum of clinical and pathological patterns manifested by focal, asymmetric, transmural, and, chronic granulomatous inflammation affecting the gastrointestinal tract with the potential for systemic and extraintestinal complications. The etiology of Crohn's disease is thought to be multifactorial, involving an interaction between genetic susceptibility, environmental triggers, and immune-mediated tissue injury. In this regard, there is considerable suggestive evidence to support an environmental factor, such as *M. avium* subsp. *paratuberculosis* infection. This evidence includes similarity of the macro and microscopic injuries, bacteriological isolation and molecular biology tests which have allowed the detection of this mycobacterium in intestine, milk and peripheral blood of

* Gilberto Chávez-Gris[2], Francisco J. García-Vázquez[3], José M. Remes-Troche[4], Luis F. Uscanga[4], Marco A. Santillán Flores[1], Fernando Paolicchi[5], Erika M. Carrillo-Casas[6], Rigoberto Hernández Castro[6]
[1] *Laboratorio de Tuberculosis. CENID-Microbiología Animal. INIFAP. México*
[2] *Centro de Enseñanza, Investigación y Extensión en Producción Animal en Altiplano, Facultad de Medicina Veterinaria y Zootecnia, Universidad Nacional Autónoma de México. Tequisquiapan, Querétaro, México*
[3] *Departamento de Patología Molecular. Instituto Nacional de Pediatría. Coyoacán 04530. México*
[4] *Departamento de Gastroenterología. Instituto Nacional de Ciencias Médicas y Nutrición "Salvador Zubirán".Tlalpan 14000. México*
[5] *Grupo de Sanidad Animal/Animal Health Group. INTA, Est Exp Agrop Balcarce - Facultad Cs Agrarias UNMdP. Casilla de Correo 276/ PO Box 276. 7620 Balcare, Argentina*
[6] *Departamento de Biología Molecular e Histocompatibilidad. Hospital General "Dr. Manuel Gea González". Tlalpan 14080 México*

patients with Crohn's disease [5, 6, 7]. Despite this; *M. avium* subsp. *paratuberculosis* is still not recognized as a human pathogen.
Cronh's disease has a high prevalence in North America, and Northern and Western Europe is less so in South Africa, Australia, and South and Middle Europe. It is considered a rare disease in Asia, Africa and Latin America. However, recently an increase in the incidence of Crohn's disease has been noted in Spain and Latin American countries, such as Puerto Rico and Brazil [10, 11]. These populations are very similar to the Mexican population, mainly composed by Mexican Mestizo individuals which have a proportion of 56% Native American Indian genes, 40% Caucasian genes (the most common European ancestry are the Spaniards), and 4% Afro-American genes [12]. In 2010, 14,706 persons were diagnosed with tuberculosis in Mexico (1.39% of them suffering meningitis), unfortunately the prevalence of other mycobacteriosis remains unknown [13]. The present study used *in situ* hybridization to detect a fraction of *M. avium* subsp. *paratuberculosis* specific sequence IS*900*, it was carried out to determine the presence of *M. avium* subsp. *paratuberculosis* on formalin fixed intestinal samples of Mexican patients with Crohn's disease, and in samples of ruminants with paratuberculosis.

2. Material and methods

2.1 Samples origin and characteristics

Twenty three paraffin blocks with intestinal samples from 14 patients with clinical and histopathological diagnosis of Crohn's disease were included. All patients underwent surgical resection of the small and/or large bowel segments for disease at the Medical Sciences and Nutrition National Institute "Salvador Zubirán". A sample of human intestine diagnosed with intestinal tuberculosis and ulcerative colitis was included as a negative control; this case was kindly facilitated by the National Institute of Pediatrics. Paraffin blocks with intestine samples from 1 bovine, 2 goats and 9 ovines, previously diagnosed with paratuberculosis by ELISA, histopathology and tissue culture were used, as controls.

2.2 Test area selection

Histopathological evaluation to characterize the inflammatory disease and select appropriate target areas for the application of the hybridisation probe was performed on all the intestine samples after staining with hematoxilin and eosin (HE); and Ziehl-Neelsen (ZN). The Criteria for group formation, was to consider the presence or absence of acid fast bacilli after ZN stain, accordingly we separated the animal tissues into two paratuberculosis groups: Group A with 8 samples showing a granulomatous reaction and ZN (+); and group B with 4 samples showing granulomatous reaction but ZN (-).
All Crohn's disease cases were negative to the ZN stain. Group C included those Crohn's disease cases in which at histopathological examination we observed transmural inflammatory infiltrate with the presence of macrophages, epitheliod cells and sometimes giant Langhans cells; and considered as granulomatous. Whereas group D consisted of those cases in which infiltration was predominantly lymphocytic with plasma cells or mixed with some granulocytes at mucosal or transmural level which were considered as non granulomatous. In a single case with multiple samples, one was classified within group C and another one in group D. Group C consisted of 7 patients and 10 samples, whereas group D comprised 8 patients with 13 samples.

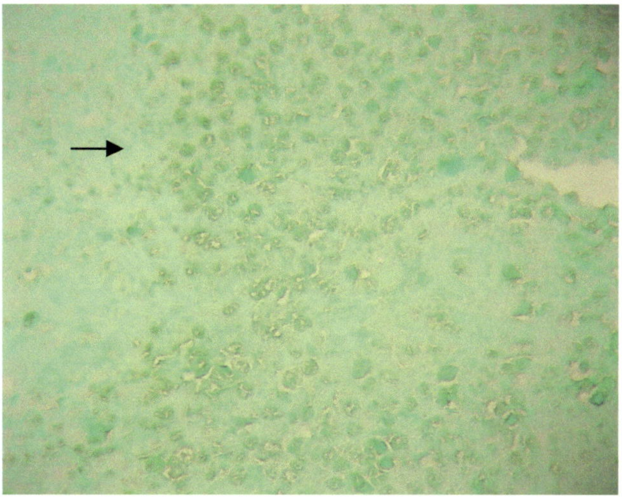

Fig. 1. Case of paratuberculosis from group A. ISH, DAB. 40x. Positive reaction inside macrophages in ileal submucosa.

2.3 In situ hybridization (ISH)

The biotinylated probe used consists in 25 bases: TAGGACTGGTCGGCTGCAAGGTAG. This sequence belongs to the region 639-664 of the 3' chain of IS*900*. Sections of 2 μm of thickness were placed in positive charged and pre-cleaned slides (FisherBiotech, USA). The slides were baked for 30 min at 60°C and submerged 5 min in xylol, rehydrated through graded alcohol (2 x 100%, 96%, 70%, 3 min each step) and air dried. Sections were incubated with proteinase K (DakoCytomation, USA) for 10 min at 42°C. Sections were washed twice with distilled water and H_2O_2 0.3% were added and placed 5 min at room temperature (RT). By capillarity, 5-10 μl of the probe at 17.04 μg/ml was added (depending on the large of the sample). Slides were placed in termoblock for 10 min at 94.5°C. Hybridization was allowed overnight at 37°C. Sections were washed 4 times with Tris Buffered Solution (TBS, pH 7.5). Immediately, 50 μl of the stringent wash solution (0.015 M NaN_3) were added on each slide and they were placed in termoblock, 30 min at 40°C and Finally TBS-washing for 4 times.

2.4 Signal detection

Two systems of signal detection were used. Catalyzed signal amplification system (CSA). 50 μl of primary streptavidin-HRP was added and slides were placed in termoblock 20 min at 37°C. Slides were washed 4 times with TBS. Then, the slides were incubated with a drop of Biotinyl-tyramide 20 min at RT. Slides were washed 4 times with TBS and a drop of secondary streptavidin-HRP was added to the sections and incubated 15 min at RT. Reaction was revealed with 20 μl of 1:50 dilution of diaminobenzidine tetrahydrochloride (DAB). The reaction was observed in the microscope and it was stopped rinsing slides with distilled water.

2.5 Alkaline peroxidase system (AP)

Alkaline streptavidin phosphatase (DakoCytomation, USA) was added and incubated 30 min at 37°C. Slides were washed 4 times with TBS and the reaction was revealed adding 2 drops of N2 N-dimethylformamide (NBT/BCIP) to the 1.7%. Every 10 min the reaction was observed in the microscope and finally stopped rinsing slides with distilled water. Finally the reaction was counterstained with light green at 3%. Slides were rinsed with alcohol 96%; air dried and submerged in xylol to adhere them a cover slip with entellan resin. The results were submitted to a difference between proportions test in the program Statistica 6.0 (Statsoft, Tulsa Ok. EU), to verify the difference between groups A and B, as well as between groups C and D, with a confidence level of 95%. A p value of less than 0.05 was considered to be significant.

3. Results

In the ruminant groups A and B, as expected, all the samples were positive by *in situ* hybridization. In humans (groups C and D), overall positivity for *M. avium* subsp. *paratuberculosis* by *in situ* hybridization was 64.28% (n= 9). According to the groups distribution, all 7 patients (100%) in group C were positive for *M. avium* subsp. *paratuberculosis* by *in situ* hybridization, compared to 3/8 (37.5%) patients in group D; this difference was statistically significant (p= 0.0239).

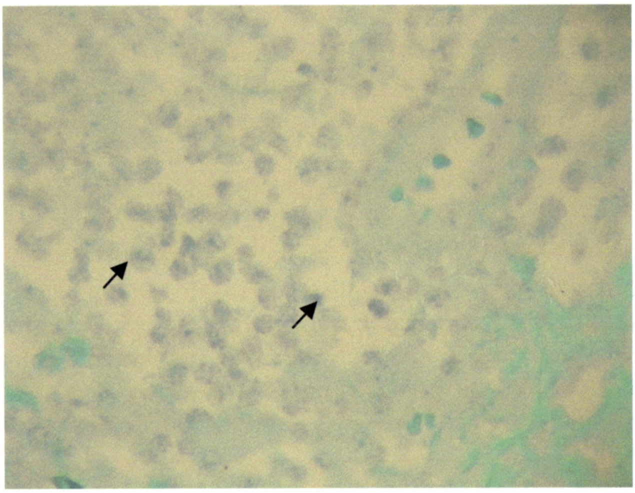

Fig. 2. Case of Crohn's disease from group C, ISH, NBCT/BCIP. 40x. Positive reaction inside macrophages in the colonic submucosa.

Of the 8 patients in which more than one sample was analyzed, 3 of them were positive, 2 (25%) showed one positive and one negative sample and in 3 cases (37.5%) all were negative.

After *in situ* hybridization *M. avium* subsp. *paratuberculosis* was observed intracellularly within macrophages, epithelioid cells and giant cells in the intestinal mucosa and submucosa. In groups A, B and C the positive signal was observed within granulomas, whereas in group D it was seen within little macrophages that contribute to the inflammatory infiltrate. The positive signals were granular and intracytoplasmatic. In group A, the cases in group A with abundant intracellular Mycobacteria; the reaction coalesces and looks diffuse in the cytoplasm.

4. Discussion

Crohn's disease is a chronic inflammatory bowel disease of as yet unknown and possibly heterogeneous etiology. Diet, infections, immune dysregulation, and other unidentified environmental factors, all working under the influence of a genetic predisposition, have been suspiciously regarded. Among these, one of the most enduring hypotheses has been that *M. avium* subsp. *paratuberculosis* could be the causative agent of Crohn's disease.

By bacteriological isolation, serology and techniques of molecular biology several authors have been able to detect the presence of *M. avium* subsp. *paratuberculosis* in a great proportion of patients with Crohn's disease [2, 3, 5-7]. Even more, some authors have reported clinical remission of Crohn's disease patients who received anti-mycobacterial therapy which included macrolide antibiotics [8].

However, early results were inconsistent so that the role of this chronic enteric pathogen in the pathogenesis of Crohn's disease is not yet clearly established. The disparity in the earlier results can be due to several factors; among them the application of different methodologies.Successful isolations have been achieved by bacteriologists in veterinary laboratories since human medicine laboratories do not routinely culture mycobactin dependent mycobacteria, and therefore, don't necessary have adequate media for the isolation of these very difficult and slow growing organisms. In addition, when culture has been successful, the primary isolation consists on ZN-negative cell wall deficient forms which require long incubation times; which can extend for years to revert to bacillary forms [1]. In this study all cases showed a granular and intracytoplasmatic stain pattern, as expected for intracellular bacteria like mycobacteria and *Chlamydophila* in agreement with the previous work described by Hulten *et al* and Meijer *et al.* [12, 14-15].

In the veterinary group A, the tissues were from multibacillary Johne's disease, with the labeled probe therefore hybridizing to the bacillary forms of *M. avium* subsp. *paratuberculosis.* In group B, as well as in the cases of Crohn's disease in groups C and D; the labeled probe hybridized *in situ* to the ZN-negative form of these versatile pathogens showing that this technique is capable of recognizing the cell wall deficient phenotype. Therefore, the protocol of *in situ* hybridization used identifies both forms of *M. avium* subsp. *paratuberculosis.* The enzymatic digestion treatment is apparently able to permeabilise the mycobacterial cellular wall without altering intestine tissue architecture in ruminants and humans.

The identification, by *in situ* hybridization of positive cases to *M. avium* subsp. *paratuberculosis* in groups B, C and D is consistent with the findings of the study of Hulten *et al* in which they identify spheroplasts of this mycobacterium in paucibacillary cases of Johne´s disease in ovines [14], as well as their later study when they demonstrated the presence of spheroplasts in 7 of 37 (18.91%) of the Crohn's disease patients [15]. In the same way, Sechi *et al* demonstrated by *in situ* hybridization, the presence of *M. avium* subsp. *paratuberculosis* spheroplasts in 35 of 48 (72.91%) of Crohn's disease patients, despite the fact that on this occasion they did not find *M. avium* subsp. *paratuberculosis* by PCR IS*900* in the same samples [17]. However, these authors did identify *M. avium* subsp. *paratuberculosis* by PCR in subsequent work using improved sample processing procedures [18].

Although some literature classifies patients with Crohn's disease according to the fistulous or obstructive phenotype, in our present series of clinical cases we observed that the same patient can demonstrate both phenotypes in different intestinal segments. The value of this method of classification is in our view uncertain. Most of the studies of the molecular pathology in Crohn's disease do not differentiate between patients with the granulomatous and non granulomatous presentation. The results obtained in the present study indicate that a greater proportion of patients with granulomatous disease are *M. avium* subsp. *paratuberculosis* positive by *in situ* hybridization. This observation agrees with those of Hulten *et al.* However; we found the positive *in situ* hybridization signal particularly in relation to the granulomas in Crohn's disease patients.

Greenstein suggested that the identification of *M. avium* subsp. *paratuberculosis* DNA in the tissues of patients with Crohn's disease cannot be taken as proof of a causal association between this mycobacterium with Crohn's disease. It could be a coincidence of *M. avium* subsp. *paratuberculosis* DNA being in the intestinal lumen of people who had ingested cow's milk containing these pathogens [19]. In the present study using an *in situ* diagnostic procedure we were able to confirm the presence of *M. avium* subsp. *paratuberculosis* within the inflamed gut wall and related to the granulomatous lesions. In this situation *M. avium* subsp. *paratuberculosis* is most unlikely to be a transient food-borne contaminant. It is much more likely that is well characterized multi-host chronic enteric pathogen is related to the causation of the chronic inflammatory intestinal disease. The exact mechanism is not know but one theory is that *M. avium* subsp. *paratuberculosis* either can infect the host and cause a primary infection responsible for the development of the disease, or it is a secondary opportunistic infection that could perpetuate the cycle of inflammation and cytokine release. Regarding the Crohn's disease pathogenesis, there is no doubt that Crohn's disease is a result of immune dysregulation, where an excessive TH1-driven, cell-mediated immune response is elicited and persists. In this context, chronic intracellular *M. avium* subsp. *paratuberculosis* infection may be the trigger for this excessive TH1 immune response that results in the clinical, endoscopic, radiological, and histological manifestation known as Crohn's disease.

Even if *M. avium* subsp. *paratuberculosis* is not causally linked with Crohn's disease, the presence of DNA from *M. avium* subsp. *paratuberculosis* and other bacteria within the mucosa might have secondary clinical implications. Some studies have proved that bacterial DNA has immunomodulatory activity by signaling via pattern recognition receptors such as toll-like receptor 9 on host epithelial cells [20]. Further studies are needed, and it is imperative that researchers adopt standardized methods and techniques, including appropriate controls, and search for intracellular bacteria other than *M. avium* subsp. *paratuberculosis.* The availability of these tests could influence the therapeutic approach of these patients; antimycobacterial therapy may include macrolide antibiotics which have been beneficial for remission of intestinal lesions [8].

Although previous epidemiological studies have suggested that the incidence of inflammatory bowel disease is lower in Latin American populations, recent studies have demonstrated that the incidence is increasing and may be higher than suspected. For example, Appleyard *et al* showed that in Puerto Rico, an Hispanic predominant population; the total incidence of IBD increased significantly between 1996 and 2000 (3.07/100,000 to 7.74/100,000; p <0.001), being significantly higher for Crohn's disease (four-fold increase, p < 0.01), but not for ulcerative colitis (1.7-fold increase) [10]. Puerto Ricans are genetically complex and comprised of various proportions of Native American, African, and European genetic origins, as our Mexican population. Although the reasons for this are unclear, the data suggest several possible explanations such as changes in health care system, movement from rural areas to urban cities, a more Westernized and fairly high carbohydrates and fat diet, and decrease in the incidence of intestinal parasites; which have a protective effect via regulation of the immune response.

5. Conclusion

In conclusion, despite the obvious need to evaluate a greater number of Mexican patients with and without inflammatory bowel disease these initial results remark the exposure of the Mexican population to *M. avium* subsp. *paratuberculosis* and provide further evidence in support of the zoonotic features of this agent. Taking on account the public health relevance of the issue as well as its economic impact, wider studies are needed in Mexico.

6. References

Chiodini RJ, Van Kruiningen HJ, Thayer WR, *et al.* Spheroplastic phase of mycobacteria isolated from patients with Crohn's disease. *J Clin Microbiol.* 1986;27:357-363.

Bull TJ, McMinn EJ, Sidi-Boumedine K, *et al.* Detection and verification of *Mycobacterium avium* subsp *paratuberculosis* in fresh ileocolonic mucosal biopsy specimens from individuals with and without Crohn's disease. *J Clin Microbiol.* 2003; 41:2915-23.

Ikonomopoulos JA, Gorgoulis VG, Kastrinakis NG, *et al.* Sensitive differential detection of genetically related mycobacterial pathogens in archival material. *Am J Clin Pathol.* 2000;114(6):940-50.

Dow CT. Paratuberculosis in Blau Syndrome tissues. Memories from the 8th International Colloquium on Paratuberculosis. August 14-18 2005. Copenhagen, Denmark.

Schwartz D, Shafran I, Romero C, *et al.* Use of short-term culture for identification of *Mycobacterium avium* subsp. *paratuberculosis* in tissue from Crohn's disease patients. *Clin Microbiol Infect.* 2000;6:303-307.

Naser SA, Schwartz D, Shafran I. Isolation of *Mycobacterium avium* subsp *paratuberculosis* from Breast Milk of Crohn's Disease Patients. *Am J Gastroenterol.* 2000;95:1094-5.

Naser SA, Ghobrial G, Romero C, *et al.* Culture *of Mycobacterium avium* subspecies *paratuberculosis* from the blood of patients with Crohn's disease. *Lancet.* 2004;364:1039-44.

Gui GP, Thomas PR, Tizard ML. Two-year outcomes analysis of Crohn's disease treated with rifabutin and macrolide antibiotic. *J Antimicrob Chemother.* 1997;39: 393-400.

Jinch H, Rojas E, De Castro R. Regional enteritis in Mexico. *Gac Med Mex.* 1967;97:681-91.

Appleyard CB, Hernandez G, Rios-Bedoya CF. Basic epidemiology of Inflammatory Bowel Disease in Puerto Rico. *Inflamm Bowel Dis.* 2004;10:106-11.

Souza MH, Troncon LE, Rodrigues CM, *et al.* Trends in the occurrence (1980-1999) and clinical features of Crohn's disease and ulcerative colitis in a university hospital in southeastern Brazil. *Arq Gastroenterol.* 2002;39:98-105.

Yamamoto-Furusho JK, Uscanga LF, Vargas-Alarcon G, *et al.* Clinical and genetic heterogeneity in Mexican patients with ulcerative colitis. *Hum Immunol.* 2003;64(1):119-23.

Sistema Nacional de Vigilancia Epidemiológica. Boletín Epidemiológico 2011;32(27) 2009. Available in: http://www.dgepi.salud.gob.mx/boletin/2010/2010/sem52.pdf.

Hulten K, Karttunen TJ, El-Zimaity HM, Naser SA, Collins MT, Graham DY, El-Zaatari FA. Identification of cell wall deficient forms of *M. avium* subsp. *paratuberculosis* in paraffin embedded tissues from animals with Johne's disease by *in situ* hybridization. *J Microbiol Methods*. 2000; 42(2):185-95.

Hulten K, El-Zimaity HM, Karttunen TJ, Almashhrawi A, Schwartz MR, Graham DY, El-Zaatari FA. Detection of *Mycobacterium avium* subspecies *paratuberculosis* in Crohn's diseased tissues by *in situ* hybridization. *Am J Gastroenterol*. 2001;96:1529-35.

Meijer A, Roholl PJ, Gielis-Proper SK, *et al. Chlamydia pneumoniae in vitro* and *in vivo*: a critical evaluation of *in situ* detection methods. *J Clin Pathol*. 2000;53(12):904-10.

Sechi LA, Mura M, Tanda F, *et al.* Identification of *Mycobacterium avium* subsp. *paratuberculosis* in biopsy specimens from patients with Crohn's disease identified by *in situ* hybridization. *J Clin Microbiol*. 2001;39:4514-7.

Sechi LA, Mura M, Tanda E, *et al. Mycobacterium avium* subsp. *paratuberculosis* in tissue samples of Crohn's disease patients. *New Microbiol.* 2004;27(1):75-7.

Greenstein RJ. Is Crohn's disease caused by a mycobacterium? Comparisons with leprosy, tuberculosis, and Johne's disease. *Lancet Infect Dis*. 2003;3:507-14.

Watson JL, McKay DM. The immunophysiological impact of bacterial CpG DNA on the gut. *Clin Chim Acta*. 2005;:1-11.

8

Mycobacterium avium ssp. *paratuberculosis* vs Crohn's Disease

Isabel Azevedo Carvalho[1], Maria de Lourdes de Abreu Ferrari[2] and Maria Aparecida Scatamburlo Moreira[1]
[1]*Federal University of Viçosa (UFV)*
[2]*Federal University of Minas Gerais (UFMG)*
Brazil

1. Introduction

Crohn's disease (CD) is a chronic inflammatory bowel disease, with the potential to affect any segment of the gastrointestinal tract. Despite the great advances in recent decades, which provided a better understanding of the pathogenesis of the disease, it is yet to be completely elucidated. Presence of genetic factors, luminal factors such as microflora and factors related to the intestinal barrier and immunoregulation are pieces that interact with each other and with environmental factors. The possibility of an infectious etiology has always been widely discussed. In this context, *Mycobacterium avium* subspecies *paratuberculosis* (MAP) has attracted the interest of many researchers because of the similarity between paratuberculosis and CD. In 1913, two decades before the description of CD in 1932, T. K. Dalziel made associations between chronic cases of enteritis in humans and paratuberculosis in cattle (Behr and Kapur, 2008).

Some genetic studies also support the role of MAP in CD and susceptibility genes have been identified, which encode proteins involved in the innate immunity defense against intracellular bacteria. However, no study is conclusive about a causal relationship. It is not possible to conclude that a single agent is solely responsible for the etiology of CD: a multifactorial cause is much more likely (Grant et al., 2001).

Whereas the causal relationship has not been established, therapeutic implications require further studies. Results of these studies could help answer questions about the role of MAP in the etiology of CD.

2. *Mycobacterium avium* subspecies *paratuberculosis*

Mycobacterium avium subspecies *paratuberculosis* (MAP) is a small bacillus, Gram-positive, intracellular, acid-resistant bacterium belonging to the Mycobacteriacea family. It grows slowly and when observed under an optic microscope, usually appears to form small clusters (Fig.1). Like other mycobacteria, this microorganism has a thick cell wall, composed mainly of lipids, which determines its acid-resistant, hydrophobicity and high resistance to chemical processes, such as chlorination of water, and physical processes, such as pasteurization (Harris and Barletta, 2001).

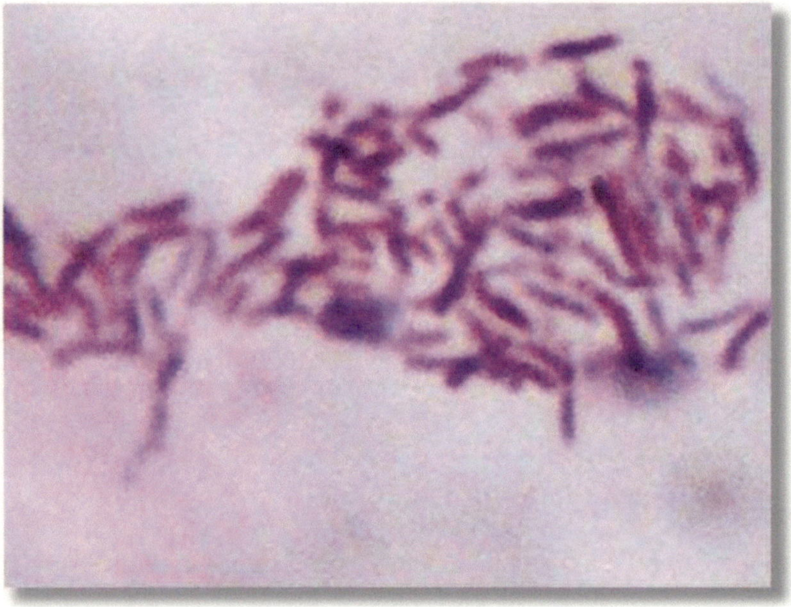

Fig. 1. *Mycobacterium avium* subspecies *paratuberculosis* (MAP) stained by Ziehl-Neelsen. Optical microscopy (1000x).

The first observation of the microorganism was made in 1895 by Johne and Frothingham, who isolated an acid-resistant bacterium from the ileum of animals with chronic granulomatous inflammation. The disease was called paratuberculosis, according to its similarity with intestinal tuberculosis. Although the disease had been reported in 1895, identification of the agent was assigned by Twort in 1910 who could grow the microorganism for the first time in laboratory (Cocito et al., 1994).

Morphology of MAP colonies depends on the medium used for growth. In Herrold Egg Yolk Medium (HEYM), colonies are small, measuring about 1 to 2 mm, generally white, convex and smooth, while in Middlebrook Agar they become more wrinkled. Even under optimal conditions, colonies may take 3 to 4 months or longer to become visible (Harris and Barletta, 2001). Other features of MAP, which serve to differentiate it from other bacteria, are its dependence on mycobactin *J* for in vitro growth, a compound extracted from mycobacterial cells that helps in iron uptake, and the presence of insertion element IS*900*, which appears as 14 to 18 copies within the genome (Green et al., 1989).

The complete genome of MAP K-10 was sequenced in 2004 by researchers at the University of Minnesota, USA. Analysis showed that MAP K-10 has a circular sequence of 4,829,781 base pairs with 69.3% G+C. When comparing the genome of MAP and other mycobacteria, researchers have suggested two hypotheses to explain the extremely slow growth of MAP. Firstly, the presence of an insertion sequence, MAP0028c/IS1311, much closer to oriC in MAP compared to *M. tuberculosis*, would be detrimental to chromosomal replication, leading to a wider range of generation. The second theory is the presence of the gene map0638, with a higher replacement rate compared to *M. tuberculosis*. This gene is responsible for regulating synthesis of purine and therefore has a role in rate of protein synthesis and cell growth (Li et al., 2005).

3. Paratuberculosis

Mycobacterium avium subspecies *paratuberculosis* (MAP) is the causative agent of paratuberculosis or Johne's disease, a chronic infectious enteritis, characterized by the presence of persistent diarrhea and progressive weight loss, which mainly affects domestic and wild ruminants worldwide and may also affect several other species of mammals, including primates.

In the USA, bovine paratuberculosis is well documented and it is estimated that economic losses for the dairy industry are of the order of millions of dollars annually. These losses are due to decreased production, reduced protein content of milk, premature culling, increased susceptibility to other diseases, reduced fertility and increased health costs (Hendrick et al., 2005).

Under natural conditions, the transmission of the microorganism is usually horizontal, by ingesting food or water contaminated with MAP. Transmission can also occur vertically by intrauterine infection, colostrum from females infected or contaminated semen.

Paratuberculosis usually manifests in young adult cattle. After an incubation period of about 2 to 5 years clinical symptoms begin to appear. However, infected animals eliminate the microorganism in their stools and in minor amounts in milk even before the onset of clinical signs, which contributes to the spread of the agent. Confinement contributes to the infection of animals and can be one of the reasons for higher prevalence of the disease in dairy cattle herds compared to meat cattle. The long incubation period has great importance in the economic impact of disease because infected animals are responsible for the unnoticed spread of the agent and, therefore, of the disease in herds.

In vivo, the primary target of MAP infection is the M cells from Peyer's patches and the primary lesions occur on the walls of the small intestine and mesenteric lymph nodes. The multiplication of the microorganism leads to the extent of injury to the ileum, jejunum, cecum and colon, interfering with the intestinal metabolism. The main gross lesions are characterized by thickening of the intestinal mucosa, which presents an aspect grid with transverse folds, well-exposed and enlarged mesenteric lymph nodes, and the main histopathological findings consist of enteritis and granulomatous lymphangitis and lymphadenitis associated with the presence of acid-fast bacilli resistant into macrophages.

Typical clinical signs of the disease are rapid and progressive weight loss (Fig. 2) and intermittent diarrhea, which becomes progressively more severe. Animals continue with a normal appetite but cannot effectively absorb nutrients. Lower body condition scores are generally found. In the final stage, chronic diarrhea of animals becomes untreatable and then, they will die in cachectic state. During the early stages of paratuberculosis, the immunity is characterized by a strong cell-mediated immune response and in the later stages there is a humoral immune response. Antibody concentrations become higher with the progression of the disease when the lesions become more extensive, reflecting the amount of antigen present.

Diagnosis can be based on the detection of the etiologic agent or detection of immune response to this agent. Several methods have been used to diagnose the disease such as fecal culture, immunological tests, histopathological tests and molecular tests.

MAP isolation by fecal culture is considered the "gold standard" for diagnosis of paratuberculosis, despite having low sensitivity and requiring up to 16 weeks until the first colonies can be seen. To detect infected animals in the early stages of the disease by this method is very difficult due to the slow growth of MAP. The agent is grown on specific medium and confirmation of the identity of the colonies is done by its dependence of micobactin J or targeting the insertion sequence IS*900* on molecular tests, an element pattern that enables the genetic identification of MAP.

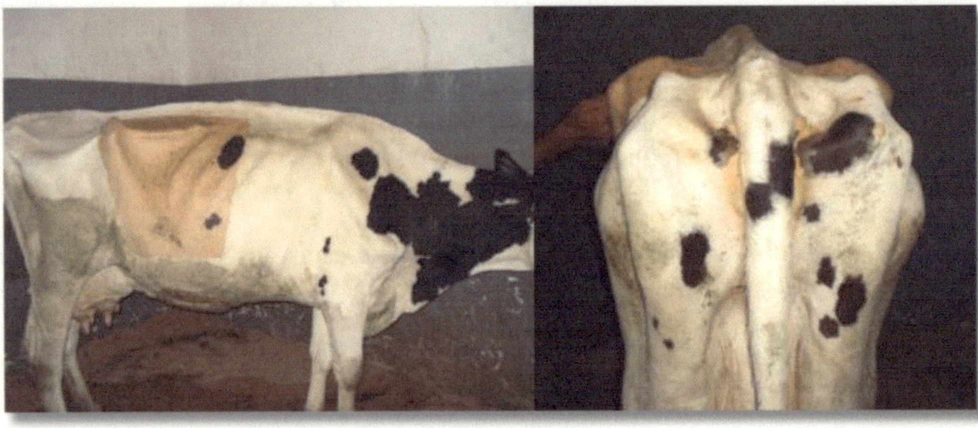

Fig. 2. Animal with paratuberculosis showing low body score

Several serological tests have been used for rapid detection of infected animals including complement fixation, agar gel immunodiffusion and ELISA. However, because disease immunity is mediated by cells in the early stages and humoral in the later stages, these tests generally have high sensitivity in infected animals showing clinical signs, and low sensitivity in animals that do not. Therefore they are most useful in the clinical stages of disease. Among the serological tests, ELISA is the most commonly used for its high sensitivity and acceptable specificity. Despite the low sensitivity and specificity, intradermal tests have also been used. Infected animals show a cellular response when in contact with purified MAP proteins. These tests are not recommended because it may cause cross-reactivity of these proteins with tuberculin during the tuberculin test, leading to false positive results. This is a test performed by control programs for diagnosis of tuberculosis, a disease caused by *M. bovis* in countries where this disease is present.

Rapid detection of microorganisms of slow growth has become possible through use of molecular biology techniques. Discovery of insertion sequence IS*900* in the MAP genome and the development of the polymerase chain reaction (PCR) revolutionized this field. PCR is used successfully to detect MAP DNA in samples of pasteurized milk and fresh milk and is more sensitive than fecal culture. Using PCR it is possible to detect concentrations as low as 10UFC/mL milk. It is a highly sensitive and specific technique for the detection of MAP, as well as fast, and can reduce diagnosis time from months to just two days. PCR is also very versatile, considering that it can be used in stool, tissues, milk, blood and semen. There is currently no satisfactory treatment for animals affected by MAP. Vaccines currently available against MAP do not protect animals completely and there is also the aforementioned problem of possible cross-reactions. Thus, vaccination is not recommended.

General management measures such as general hygiene facilities, separating animals by age, and identification and disposal of infected animals can be cited as preventative measures.

3.1 Paratuberculosis in Brazil

In Brazil, the first notification of paratuberculosis occurred in Rio de Janeiro, in an imported animal (Dupont, 1915). Afterwards, the disease was reported in the Southeastern (Santos and Silva, 1956; Dacorso Filho et al., 1960; Silva, 1961; Nakajima et al., 1991; Ristow et al., 2007; Costa et al., 2010), Southern (Portugal et al., 1979; Ramos et al., 1986; Driemeier et al., 1999), Mid-western (Brautingam et al., 1996; Acypreste et al., 2005), and Northeastern (Mota et al., 2010; Oliveira et al., 2010) regions of the country in animals born and raised in Brazil. The first report in raw milk samples is recent (Carvalho et al., 2009).

The first report of the presence of MAP in milk samples in the country was fairly recent. Although researches on paratuberculosis in Brazil have increased considerably, the studies published in the area are still few and the economic impact of the disease has not been measured in the country. In Brazil, the estimated prevalence of paratuberculosis is higher than in other countries. Further studies are needed to subsidize control measures in the national herd, since, in Brazil, there is no health program for this disease.

4. Crohn's disease

Crohn's disease (CD) is an inflammatory bowel disease of unknown etiology, which is characterized by chronic, focal, asymmetric, transmural and granulomatous inflammation, and can affect any segment of the digestive tract, from mouth to anus, although with preference for the distal small intestine and proximal large intestine. The disease has three phenotypes which are: stenosing, penetrating, and not stenotic and non-penetrating.

Incidence and prevalence of CD varies greatly with geographic location. USA, Britain, Scandinavia (especially Norway and Sweden), Italy and countries of northern Europe are considered areas with greater impact. Intermediate incidence areas are represented by the countries of southern Europe, South Africa, Australia and New Zealand. Low incidence is reported in Asia and South America.

The disease can affect individuals of any age, but occurs with greater frequency in patients between 20 and 40 years old. It affects people in their most productive period, with an enormous impact on quality of life of patients. A second peak in incidence, less obvious, is described in patients between 60 and 80 years old, setting a bimodal presentation. The disease has no predilection for sex.

Pathogenesis of CD, although not fully understood, fundamentally involves four aspects that interact with each other and with environmental factors: a) genetic factors; b) luminal factors related to the intestinal microbiota, its antigens, metabolic products and food antigens; c) factors related to the intestinal barrier, including aspects related to innate immunity and intestinal permeability; and d) factors related to immunoregulation, based on the adaptive or acquired immunity.

CD is characterized by periods when the disease is active and others where it is in remission. Symptoms depend on the severity and location of intestinal involvement. In approximately one third of patients, CD involves the small intestine, especially ileum, and in some cases the jejunum. About 20% to 25% of cases present only colonic lesions. The isolated involvement of the jejunum is rare, as well as cases involving the esophagus, stomach and duodenum. The most common clinical manifestations are abdominal pain, diarrhea and weight loss. CD progresses with periods of remission and exacerbation, even after surgical resection of the affected areas. It has a high percentage of complications with formation of abscesses, fistulas, stenosis, cavity free perforation and anoperineal involvement (Fig. 3). About 70% of individuals affected by the CD undergo surgery and 30% suffer from repeated bowel resections. This disease may be associated with extraintestinal manifestations, and rheumatological, dermatological, ophthalmological, and hepatobiliary nephrology manifestations are the most frequent.

Diagnosis of the disease represents a major challenge, especially when it comes to early diagnosis. It is based on a combination of clinical, laboratory, radiological, endoscopic and histopathological findings. There is no pathognomonic test for the diagnosis of CD.

To date there is no medical or surgical treatment that provides healing of CD. As inflammation is the maximum expression of the disease pathophysiology, clinical therapy, which involves different groups of medications such as aminosalicylates, corticosteroids, immunomodulators and biologic therapy are aimed at blocking the inflammatory cascade and ending the inflammation and scarring of the intestinal mucosa.

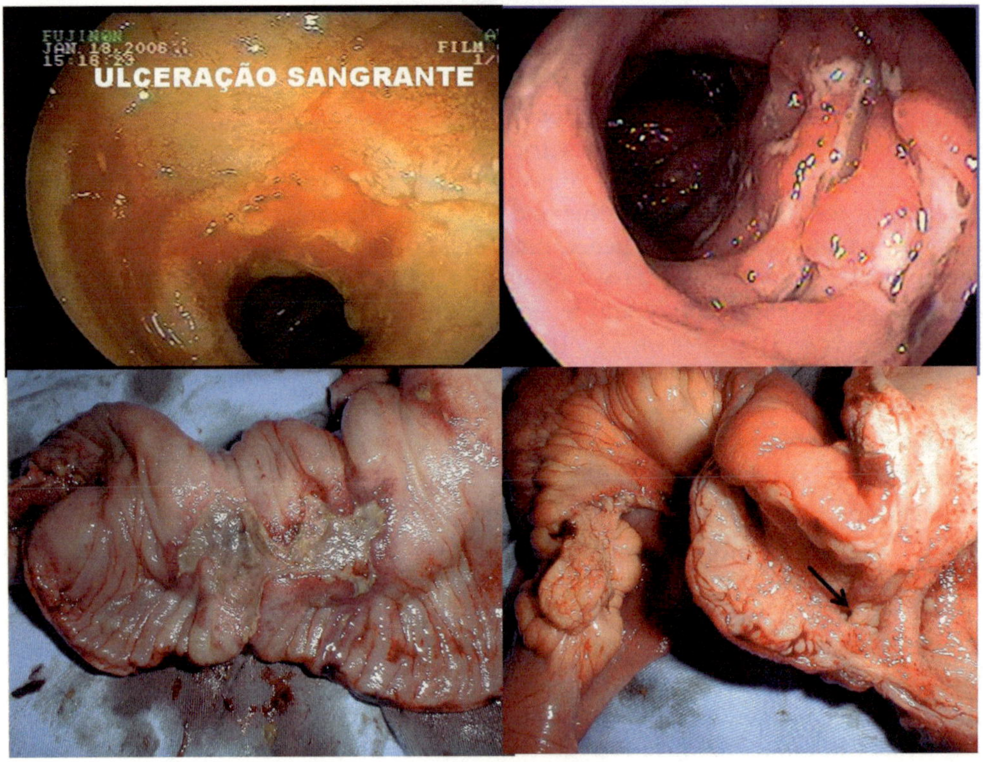

Fig. 3. Endoscopic appearance of Crohn's disease (CD). A: bleeding ulcerated lesion; B: serpiginous ulcerations in the mucosa showing cobblestones appearence. Surgical specimens. C: ileum with extensive ulcerated lesion, D: intestinal wall thickening and opening of the fistulous orifice (arrow).

Although it is a benign disease with low mortality rate, CD is accompanied by high morbidity, with an unpredictable course and the phases of activity, exteriorized through uncomfortable manifestations and/or complications, even when the best care and treatments are implemented. Patients have to live for a long time with limitations that affect directly their daily lives, impacting greatly on the quality of life (Sands, 2006; Brand, 2009).

4.1 Crohn's disease in Brazil

Brazil is located in South America, a region considered to have a low incidence of CD. Despite the paucity of epidemiological studies that allow us to know the real incidence and prevalence of the disease, reports of cases, predominantly from universities, have shown that this disease is not rare, and that its incidence had increased in recent decades. This epidemiological profile, now recognized in Brazil, has been previously observed in different countries with a high incidence. Nowadays, these countries have been evolving for stability in the frequency of the disease. For the different areas of Brazil, CD is most frequently observed in states located in the south and southeast, areas with higher socioeconomic development. Currently, there is a joint effort of hospitals for inflammatory bowel diseases to collect reliable statistical data that would serve as an international database.

In one follow up study, researchers evaluated 100 patients with CD in university referral center for inflammatory bowel disease. The mean follow-up was 47.3 months, with variations from one month to 9.5 years. As for gender distribution, 59% were female and 41% male. Age of patients ranged from 16 to 69 years old, with an average of 29.9 and a median of 27 years old. 5% of patients had a family history of ulcerative colitis or CD. Among the clinical manifestations, abdominal pain was the most common symptom observed in 98% of cases, followed by chronic diarrhea in 83% and weight loss in 82% of patients. Regarding the behavior of the disease, stenosing form was observed in 35% of cases, followed by non-penetrating and not stenosing form in 34% of cases and fistulizing form was described in 31% of cases. Of the extraintestinal manifestations, rheumatological manifestation was the most frequently observed, followed by skin and eyes manifestations. 50% of patients underwent surgical procedures and 63% were hospitalized at least once. The authors conclude that the profile of CD in evaluated patients was similar to that described in the literature, and these data were corroborated by other Brazilian authors (Faria et al., 2004; Santana et al., 2008; Torres et al., 2010).

5. *Mycobacetrium avium* subspecies *paratuberculosis* vs Crohn's disease

Paratuberculosis and Crohn's disease (CD) are two diseases that share many clinical and histopathological similarities. Both diseases are characterized by chronic inflammation, weight loss and there is no cure.

While there have been, in recent years, various hypotheses about the etiology of CD and the mechanisms that trigger it may be cited as diet, environmental factors, genetic predisposition and autoimmune responses, the two main causal theories are infection and the autoimmune response. *Mycobacterium avium* subspecies *paratuberculosis* (MAP) has been cited as the leading candidate from the point of view of infection.

Considering the high prevalence of MAP in dairy herds and the resistance of microorganisms to disinfectants and pasteurization, several countries have created programs to control the disease considering its possible zoonotic potential.

5.1 Facts that support MAP in Crohn's disease

Despite extensive research and large and important advances in the past few decades, the etiology of Crohn's disease (CD) remains unknown, hindering the development of a specific therapy. Due to the similarity of clinical signs and histopathological findings between the two diseases, associations between paratuberculosis in cattle and chronic ileocolitis in humans have been made. Interest in participation in the infectious etiology of CD has increased with the isolation and detection of DNA of *Mycobacterium avium* subspecies *paratuberculosis* (MAP) in samples from patients with the disease. MAP is not classified as a zoonotic agent, but it represents a major concern in the field of public health because of the associations that have been made.

The controversial zoonotic potential of CD grows as more research has been seeking an association between MAP and CD. In recent studies, MAP strains were isolated from human intestinal tissues and blood from patients with CD. It is known that patients with CD are substantially more positive for MAP, regardless of method used, when compared with individuals with ulcerative colitis or individuals without inflammatory bowel disease. The isolation of MAP and detection of MAP DNA from breast milk of nursing mothers with a diagnosis of CD has also been reported and a possible maternal-fetal transmission of MAP may be suggested. These results, however, were not replicated by other researchers and there is no evidence of increased frequency of CD in children of mothers with CD (Naser et al., 2000; Schwartz et al., 2000; Bull et al., 2003; Naser et al., 2004).

In several published reports, presence of antibodies against MAP has also been demonstrated in serum samples from patients with CD by serological tests. Using these tests, there are also significant differences when compared with sera from patients with CD, ulcerative colitis and control patients. This is another fact that supports the association of MAP with CD (Olsen et al., 2009; Rosenfeld and Bressler, 2010).

Molecular techniques have been used for providing faster results than conventional diagnostic techniques. Using PCR-based sequence IS*900*, MAP DNA has also been found in a significantly higher proportion of patients with CD than in patients with ulcerative colitis or patients without inflammatory bowel disease (Abubakar et al., 2008).

Besides all this evidence, CD's patients have been treated successfully using antimycobacterial drugs. If MAP is involved in the etiology of CD, it is expected that antimycobacterial drugs should improve the clinical status of affected patients (Hermon-Taylor, 2002).

Contaminated milk would be the main, but not the only, vehicle of transmission of MAP from animals to human beings. Infected animals can eliminate the organism in this way and furthermore can occur a milk contamination with via fecal material, a route through which the organism is eliminated at higher concentrations. It is known that occurrence of MAP in milk is well documented and several studies have shown that the microorganism can remain viable after being subjected to standard conditions of pasteurization and processes used to produce cheese if it is present in large concentrations. In addition, although not recommended, it is known that raw milk is consumed fresh in many parts of the world, besides being used for the manufacture of several dairy products. A causal association of MAP with CD would have important implications for the processing of milk and other dairy products (Grant et al., 2001).

There is no doubt therefore that there is a potential source of zoonotic infection, considering (1) the widespread dissemination of MAP in dairy herds in Europe, America and Australia, (2) the elimination of MAP in milk of infected animals, (3) the relative strength of MAP to pasteurization process used currently and (4) the recovery of viable MAP in milk samples, water and beef, other potential sources of transmission of MAP. So, considering the association between CD and MAP infection to be correct, the fact that MAP has been detected in foods could be a public health problem.

It is known that the vast majority of studies using many different techniques have detected MAP DNA or cultured the microorganism most frequently in tissue from patients with CD, rather than in those with ulcerative colitis and other disorders. These results are consistent with two possibilities: either MAP infection could cause CD in a subgroup of patients that are selectively exposed to this microorganism or are genetically susceptible to infection, or alternatively, this microorganism, relatively common in the diet, can colonize selectively to ulcerated mucosa of patients with CD, but not initiate or perpetuate intestinal inflammation (Behr and Kapur, 2008; Hermon-Taylor, 2009; Rosenfeld and Bressler, 2010).

The most plausible theory that would explain a role for MAP in the etiology of CD is related to the recipient NOD2/CARD15. NOD2/CARD15 is an intracellular receptor for muramyl dipeptide (MDP), the smallest immunologically active component of bacterial peptidoglycan. The binding of MDP to the receiver NOD2/CARD15 activates nuclear factor kB. This may contribute to the elimination of intracellular bacterial infection and secretion of α defensins by Paneth cells, which constitutively express NOD2/CARD15. The three most common polymorphisms of this gene lead to a defective activation of nuclear factor kB by the MDP and they are found in 35% of Caucasian patients with CD. NOD2/CARD15 mutations in CD are associated with a decreased expression of α defensins in the mucosa. Thus, a plausible explanation linking NOD2/CARD15 to CD is that a defect in this gene could not result in elimination of intracellular infection by MAP and decreased secretion of luminal α defensins in the mucosa, allowing a greater adhesion and epithelial invasion by the microorganisms ingested (Sartor, 2005).

Despite all the evidence implying an association of MAP with CD, it is not possible to conclude that a single agent is solely responsible for the cause of CD - a multifactorial cause is more likely. The role of MAP in the etiology of CD cannot yet be confirmed or refuted with certainty. The organism can act as a causative agent, it may have a role in the context of infection, it can exacerbate the disease, or it may be non-pathogenic. Clearly, more studies are needed to determine whether MAP infection causes the disease or whether this environmental contaminant innocently lodges in ulcerated mucosa. Well-designed studies are needed to definitively resolve this debate.

5.2 Facts that do not support MAP in Crohn's disease

It has been suggested that a relationship between MAP infection and Crohn's exists due to the clinical and pathological similarities between Crohn's disease (CD) in human patients and paratuberculosis in animals. However, there are also many arguments against MAP being the causative agent of CD. Despite the similarities between clinical signs and histopathological features of both diseases, there may be differences in clinical and pathological responses between both diseases, which are not expected if both diseases are caused by the same microorganism.

Another important factor to be considered is the lack of epidemiological support considering the infection's transmission. If animals eliminate MAP in large quantities in feces and milk, it would be expected that the prevalence of CD in people in direct contact with animals infected with MAP was great if the association between the CD and paratuberculosis is true. These facts have not yet been reported (Jones et al., 2006).

Not all patients with CD respond well to treatment with anti-MAP. The failure of treatment in such cases can be attributed to the fact that CD can exist in two forms: one form caused or triggered by infection with MAP and otherwise, induced by some other unknown cause. If this is true, the treatment may be ineffective due to inability to identify patients infected with MAP before the start of treatment. There is not enough evidence to assert the effects of antimycobacterial therapy in patients with CD, but it is suggested that this therapy can help maintain remission of clinical signs of disease (Selby et al., 2007).

Genetic profiles of different strains already isolated have been outlined and possible epidemiological associations between the species from which they were isolated has been studied. Studies have shown that human isolates have profiles more similar to those isolated from sheep and goats than to those isolated from cattle. This fact also contrasts with the idea that cow's milk would be the main source of transmission of MAP from cattle to human beings. In contrast to this fact, there are studies reporting that both animals and humans are susceptible to infection by MAP isolates with similar genotypes (Jones et al., 2006).

Just as there are several research groups associating MAP to CD using detection of MAP DNA in samples of intestinal tissues and blood of patients with CD, other groups have shown the opposite: the same levels of detection of MAP in patients with CD compared with patients with ulcerative colitis or patients without inflammatory bowel diseases. Moreover, the absence of MAP DNA in patients with CD was also reported. Data are very variable for all groups. There is a variation from 0 to 100% of MAP by PCR detection (Abubakar et al., 2008).

Another argument against a possible etiology of MAP in CD is related to the observation of a good response from patients with CD undergoing immunosuppressive therapy.

5.3 Conditions in Brazil that could facilitate the transmission from MAP to humans

MAP has been detected in several states in the Southeast, South, Midwest and Northeast regions of Brazil. Despite reports of paratuberculosis in several states, few research groups working in this field are still doing surveys on the disease. In addition to bovine paratuberculosis, there are some groups in the country researching the presence of MAP in goats and sheep.

Although there is a strong and effective control program for tuberculosis in the country, there is not a control program for paratuberculosis. Research into this disease is still preliminary and there has been no survey even made, even superficially, about the economic losses caused by the disease.

Currently, Brazil is the sixth largest milk producing country, with a volume that corresponds to approximately 4.5% of world production (IBGE, 2006). The Southeast region is the largest producing region, accounting for 38.4% of all domestic production. Despite the high production, productivity of dairy herds in Brazil is low. The milk industrial chain is important from the standpoint of economic and social development, generating significant income and jobs in all sectors. Despite all these factors, no studies in the country are aimed at detection of MAP in dairy products and the first detection of MAP in milk was quite recent. MAP was detected by PCR using primers based on the IS*900* sequence in an initial survey about the disease in the Southeast region (Carvalho et al., 2009).

Brazil has also not been reported the presence of MAP in pasteurized milk. A survey in this sense, in the same region where it was detected MAP DNA in raw milk samples, is already in the early stages. In parallel, the resistance of MAP to pasteurization temperatures in the laboratory is being tested.

Brazil has a volume estimated at around 112 billion cubic meters of fresh water of the planet. Moreover, in Brazilian subsoil there is the Brazilian Guarani aquifer, the largest subsoil reservoir of freshwater on the planet. This enormous underground wealth extends over an area of 1.6 million square kilometers, of which two thirds are in Brazilian territory. Even with all that water, there have been no studies in the country to verify the presence of MAP in water.

There are no studies about the possible association between MAP infection and Crohn's disease (CD). A first attempt of an association between MAP infection and CD is being performed. Intestinal biopsies of patients with CD, ulcerative colitis patients and patients without inflammatory bowel disease are being collected with the aim of isolating MAP and/or detection of DNA of the microorganism for molecular tests.

6. Future prospects

Historically, one of the ways to make the connection between a potential agent of an infectious disease and the disease itself was considering whether Koch's postulates were true. For the relationship between MAP infection and Crohn's disease (CD), postulates "The organism can be isolated from a sick patient" and "The organism can be cultured in the laboratory" can still be controversial, but are true. "If the causative microorganism is introduced into another susceptible host, the same disease should be generated" is a postulate a little harder to prove. Disease results from interaction between infection and immune response by the microorganism that causes it. Clinical manifestations of infection depend on several variables such as genetics of the host and the state of the immune system, among others (Rosenfeld and Bressler, 2010).

CD certainly involves host genetic influences and environmental influences that interact to cause clinically evident disease. It is known that MAP is widely present in the human food chain and that MAP DNA can be recovered from intestinal samples of patients with CD. Although existing data do not necessarily involve MAP as a causative agent of CD, this possibility cannot be definitively excluded.

Besides this, there is the difficulty in obtaining experimental models for studies involving human pathogens or potential human pathogens. Such studies are complicated to performed, since although the relationship between MAP and CD is not yet established, it is reckless inoculate MAP in human patients for testing.

There is still much to be learned about MAP and diseases that it can cause in humans. CD may be a syndrome with multiple etiologies that result in clinical, endoscopic, radiological and pathological findings that define the disease. MAP may be one of the etiologies of this syndrome.

7. Conclusion

Some studies have shown that the etiology of Crohn's disease (CD) may involve a variety of viral and bacterial agents, including MAP, or an immunological origin. Evidence supports an interaction between a persistent environmental stimulus, such as a microbial antigen, and genetic factors that regulate an immune response or a function of the intestinal mucosa. Recent discoveries in many research fields have generated favorable results suggesting an association between CD and MAP, but that does not necessarily indicate that the microorganism is involved in the etiology of the disease. It is not possible to conclude that a single agent is solely responsible for the cause of CD as a multifactorial cause is more likely. For patients and their physicians, a clear answer on this association is an important step toward establishing control measures and treatment for this debilitating disease. Theories of mycobacterial and autoimmune etiologies of CD should be seen as complementary rather than mutually exclusive. The causal association between CD and MAP infection remains unanswered.

If MAP is responsible for a subset of CD, public health measures should be implemented to eliminate the source of infection in the human food chain and food processing practices must be modified. If there is no evidence of a causal association of MAP and CD, we must direct resources to other research fields. This controversy has persisted for too long and needs to be resolved.

When appropriate methods are used, most patients with CD are detected and there is no data showing that MAP is harmless to human patients. More epidemiological studies seeking to rigorously analyze both diseases are needed. While CD is likely to be a multifactorial condition, MAP can be a primary etiologic agent or a significant secondary invading agent. It is well documented that MAP is present in humans and that there are many routes of transmission and consumption of milk and dairy products are the main, and perhaps the biggest, problem link on the subject, since it has been shown that the microorganism can resist milk pasteurization processes and also the chlorination processes of drinking water. Therefore, until MAP is declared as a non-pathogenic agent for humans, it should be treated as such.

8. Acknowledgments

The authors would like to thank Pró-Reitoria de Extensão e Cultura from Federal University of Viçosa (UFV), CNPq (Conselho Nacional de Desenvolvimento Científico e Tecnológico), CAPES (Coordenação de Aperfeiçoamento de Pessoal de Nível Superior) and FAPEMIG (Fundação de Amparo à Pesquisa do Estado de Minas Gerais) for financial support.

9. References

Abubakar, I., Myhill, D., Aliyu, S.H.& Hunter, P.R. (2008). Detection of *Mycobacterium avium* subspecies *paratuberculosis* from patients with Crohn's disease using nucleic acid-based techniques: A systematic review and meta-analysis. *Inflammatory Bowel Diseases*, Vol.14, No.3, pp.401-410

Acypreste, C.S., Juliano, R.S., Riveira, F.E.B., Silva, L.A.F., Fioravanti, M.C.S.& Filho, F.C.D. (2005). Uso da técnica do ELISA indireto na detecção de anticorpos anti-*Mycobacterium paratuberculosis* em vacas em lactação. *Ciência Animal Brasileira*, Vol.6, pp. 41-45

Behr, M.A.& Kapur, V. (2008). The evidence for Mycobacterium paratuberculosis in Crohn's disease. *Current Opinion in Gastroenterology*, Vol.24, No.1, pp.17-21

Brand, S. (2009). Crohn's disease: Th1, Th17 or both? The change of a paradigm: new immunological and genetic insights implicate Th17 cells in the pathogenesis of Crohn's disease. *Gut*, Vol.58, No.8, pp.1152-1167 1468-3288 (Electronic) 0017-5749 (Linking)

Brautingam, F.E., Glass, R.& Mendy, W., 1996. Levantamento sorológico utilizando a técnica de ELISA para paratuberculose em cinco rebanhos de corte do Mato Grosso do Sul e quatro rebanhos de leite do Estado de São Paulo. In: XV Congresso Panamericano de Ciências Veterinárias, Campo Grande, MT, p. 271.

Bull, T.J., McMinn, E.J., Sidi-Boumedine, K., Skull, A., Durkin, D., Neild, P., Rhodes, G., Pickup, R.& Hermon-Taylor, J. (2003). Detection and verification of Mycobacterium avium subsp. paratuberculosis in fresh ileocolonic mucosal biopsy specimens from individuals with and without Crohn's disease. *Journal of Clinical Microbiology*, Vol.41, No.7, pp.2915-2923

Carvalho, I.A., Silva, A., Jr., Campos, V.E.& Moreira, M.A. (2009). Short communication: detection of *Mycobacterium avium* subspecies *paratuberculosis* by polymerase chain reaction in bovine milk in Brazil. *Journal of Dairy Science*, Vol.92, No.11, pp.5408-5410, ISSN 1525-3198 (Electronic) 0022-0302 (Linking)

Cocito, C., Gilot, P., Coene, M., de Kesel, M., Poupart, P.& Vannuffel, P. (1994). Paratuberculosis. *Clinical Microbiology Reviews*, Vol.7, No.3, pp.328-345

Costa, J.C.M., Pieri, F.A., Souza, C.F., Espeschit, I.F., Felippe, A.G., Santos, G.M., Tobia, F.L., Silva Jr., A.& Moreira, M.A.S. (2010). Levantamento sorológico de *Mycobacterium avium* subesp. *paratuberculosis* em bovinos leiteiros no estado do Espírito Santo. *Arquivo Brasileiro de Medicina Veterinária e Zootecnia*, Vol.62, No.6, pp.1491-1494

Dacorso Filho, P., Campos, I.O.N., Faria, J.F.& Langenegger, J. (1960). Doença de Johne (Paratuberculose) em bovinos nacionais. *Arquivos do Instituto Biológico*, Vol.3, pp.129-139

Driemeier, D., Cruz, C.E.F., Gomes, M.J.P., Corbellini, L.G., Lorett, A.P.& Colodel, E.M. (1999). Aspectos clínicos e patológicos da paratuberculose em bovinos no Rio Grande do Sul. *Pesquisa Veterinária Brasileira*, Vol.19, No.3/4, pp.109-115

Dupont, O. (1915). *Jornal do Commercio*, pp.8

Faria, L.C., Ferrari, M.L.A.& Cunha, A.S. (2004). Aspectos clínicos da doença de Crohn em um centro de referência para doenças intestinais *GED Gastroenterologia e Endoscopia Digestiva*, Vol.23, No.4, pp.151-163

Grant, I.R., Rowe, M., Dundee, L.& Hitchings, E. (2001). *Mycobacterium avium* ssp. *paratuberculosis*: its incidence, heat resistance and detection in milk and dairy products. *International Journal of Dairy Technology*, Vol.54, No.1,

Green, E.P., Tizard, M.L., Moss, M.T., Thompson, J., Winterbourne, D.J., McFadden, J.J.& Hermon-Taylor, J. (1989). Sequence and characteristics of IS*900*, an insertion element identified in a human Crohn's disease isolate of *Mycobacterium paratuberculosis*. *Nucleic Acids Research*, Vol.17, No.22, pp.9063-9073

Harris, N.B.& Barletta, R.G. (2001). *Mycobacterium avium* subsp. *paratuberculosis* in Veterinary Medicine. *Clinical Microbiology Reviews*, Vol.14, No.3, pp.489-512

Hendrick, S.H., Kelton, D.F., Leslie, K.E., Lissemore, K.D., Archambault, M.& Duffield, T.F. (2005). Effect of paratuberculosis on culling, milk production, and milk quality in dairy herds. *Journal of the American Veterinary Medical Association*, Vol.227, No.8, pp.1302-1308 0003-1488 (Print) 0003-1488 (Linking)

Hermon-Taylor, J. (2002). Treatment with drugs active against *Mycobacterium avium* subspecies *paratuberculosis* can heal Crohn's disease: more evidence for a neglected public health tragedy. *Digestive and Liver Disease*, Vol.34, No.1, pp.9-12

Hermon-Taylor, J. (2009). *Mycobacterium avium* subspecies *paratuberculosis*, Crohn's disease and the Doomsday scenario. *Gut Pathogens*, Vol.1, No.1, pp.15 1757-4749 (Electronic) IBGE, 2006. Produção da Pecuária Municipal. Online available: http://www.cnpgl.embrapa.br/nova/informacoes/estatisticas/producao_leite/index.php. Acessed: 5 Nov 2006

Jones, P.H., Farver, T.B., Beaman, B., Cetinkaya, B.& Morgan, K.L. (2006). Crohn's disease in people exposed to clinical cases of bovine paratuberculosis. *Epidemiology and Infection*, Vol.134, No.1, pp.49-56 0950-2688 (Print) 0950-2688 (Linking)

Li, L., Bannantine, J.P., Zhang, Q., Amonsin, A., May, B.J., Alt, D., Banerji, N., Kanjilal, S.& Kapur, V. (2005). The complete genome sequence of *Mycobacterium avium* subspecies *paratuberculosis*. *Proceedings of the National Academy of Sciences of the United States of America*, Vol.102, No.35, pp.12344-12349

Mota, R.A., Peixoto, P.V., Yamasaki, E.M., Medeiros, E.S., Costa, M.M., Peixoto, R.M.& Brito, M.F. (2010). Ocorrência de paratuberculose em búfalos (*Bubalus bubalis*) em Pernambuco. *Pesquisa Veterinária Brasileira*, Vol.30, No.3,

Nakajima, M., Maia, F.C.L.& Mota, P.M.P.C., 1991. Diagnóstico da Paratuberculose em Minas Gerais. In: IV Simpósio Brasileiro em Micobactérias, Bauru, São Paulo.

Naser, S.A., Ghobrial, G., Romero, C.& Valentine, J.F. (2004). Culture of *Mycobacterium avium* subspecies *paratuberculosis* from the blood of patients with Crohn's disease. *The Lancet Infectious Diseases*, Vol.364, No.9439, pp.1039-1044

Naser, S.A., Schwartz, D.& Shafran, I. (2000). Isolation of *Mycobacterium avium* subsp *paratuberculosis* from breast milk of Crohn's disease patients. *American Journal of Gastroenterology*, Vol.95, No.4, pp.1094-1095

Oliveira, D.M., Riet-Correa, F., Galiza, G.J.N., Assis, A.C.O., Dantas, A.F.M., Bandarra, P.M.& Garino Jr, F. (2010). Paratuberculose em caprinos e ovinos no Brasil. *Pesquisa Veterinária Brasileira*, Vol.30, No.1,

Olsen, I., Tollefsen, S., Aagaard, C., Reitan, L.J., Bannantine, J.P., Andersen, P., Sollid, L.M.& Lundin, K.E. (2009). Isolation of *Mycobacterium avium* subspecies *paratuberculosis* reactive CD4 T cells from intestinal biopsies of Crohn's disease patients. *PLoS ONE*, Vol.4, No.5, pp.e5641 1932-6203 (Electronic)

Portugal, M.A.S.C., Pimentel, J.N., Saliba, A.M., Baldassi, L.& Sandoval, E.F.D. (1979). Ocorrência de paratuberculose no estado de Santa Catarina. *O Biológico*, Vol.4, No.1/2, pp.19-24

Ramos, E.T., Poester, F.P., Correa, B.L., Oliveira, S.J., Rodrigues, N.C.& Canabarro, C.E. (1986). Paratuberculose em bovinos no Estado do Rio Grande do Sul. *A Hora Veterinária*, Vol.34, No.6, pp.28-32

Ristow, P., Marassi, C.D., Rodrigues, A.B., Oelemann, W.M., Rocha, F., Santos, A.S., Carvalho, E.C., Carvalho, C.B., Ferreira, R., Fonseca, L.S.& Lilenbaum, W. (2007). Diagnosis of paratuberculosis in a dairy herd native to Brazil. *The Veterinary Journal*, Vol.174, No.2, pp.432-434

Rosenfeld, G.& Bressler, B. (2010). *Mycobacterium avium paratuberculosis* and the etiology of Crohn's disease: a review of the controversy from the clinician's perspective. *The Canadian Journal of Gastroenterology*, Vol.24, No.10, pp.619-624 0835-7900 (Print) 0835-7900 (Linking)

Sands, B.E., 2006, Crohn's Disease, In: Feldman, M.e.a. (Ed.), Sleisenger and Fordtran's Gastrointestinal and liver Disease, Saunders Elsevier, Philadelphia, pp. 2459-2498.

Santana, G.O., Souza, L.R., Azevedo, M., Sá, A.C., Bastos, C.M.& Lyra, A.C. (2008). Application of the Vienna classification for Crohn's disease to a single center from Brazil. *Arquivos de Gastroenterologia*, Vol.45, pp.64-68

Santos, J.A.& Silva, N.L. (1956). Sobre a 1ª observação da paratuberculose no Brasil. *Boletim da Sociedade Brasielira de Medicina Veterinária*, Vol.24, pp.5-14

Sartor, R.B. (2005). Does *Mycobacterium avium* subspecies *paratuberculosis* cause Crohn's disease? *Gut*, Vol.54, No.7, pp.896-898, ISSN 0017-5749 (Print) 0017-5749 (Linking)

Schwartz, D., Shafran, I., Romero, C., Piromalli, C., Biggerstaff, J., Naser, N., Chamberlin, W.& Naser, S.A. (2000). Use of short-term culture for identification of *Mycobacterium avium* subsp. *paratuberculosis* in tissue from Crohn's disease patients. *Clinical Microbiology and Infection*, Vol.6, No.6, pp.303-307 1198-743X (Print) 1198-743X (Linking)

Selby, W., Pavli, P., Crotty, B., Florin, T., Radford-Smith, G., Gibson, P., Mitchell, B., Connell, W., Read, R., Merrett, M., Ee, H.& Hetzel, D. (2007). Two-year combination antibiotic therapy with clarithromycin, rifabutin, and clofazimine for Crohn's disease. *Gastroenterology*, Vol.132, No.7, pp.2313-2319

Silva, N.M. (1961). Estudos sôbre a paratuberculose. *Arquivos do Instituto Biológico*, Vol.4, pp.169-173

Torres, U.S., Rodrigues, J.O., Junqueira, M.S., Uezato, S.& Netinho, J.G. (2010). The Montreal classification for Crohn's disease: Clinical application to a Brazilian single-center cohort of 90 consecutive patients. *Arquivos de Gastroenterologia*, Vol.47, No.3, pp.279-284

Part 3

Treatment of Crohn's Disease

9

Manipulation of Intestinal Flora as a Way to Treat Crohn's Disease: The Role of Probiotics, Prebiotics and Antibiotics

Petra Zadravec, Borut Štrukelj and Aleš Berlec
Jožef Stefan Institute
Slovenia

1. Introduction

Crohn's disease (CD) is a chronic gastrointestinal disorder which, together with ulcerative colitis, is known as Inflammatory Bowel Disease (IBD). CD is characterized by transmural inflammation of the entire gastrointestinal tract, from oral cavity to anus. The most common symptoms are chronic diarrhea and abdominal pain, which are often accompanied by anorexia, malaise, weight loss, fever and extra-intestinal manifestations. The latter can involve almost every organ system (Macfarlane et al., 2009). CD can cause the formation of strictures, abscesses or fistulas. For that reason, surgical resection in CD patients is very common.

Regardless of the vast amount of data gathered on the etiology and the course of CD, the actual cause is still unknown. The interplay of various factors is blamed for the disease outbreak. These factors include genetic predisposition, environmental influences (e.g. smoking), imbalance in immune response and changes in intestinal flora. Given the complexity of the disease, some factors may be the consequence of others.

Genetic predisposition has received the most research attention in recent years. Family studies have shown that more than 50% concordance of CD can be expected in monozygotic twins. These findings indicate that the pathogenesis of CD is not based only on one gene but on a polygenic risk profile (Vavricka & Rogler, 2009). In 2001, two independent groups of researchers discovered one of the most important susceptibility genes for CD, a gene for NOD2/CARD15 (Hugot et al., 2001; Ogura et al., 2001). Its mutation is present in about one third of all CD patients. Patients with mutated NOD2/CARD15 variants could have a deficient response to bacterial LPS which could lead to the development of CD (Ogura et al., 2001). Several other genes that can contribute to susceptibility to CD have been identified. These include IBD5, IL23R, ATG16L1, Chr5p13.1, Chr5q33.1 and Chr10q21.1 (Xavier & Podolsky, 2007). They are involved in the maintenance of barrier function and regulation of innate and adaptive immunity.

There are several environmental factors that have been predicted to be involved in the development of CD. The single most important environmental risk factor for the development of CD is tobacco smoking. Further environmental risk factors are related to living in urban areas of developed western countries with stressful lifestyle. There is also some evidence that diet could influence the risk for CD. Uptake of fatty acids and sugar, which has increased in the last decades in developed countries, has been linked to an increase in the incidence of CD (Hanauer, 2006).

Dysregulated immune response and exaggerated response to exogenous factors, including the intestinal microbiota, is also an important contributor to CD. Immune response at the intestinal mucosa is mediated by epithelial and mucosal immune cells. They recognize molecules of bacterial origin via Toll-like and NOD-like receptors. Receptor binding leads to activation of the NF-κB pathway, which is a crucial regulator of the inflammatory response. In epithelial Paneth cells, NF-κB activation leads to the production of defensins. In antigen presenting cells, activation of NF-κB leads, with the involvement of procaspase 1, to the production of proinflammatory cytokines, which stimulate further inflammation events (Xavier & Podolsky, 2007). Increased expression of Th1 cytokines, mainly IFNγ, IL-12, TNFα, IL-1β and IL-6, has been considered fundamental in maintaining the inflammation. Other cytokines, such as IL-8, IL-18 and IL-23 have also been involved (Dharmani & Chadee, 2008).

Even though the actual role of bacteria in the pathogenesis of CD is still unknown, the differences in the composition of intestinal flora between healthy individuals and CD patients are today a well established fact. They have recently been confirmed by the metagenomic sequencing of the intestinal microbiome (Manichanh et al., 2006; Qin et al., 2010). The difference is characterized by the reduction of species diversity from the phylum *Firmicutes* and an increase in the concentration of enterobacteriaceae, especially *Escherichia coli*. Interestingly, no significant differences in flora composition were observed between inflamed and non-inflamed intestinal mucosa of CD patients (Vasquez et al., 2007). CD is often associated with the presence of specific microorganisms (adherent and invasive *E. coli*, *Mycobacterium avium* subsp. *paratuberculosis*; described below) and lack of others (*Faecalibacterium prausnitzii*). *F. prausnitzii* is a member of *Firmicutes* which has been observed to be present in lower quantities in patients with endoscopic recurrence of CD six months after the surgery, in comparison to patients that were still in remission after surgery. Anti-inflammatory effects of *F. prausnitzii* have been demonstrated in *in vitro* and *in vivo* mouse models (Sokol et al., 2008). Taken together, it has been hypothesized that either a single pathogen, increased mucosal permeability, or imbalance between "good" and "bad" bacteria (dysbiosis) contribute to the CD onset.

The hypothesis of a single pathogen is based on the assumption that *M. avium* subsp. *paratuberculosis* (MAP) could be the causative agent of CD, and has been supported by a considerable body of evidence. Investigators were able to isolate MAP from the inflamed tissue and peripheral blood of CD patients, detect anti-MAP antibodies and also prove its presence using molecular analysis (De Hertogh et al., 2008; Macfarlane et al., 2009). However, this was not enough to prove MAP as causative agent of CD, especially since treatment with drugs against MAP had no effect on the improvement of CD. Several other bacteria have also been associated with CD pathogenesis. These include *Listeria monocytogenes, Pseudomonas maltophilia, M. kansasii, Bacteroides fragilis* and adherent invasive *E. coli* (AIEC) (De Hertogh et al., 2008; Macfarlane et al., 2009). The latter is a specific pathovar that has been shown to colonize intestinal mucosa of 36.4% of patients with ileal CD. It is able to replicate in macrophages and cause the release of large amounts of TNFα (Rolhion & Darfeuille-Michaud, 2007). There is also evidence that AIEC plays an important role in the formation of granulomas which are a histological characteristic of CD. Colonization with AIEC was recently linked to the previously mentioned NOD2/CARD15 mutation, (Barnich & Darfeuille-Michaud, 2007; Rolhion & Darfeuille-Michaud, 2007).

A second hypothesis is based on an increased permeability of intestinal mucosa which can cause translocation of bacteria and their metabolites from the gastrointestinal tract to mesenteric lymph nodes and other internal organs (De Hertogh et al., 2008). Occurrence of such bacterial translocation in patients with CD after surgery has been documented and has caused systemic inflammatory septic response. *E. coli*, *Enteroccoccus* ssp, *Bact. fragilis*, and *Klebsiella pneumoniae* were among the bacterial species which translocated to the greatest extent (Takesue et al., 2002).

A third, dysbiosis theory suggests a broken equilibrium between "good" and "bad" intestinal bacteria as a cause of CD (Tamboli et al., 2004). The hypothesis is based on a number of studies of faecal and mucosal associated microflora which were found to differ between CD patients and healthy individuals (reviewed by Tamboli et al., (2004)). The data obtained with classic bacteriological culturing techniques was recently substantiated by metagenomic sequencing (Qin et al., 2010). Faecal microflora from patients with CD contains decreased numbers of butyrate producing *Firmicutes*, especially the *Clostridium leptum* group (Manichanh et al., 2006). Ribosomal DNA sequence analysis of mucosa associated bacteria in patients with CD has shown increased levels of facultative bacteria (e. g. *E. coli*) in colonic mucosa. In small intestinal mucosa, decreased levels of *C. leptum* and *Prevotella nigrescens* subgroups were observed, as well as increased level of the *Ruminococcus gnavus* subgroup (Prindiville et al., 2006). These results speak in favor of the dysbiosis theory and make the single pathogen theory less likely.

The aim of this chapter is to introduce ways of interference with the diversity and abundance of intestinal bacteria, which are important in CD pathogenesis. Clinical efficacy of various strategies will also be presented.

2. Probiotics

The Food and Agriculture Organization and the World Health Organization have defined probiotics as "live microorganisms which, when administrated in adequate amounts as part of food, confer a health benefit on the host". Probiotics usually belong to the genera *Lactobacillus* or *Bifidobacterium.* These are gram positive bacteria with fermentative metabolism, in which lactic acid is a major product. They are obligatory or facultative anaerobes and are non-motile. Among lactobacilli, strains with probiotic properties are *Lb. acidophilus,* including strain LA-5, *Lb. crispatus, Lb. johnsonii* LA1, *Lb. gasseri* PA16, *Lb. casei, Lb. paracasei,* strains *"shirota"* and *"defensis", Lb. rhamnosus* GG, *Lb. reuteri* and *Lb. plantarum.* Among bifidobacteria, *B. longum,* strains BB536 and SP07/3, *B. bifidum* MF20/5, *B. infantis, B. animalis, B. adolescentis* and *B. breve,* have been considered probiotic. Some other bacteria and yeasts can also have probiotic properties. These include *Enterococcus faecalis, Streptococcus thermophilus, Propionibacteria, E. coli* Nissle 1917 and yeast *Saccharomyces boulardii* (de Vrese & Schrezenmeir 2008). Probiotics have many potential beneficial health effects, which are more or less well documented. The effective use of probiotics for significant improvement of lactose digestibility, childhood infectious gastroenteritis, diarrhea associated with either antibiotics, rotavirus infection, or chemotherapy, as well as traveller's diarrhea has been well documented (Schrezenmeir & de Vrese, 2001; Walker et al., 2006). Probiotics can stimulate humoral or cellular immune systems. They can cause a decrease in unfavourable metabolites (e. g. ammonium) in the colon. There are fewer reports of other possibilities of the use of probiotics for health improvement, which are limited to a

specific probiotic strain, or to a combination of two or more strains (Schrezenmeir & de Vrese, 2001; Walker et al., 2006; Thomas & Greer, 2010).
Due to the implication of intestinal bacteria in the CD, probiotics were also suggested as a possible treatment for CD. Among probiotics, *Lb. rhamnosus* GG, *Lb. johnsonii* LA1, *B. lactis*, *Str. thermophilus*, *E. coli* Nissle 1917 and yeast *S. boulardii* have been tested for the treatment of CD.

2.1 Mechanism of action

Several mechanisms by which probiotics exert beneficial effects in treatment of CD have been suggested (Boirivant & Strober, 2007; Dharmani & Chadee, 2008; Guandalini, 2010; Ng et al., 2009). Probiotics are supposed to improve the epithelial cell barrier function, decrease the load of "bad" bacteria by direct or indirect antibacterial effects or exert direct effects on epithelial and immune cells by, among other things, affecting their cytokine expression profiles. These effects are intertwined to a large extent and the contribution of an individual effect is therefore hard to establish. Besides, an individual probiotic bacterium is probably not capable of exerting the entire spectrum of activities. Instead, it is more likely to be responsible for a specific effect.

2.1.1 Effects on epithelial cell barrier function

The layer of epithelial cells that lines the intestinal tract constitutes a physical barrier that prevents intestinal bacteria from entering into the organism. The mix of probiotic organisms, VSL#3, was able to normalize barrier integrity in IL-10 deficient mice, as shown by the measurements of several parameters (conductivity, mannitol flux) on excised tissue (Madsen et al., 2001). Barrier function is reinforced by the layer of mucus, which is secreted by goblet epithelial cells. It has been shown that some probiotic bacteria are capable of modifying the expression of proteins that are involved in mucin production. *Lb. plantarum* 299v was able to increase MUC2 and MUC3 mRNA expression in the epithelial cell line (Mack et al., 1999), while VSL#3 and *E. coli* Nissle 1917 increased MUC2, MUC3 and MUC5AC protein expression (Otte & Podolsky, 2004). The epithelial layer is also responsible for the active transport of nutrients, electrolytes and water. Impaired ability for reabsorption of sodium and water from the distal colon leads to diarrhea that usually accompanies CD (Zeissig et al., 2007). *Str. thermophilus* and *Lb. acidophilus* were able to increase trans-epithelial resistance, but also alleviate electrolyte transport by increasing chloride secretion (Resta-Lenert & Barrett, 2009). Probiotics were also reported to influence the maintenance of tight junction proteins by influencing the cytoskeleton architecture. VSL#3 prevented the redistribution of tight junction protein ZO-1 (Otte & Podolsky, 2004) and *Lb. acidophilus* was able to prevent the rearrangement of F-actin upon exposure to pathogenic *E. coli* (Liévin-Le Moal et al., 2002). Probiotics can even prevent apoptosis of epithelial cells, as was shown for *Lb. rhamnosus* GG, which was able to activate anti-apoptotic and inhibit pro-apoptotic proteins (Yan & Polk, 2002).

2.1.2 Antibacterial effects

Probiotics influence the composition of intestinal flora by competing for the available space (e. g. available binding sites for adhesion) and for available essential nutrients. They can also exert antimicrobial effects by either direct or indirect means. Direct means include productions of inhibitory substances like bacteriocins, hydrogen peroxide and organic acids.

Bacteriocins are diverse group of low molecular weight peptides, usually produced by strains from genus *Lactobacillus*, and by some other lactic acid bacteria, including *Lactoccocus lactis*. Bacteriocins have antimicrobial activity against several bacteria, but are especially effective against Gram positive bacteria. Similar substances are produced in probiotic strains of *Bifidobacteria*, and are active against both Gram negative and Gram positive bacteria (Guandalini, 2010). Organic acids such as lactic acid, propionic acid and butyric acid are produced in fermentative metabolism of probiotics and are responsible for a decrease in pH in the gastrointestinal tract, which is harmful to acid sensitive intestinal bacteria. Probiotics can also exert indirect antibacterial effects, by stimulating the production of defensins. Defensins are human endogenous cationic antimicrobial peptides with antimicrobial activity against Gram negative and Gram positive bacteria. They are secreted by specialized epithelial Paneth cells. Deficiency in defensins could play an important role in the pathogenesis of colonic and ileal CD (Wehkamp et al., 2009). Low expression of β-defensin occurs in patients with colonic CD and affects the structure of colonic mucosa. In patients with ileal CD, decreased level of Paneth cells α-defensin has been observed and these patients also had the NOD2 mutation. These results suggest that there is a connection between NOD2 function and expression of α-defensin and that this connection has an important implication in the development of ileal CD (Wehkamp et al., 2009).

2.1.3 Immunomodulative effects on epithelial and immune cells

Probiotic bacteria can modulate the activity of epithelial and immune cells including dendritic cells, monocytes, macrophages, T cells, B cells and NK cells. The immune response is mediated by pattern recognition receptors, such as toll-like receptors, which recognize specific bacterial features, termed pathogen-associated molecular patterns. These include peptidoglycan, lipopolysaccharides, flagellin and DNA variants, such as unmethylated CpG motifs. Probiotic bacteria can induce regulatory T cells by stimulating the dendritic cells to produce anti-inflammatory cytokines IL-10 and TGFβ, as was demonstrated with the treatment with VSL#3 (Hart et al., 2004) and with several other bifidobacterial strains (Young et al., 2004). The activation of regulatory T cells can be initiated by direct binding of probiotics to dendritic cells via the DC-SIGN molecule (Smits et al., 2005). This can cause the diversion of the immune response toward noninflammatory tolerogenic pattern. Probiotics can downregulate the Th1 response by inhibition of the production of proinflammatory cytokines by dendritic cells, including the production of IL-12, TNFα and IFNγ. Downregulation of the production of TNFα was demonstrated in *ex vivo* treatment of intestinal tissue from CD patients with probiotics (Borruel et al., 2002). Probiotics can also decrease T cell proliferation and their production of IL-2, IL-4 and IL-10 cytokines, as demonstrated with *Lb. rhamnosus*. This increased T cell hypo-responsiveness was also induced *in vivo* in CD patients and in healthy individuals (Braat et al., 2004). Involvement of different mechanisms of action is highlighted by the fact that some strains of lactobacilli not only downregulate, but also upregulate the production of IL-12 (Mohamadzadeh et al., 2005) and switch towards the Th1 response.

2.2 Clinical trials with probiotics for the treatment of CD

Probiotics have been tested for their ability to treat CD in several clinical trial settings. Some basic data on clinical trials is summarized in Table 1. Some probiotic strains or mixtures of strains (*E. coli* Nissle 1917, *S. boulardii*, VSL#3, *Lb. rhamnosus* GG and *Lb. johnsonii* LA1) were tested in more than one clinical trial. Almost all the trials were designed to be randomized and placebo controlled, and more than half were double blind. Four studies were designed for the maintenance of remission in CD and five for the prevention of postoperative recurrence of CD. One study was designed for the treatment of one of the common extra-intestinal manifestations of CD, arthralgia, and one for evaluation of the impact of intestinal permeability in patients with CD.

Author	**Year**	**Probiotics and dose**	**n**	**Study design**	**Study duration**	**Study purpose**	**Outcomes**
Malchow	1997	*E. coli* Nissle 1917 $5x10^{10}$/day	28	Randomized, placebo controlled, single center	12 months	Maintenance of remission of colonic CD	Better outcome in probiotic group, not significant
Guslandi	2000	*S. boulardii* 1g/day	32	Randomized, single center	6 months	Maintenance of remission of CD	Significant difference between probiotic and mesalazine group
Campieri	2000	VSL#3 6g/day + rifaximin 1,8 g/day	40	Randomized, controlled	12 months	Prevention of postoperative recurrence of CD	Efficacy of combination of antibiotic and probiotic
Prantera	2002	*Lb. rhamnosus* GG $12x10^9$ CFU/day	45	Randomized, double blind, placebo controlled, single center	12 months	Prevention of recurrence of CD after surgery	No difference
Schultz	2004	*Lb. rhamnosus* GG $2x10^9$ CFU/day	11	Randomized, double blind, placebo controlled, single center	6 months	Maintenance of remission of CD	No difference, small number of patients
Bousvaros	2005	*Lb. rhamnosus* GG $2x10^9$ CFU/day + 295 mg inulin/day	75	Randomized, double blind, placebo controlled, multicenter	24 months	Maintenance of remission of CD in children	No difference
Karimi	2005	VSL#3 450 bilion bacteria twice a day	29	Open labeled, pilot study	3 months	Treatment of arthralgia in patients with ulcerative colitis and CD	Significant improvement

Marteau	2006	*Lb. johnsonii* LA1 $2x10^9$ CFU twice a day	98	Randomized, double blind, placebo controlled, multicenter	6 months	Prevention of postoperative recurrence of CD	No difference
Van Gossum	2007	*Lb. johnsonii* LA1 $1x10^{10}$ CFU/day	70	Randomized, double blind, placebo controlled, multicenter	3 months	Prevention of postoperative recurrence of CD	No difference
Garcia Vilela	2008	*S. boulardii*	34	Randomized, placebo controlled	3 months	Influence on intestinal permeability of patients with CD	Improvement of intestinal permeability
Madsen	2008	VSL#3 900 billion bacteria twice a day	120	Randomized, double blind, placebo controlled, multicenter	3 months	Prevention of postoperative recurrence of CD	Less endoscopic recurrence comparing to placebo

Table 1. Clinical studies investigating the effects of probiotics in the maintenance of remission in CD or in the prevention of postoperative recurrence of CD (adapted from (Isaacs & Herfarth, 2008)).

For maintenance of remission of the CD, 28 patients with active colonic CD were treated with synthetic corticosteroid prednisone and non-pathogenic probiotic *E. coli* strain Nissle 1917, or with placebo (Malchow, 1997). From the results of remission rate we can conclude that a similar proportion of patients entered in remission in the two groups. More patients from the placebo group (63.6%) had relapse, when compared with the probiotic group, in which 33.3% of patients relapsed after 12 months of treatment. Even though these results were not statistically significant, a better outcome was reached in the probiotic group, which indicated some beneficial effect of *E. coli* Nissle 1917 on the maintenance of remission in colonic CD. Because of the small number of participants in this study, the authors suggested that larger study should be performed.

Guslandi et al. investigated possible therapeutic benefits of non-pathogenic yeast *S. boulardii* in the maintenance of remission in CD (Guslandi et al., 2000). In this study, 32 patients with CD in clinical remission were divided randomly into two groups. The first group was treated with mesalamine two times a day and with *S. boulardii* once a day. The second group was treated only with mesalamine three times a day. The study was ended after 6 months of treatment. In the mesalamine group, 6 of 16 (37.5%) patients had clinical relapse after 6 months while, in the group treated with mesalamine and *S. boulardi*, only 1 patient in 16 (6.25%) had clinical relapse. This difference is statistically significant and demonstrates that *S. boulardii*, in combination with anti-inflammatory drug, could have beneficial effects in the maintenance of remission in CD.

The efficacy of *S. boulardii* in the treatment of CD was again evaluated in a study of the influence of *S. boulardii* on intestinal permeability in patients with CD in remission (Garcia

Vilela et al., 2008). The study was carried out on 34 patients who received either placebo or *S. boulardii* for 3 months. Additionally, patients received standard therapy with corticosteroids, anti-inflammatory drugs or antibiotics. Intestinal permeability was evaluated by measuring lactulose/mannitol ratio. The ratio was 0.005 +/- 0.0037 in healthy volunteers, and 0.021 +/- 0.01 in patients with CD. After 3 months of treatment, lactulose/mannitol ratio increased by 0.004 +/- 0.010 in the placebo group and decreased by 0.008 +/- 0.006 in the *S. boulardii* group. These results demonstrated that *S. boulardii*, in combination with standard therapy for CD, could improve intestinal integrity in patients with CD.

Probiotic *Lb. rhamnosus* GG was also tested for the ability to maintain the remission of CD (Schultz et al., 2004). Probiotic therapy with *Lb. rhamnosus* GG was tested in eleven patients with moderate to active CD. Patients were first treated with antibiotics for two weeks, followed by probiotic therapy for 6 months. Relapse occurred in 2 of 5 patients in the probiotic group, as well as in 2 of 6 patients in the placebo group. Two patients from each group achieved and maintained remission. No difference between probiotic and placebo group was thus observed and no benefit of *Lb. rhamnosus* GG could be reported. Small sample size was suggested as a reason why no difference was observed.

More than 70% of CD patients will undergo at least one surgery in their life, and recurrence of CD in patients after surgical intestinal resection is very common (Marteau et al., 2006). Endoscopic recurrence of CD in patients is usually observed within one year after surgery and is followed by clinical recurrence. Around one quarter of patients will require further surgery in the following years, if no postoperative treatment of the disease will take place (Doherty et al., 2009). Prevention of postoperative CD is therefore another important target of probiotic treatment. This approach was first tested with probiotic mixture VSL#3 in combination with antibiotic rifaximin in a randomized controlled clinical trial with 28 patients (Campieri et al., 2000). Half of the patients received rifaximin dose for the first three months, which was followed by probiotic dose for the next 9 months. The control group received 4 g of mesalamine per day for 12 months. Probiotic mixture VSL#3 contains 4 strains of lactobacilli, 3 strains of bifidobacteria and *Str. thermophilus*. No side effects were reported during the study. At the end of the treatment, 4 of 20 patients had endoscopic recurrence, while in the placebo group, 8 patients had endoscopic recurrence. The authors concluded that the combination of VSL#3 and rifaximin is effective in preventing postoperative endoscopic recurrence of CD. The effectiveness of probiotic mixture VSL#3 alone in preventing postoperative recurrence of CD was later confirmed in a larger randomized, double blind, placebo controlled multicenter study on 120 patients (Madsen et al., 2008). Patients receiving VSL#3 for 3 months showed less endoscopic recurrence (9,3% of patients) compared with placebo group (15,7% recurrence). Results were substantiated with measurements of mucosal pro-inflammatory cytokine levels.

Beside VSL#3, which is a mixture of probiotic strains, some *Lactobacillus* strains were tested by themselves for the ability to prevent postoperative recurrence of CD. Probiotic strain *Lactobacillus rhamnosus* GG was tested for prevention of postoperative recurrence in a randomized double blind and placebo controlled study (Prantera et al., 2002). 23 patients received *Lb. rhamnosus* GG and 22 received placebo daily for one year. No side effects were reported, however 13 patients, from the two groups, did not finish the study. At the end of the study, 15 patients from *Lb. rhamnosus* GG group and 17 patients from the placebo group showed clinical remission. Among the patients with clinical remission, 9 of 15 patients in the probiotic group, and 6 of 17 patients in the placebo group had endoscopic recurrence of CD.

Clinical recurrence was observed in 3 patients from the *Lactobacillus* GG group and in two from the placebo group. No benefit of *Lactobacillus rhamnosus* GG in the postoperative treatment of CD could thus be observed. It was suggested that the study should be considered as a pilot one because of small number of patients, different demographic and different disease background.

Lb. johnsonii LA1 is another *Lactobacillus* strain that was used in clinical trials for the prevention of postoperative CD. The first double blind, placebo controlled clinical trial with *Lb. johnsonii* LA1 was reported in 2006 (Marteau et al., 2006). 98 patients that underwent ileocolonic, colonic or ileal CD surgery were involved. Patients were administered $2x10^9$ colony forming units (CFU) *Lb. johnsonii* LA1 or placebo twice a day for 6 months. Endoscopic recurrence was observed in 49% of patients in the probiotic group and in 64% of patients in the placebo group. Clinical recurrence was noted in four patients in the probiotic group and in three in the placebo group. Results were not statistically significant and beneficial effects of *Lb. johnsonii* LA1 on postoperative recurrence in patients with CD could not be established.

A second clinical trial of the effectiveness of probiotic *Lb. johnsonii* LA1 in preventing endoscopic postoperative recurrence of CD was conducted with 70 patients that underwent curative ileo-caecal resection (Van Gossum et al., 2007). Clinical trial was designed as a randomized, double blind, placebo controlled multicenter study. Patients were treated either with $1x10^{10}$ CFU *Lb. johnsonii* LA1 daily or with placebo for 12 weeks. No difference in measured parameters or in clinical relapse between placebo group and *Lb. johnsonii* group was observed. Clinical relapse was observed in 4 patients in *Lb. johnsonii* group and in 2 patients in the placebo group after 12 weeks of treatment.

Some limited research has also been done on the use of probiotics in pediatric CD. A small pilot study was conducted with *Lb. rhamnosus* GG in children with active CD (Gupta et al., 2000). Four patients were involved in the study, two with ileocolonic CD and two with gastrocolonic CD. Report has shown significant improvement after treatment with 10^{10} CFU of probiotic. Patients were also receiving standard therapy for CD. This study was later followed by a randomized, double blind, placebo controlled trial with *Lb. rhamnosus* GG strain which was given in addition to standard therapy for the maintenance of remission in children with CD (Bousvaros et al., 2005). 75 children with CD in remission were involved in the study for the period of two years. Results of the study have shown no significant difference between probiotic and placebo group in the time of relapse of CD. These results substantiated the results of a previous study on adults which also showed the ineffectiveness of *Lb. rhamnosus* GG in maintaining remission in CD. Because the effectiveness of probiotics in the treatment of CD was not established, treatment of CD with probiotics is not recommended for children (Thomas & Greer, 2010).

Extra-intestinal manifestations like arthralgia and arthritis are common complications of CD. They are reported to occur in 10-35% of patients. Since beneficial effects of probiotics were observed in the treatment of ulcerative colitis and sometimes of CD, the treatment of arthralgia with probiotics mixture VSL#3 was also suggested (Karimi et al., 2005). Of 29 patients with IBD involved in the study, only 16 patients ended the 3 months study and 9 of them were CD patients. After three months of treatment, the status of arthralgia differed between patients with peripheral arthralgia and axial arthralgia. Only patients with peripheral arthralgia reported improvements in their general well being and joint complaints. There was no relapse reported in patients after 3 months of treatment. The results of the study were shown for all IBD patients together. The results for patients with CD therefore cannot be discerned from those of patients with ulcerative colitis. From that it can only be concluded that probiotic mixture VSL#3 had beneficial effects on arthralgia in patients with IBD, and possibly also in the subgroup of patients with CD.

2.3 Recombinant probiotic bacteria for the treatment of CD

Health effects of probiotic bacteria can be strengthened by genetic engineering which enables incorporation of new, defined traits into the existing bacterial repertoire. Recombinant bacteria can be used as a vector for the delivery of therapeutic proteins to the intestinal mucosa. Potential synergistic effects between existing probiotic and introduced therapeutic properties can be envisaged. Genetically modified probiotics will enable the selection of the desired protein, selection of the localization of protein expression (intracellular, secreted) and selection of the conditions required for the induction of the expression. It may also be possible to obtain a long term effect with colonizing strains (Marteau et al., 2009).

To date, the focus has been on lactic acid bacterium *Lactococcus lactis*. It does not have a probiotic status and does not colonize the intestine, but is well studied and is readily amenable for genetic modification. *L. lactis* strains with the ability to produce anti-inflammatory cytokine IL-10 or to bind pro-inflammatory cytokine TNFα have been constructed.

Genetically modified *L. lactis* secreting cytokine IL-10 was engineered and tested in two murine colitis mouse models (Steidler et al., 2000). Results of intragastric administration of L. lactis secreting IL-10 showed 50% reduction in DSS-induced colitis and prevention of colitis in IL-10 knockout mice. In further research, the authors presented genetically modified *L. lactis*, which was engineered by replacing the thymidylate synthase gene *thyA* with synthetic human IL-10 gene (Steidler et al., 2003). This recombinant bacterium (*LL-Thy12*) was able to produce human IL-10 and was not able to survive in the environment without thymidine or thymine. This enabled the biological containment of the bacterium and markedly decreased the safety concerns. Such a strain is appropriate for human use and the effectiveness of *LL-Thy12* was investigated in a phase I trial on patients with CD (Braat et al., 2006). Results of the trial have demonstrated safety of the strain. Only minor adverse effects were noted and some beneficial effects on the disease activity were observed.

Two recent studies have introduced another approach for the treatment of intestinal inflammations by binding the pro-inflammatory cytokine TNFα. The first study used engineered *L. lactis* which secreted TNFα-neutralizing nanobody (camelid heavy chain fragment). Its efficacy was demonstrated in two mouse models of colitis (Vandenbroucke et al., 2010). In another study, different binding TNFα-binding molecule was applied. TNFα-binding affibody was expressed and immobilized on the surface of engineered *L. lactis* (Ravnikar et al., 2010).

As noted earlier, besides IL-10, transforming growth factor beta (TGFβ) has often been described as an anti-inflammatory cytokine in CD. Commensal gut Gram-negative bacterium *Bact. ovatus* was engineered to express $TGF\beta_1$ under the control of xylan. Xylan is a dietary fiber which is important for the safety of this system. Results of the study have shown significant improvement of acute colitis in mice (Hamady et al., 2010).

Initial studies of the concept of recombinant probiotic bacteria have shown promising results, but were mostly obtained in the animal studies of the treatment of ulcerative colitis. Further research will show whether recombinant probiotics have the capacity to be considered as an alternative in the treatment of CD.

3. Prebiotics

Prebiotics were first defined by Gibson and Roberfroid as "nondigestible food ingredients that beneficially affect the host by selectively stimulating the growth and/or activity of one or a limited number of bacteria in the colon and thus improve host health" (Gibson & Roberfroid, 1995). An updated definition of probiotics was later suggested as follows: "A prebiotic is a selectively fermented ingredient that allows specific changes, both in the composition and/or activity of the gastrointestinal microflora, that confers benefits upon host wellbeing and health" (Gibson et al., 2004). In the past, many food ingredients were classified as potential prebiotics. However, in *sensu stricto*, the following criteria have to be fulfilled for a substance to be classified as prebiotic (Gibson et al., 2004):

- resistance to gastric acidity, to hydrolysis by mammalian enzymes and to gastrointestinal absorption;
- fermentability by intestinal microflora;
- selective stimulation of the growth and/or activity of intestinal bacteria associated with health and wellbeing.

These criteria are fulfilled by only three food ingredients that were marked as prebiotics: fructo-oligosaccharides (inulin and oligofructose), transgalacto-oligosaccharides and lactulose. All three prebiotics are carbohydrates; however, according to the definition, non-carbohydrates can also be classified as prebiotics. According to other authors, even the prebiotic status of lactulose can be opposed, because the first criterion for prebiotic classification is not totally fulfilled (Roberfroid, 2007). Nevertheless, lactulose prebiotic status is substantiated by a lot of data from human studies. Other carbohydrates that are good candidates for prebiotics are isomalto-oligosaccharides, lactosucrose, xylo-oligosaccharides, soybean oligosaccharides and gluco-oligosaccharides (Gibson et al., 2004; Roberfroid, 2007). These are already considered as probiotics by some authors.
Fructo-oligosaccharides, which are represented by inulin and oligofructose, occur in nature in different plants, such as chicory, leek, onion, garlic, and asparagus (Leenen & Dieleman, 2007). In 2006, results of a small study on clinical, immunological and microbiological effects of fructo-oligosaccharides in patients with active CD were published (Lindsay et al., 2006). In this study, 10 patients with active ileocolonic CD were treated with 15 g of fructo-oligosaccharides per day for 21 days. The results of the study showed that prebiotics oligofructose and inulin have beneficial effects on the activity of CD. This was demonstrated by increased intestinal bifidobacterial content and by enhanced expression of IL-10 and TLRs in dendritic cells. The authors suggested further investigation of immunological and microbiological effects of these prebiotics, and a larger randomized double-blind placebo-controlled trial was indeed published in 2011. 103 patients with active CD were enrolled. They received 15 g of fructo-oligosaccharides or placebo per day in a period of 4 weeks (Benjamin et al., 2011). No significant differences in faecal bifidobacteria concentration between the placebo and prebiotic groups after 28 day of prebiotic treatment could be observed and no clinical benefits could be recorded. The results of the pilot study therefore could not be reproduced in the larger setting.
The use of prebiotics is usually focused on stimulation of the growth or activity of bifidobacteria and lactobacilli because of their well known beneficial health effects. For that reason, probiotics and prebiotics are often used together in the treatment of active CD and other gastrointestinal disorders. The product that contains both probiotics and prebiotics is called synbiotic. An example of a synbiotic is Synbiotic 2000, which was used in a small,

multicenter, randomized, double-blind, placebo-controlled study to prevent postoperative recurrence of CD (Chermesh et al., 2007). Synbiotic 2000 is composed of 4 probiotics (10^{10} *Pediacoccus pentoseceus*, 10^{10} *Lb. raffinolactis*, 10^{10} *Lb. paracasei* subsp. *paracasei* 19, and 10^{10} *Lb. plantarum* 2362) and 4 prebiotics (2.5 g β-glucans, 2.5 g inulin, 2.5 g pectin and 2.5 g resistant starch). The clinical trial involved 30 patients with CD who were treated, after surgery, either with Synbiotic 2000 or with placebo once a day for up to 24 months. Only 9 patients completed the study, 7 from Synbiotic 2000 group and 2 from placebo group. No difference between the two groups in clinical, laboratory and endoscopic results could be confirmed and it was concluded that Synbiotic 2000 is not effective in preventing postsurgical recurrence of CD (Chermesh et al., 2007). Because of relatively small group of patients involved in this clinical trial more research was suggested, involving a larger setup and different synbiotic mixtures.

Another synbiotic therapy was reported in a clinical trial with 35 patients with active CD (Steed et al., 2010). The synbiotic product in this instance contained $2x10^{11}$ CFU of probiotic bacterium *B. longum* and 6 g of prebiotic Synergy 1, which is the commercial name for oligofructose-enriched inulin. Patients had received synbiotic or placebo twice a day for six months. Treatment with synbiotic improved clinical symptoms and histological score in treated patients with active CD. A significant reduction of TNFα expression in patient treated with synbiotic was observed after three months, however after six months, the reduction was no longer significant. A beneficial effect of synbiotic could also be observed in the significant increase of the level of bifidobacteria in treated patients.

4. Antibiotics

The use of antibiotics in the primary treatment of CD is again based on the theory of involvement of bacteria in the pathogenesis of the disease (Lal & Steinhart, 2006). CD could be caused by an aggressive immune response to antigens in the gut of genetically susceptible individuals (Prantera, 2009). Antibiotics in CD have been used for the nonspecific reduction of intestinal bacterial load. In clinical trials, several antibiotics were used for the treatment of CD (Prantera, 2009):

- antibiotics with antimycobacterial activity (clofazimin, clarithromycin, rifabutin)
- metronidazole (active against anaerobic bacteria)
- ciprofloxacin (active against *E. coli)*
- rifaximin.

Antibiotics have shown some effectiveness in the treatment of CD, mostly in reducing post-operative recurrence of CD. Their benefits however have to be balanced by the side effects they cause (Doherty et al., 2010).

4.1 Antimycobacterial therapy

The earlier described single pathogen hypothesis suggests *M. avium* subsp. *paratuberculosis* as a causative agent for CD. For that reason, antibiotics against mycobacteria have been tested in the treatment of CD. In 2007, a prospective, parallel, placebo-controlled, double-blind, randomized clinical trial in patients with active CD was reported. The authors used the combination of clarithromycin, rifabutin, and clofazimine for two years (Selby et al., 2007). They concluded that this combination of antibiotics against *M. paratuberculosis* showed no benefits in the treatment of CD. This could serve as another piece of evidence against the single pathogen hypothesis with *M. avium* subsp. *paratubercolosis*. Nevertheless, further studies should be performed to confirm or disprove these findings.

4.2 Metronidazole and ciprofloxacin

Metronidazole and ciprofloxacin are the most popular antimicrobial drugs used in the treatment of CD. They exert antimicrobial activity against Gram negative and Gram positive bacteria (Dharmani & Chadee, 2008). Metronidazole is a nitromidazole antibiotic, and ciprofloxacin belongs to a group of fluoroquinolone antibiotics. Both antibiotics, alone or in combination, were used in several clinical trials for active CD treatment. Antibiotics have been effective in preventing the remission of CD; however their benefits have to be balanced by the side effects they cause. One of the reports describes the use of a combination of metronidazole and ciprofloxacin therapy in patients with active ileal or colonic CD. The therapy was well tolerated and showed beneficial effects with symptomatic improvement in patients with active CD, especially in the colon (Greenbloom et al., 1998). Only five of 72 patients required withdrawal of the therapy because of side effects. The authors speculated that only metronidazole is to be held responsible for side effects (e. g. neuropathy, nausea and anorexia), as those have already been reported in previous studies on metronidazole treatment of CD (Greenbloom et al., 1998; Prantera et al., 1996).

4.3 Rifaximin

Rifaximin is a rifamycin-based antibiotic with a broad spectrum of antimicrobial activity. This covers Gram positive and Gram negative bacteria, and includes both aerobic and anaerobic bacteria. Rifaximin is poorly absorbed from the gastrointestinal tract and therefore has less systemic effects. It has an excellent safety profile, minimal drug interaction, and negligible impact on the intestinal microbiome. For those reasons, it has a great potential in the treatment of gastrointestinal diseases, including active CD. Rifaximin is approved in more than 30 countries for a variety of gastrointestinal disorders, including the treatment of traveler's diarrhea, caused by noninvasive diarreagenic *E. coli* (Koo & DuPont, 2010).
In recent years, several studies have reported rifaximin effectiveness in the treatment of CD. In 2006, a multicenter, double blind, randomized, placebo-controlled study was reported. Rifaximin gastroresistant granules (800 mg once a day or 800 mg twice a day) were given orally to 83 patients with mildly to moderately active CD for 12 weeks (Prantera et al., 2006). Rifaximin gastroresistant granules were designed specifically for CD treatment. They were coated with a co-polymer, which was designed to by-pass the stomach and dissolve in the duodenum-jejunum, thereby concentrating the active rifaximin in the small intestine. In the study, the clinical remission was achieved in 52% of the group who received rifaximin twice a day, in 32% of the group who received rifaximin once a day, and in 33% of the group who received a placebo dose twice a day. In comparison to the placebo group, the rifaximin group was superior in inducing clinical remission of mildly to moderately active CD, although the difference was not statistically significant. Nevertheless, the results were encouraging and a larger randomized placebo-controlled study is justified.
In 2008, Shafran and Burgunder reported the treatment of five patients with newly diagnosed mild CD with 400 mg rifaximin dose twice daily for 3 months. This was the patients' first therapy without prior biologic or immunomodulatory treatment. The therapy was successful in 3 patients and substantial endoscopic and clinical improvements were observed. The authors suggested that rifaximin therapy could be an effective first-line treatment in patients with small intestinal CD (Shafran & Burgunder, 2008).

The same authors performed a retrospective analysis of 68 patients with CD, who were treated with rifaximin between 2001 and 2005. Patients had CD localized to the small or large intestine, and 56% of patients had previously undergone surgery. Most of the patients were treated with rifaximin dose 600 mg/day. Almost half of them were also receiving steroids, and some of them were also treated with anti-inflammatory agents, biologics (e.g. infliximab), antidiarrheal agents, and immunomodulators. The retrospective analysis showed that clinical remission was achieved in 65% of the patients with CD. Interestingly, this percentage was a little higher in patients who were not treated with steroids. Among the patients who received only rifaximin therapy, 67% achieved remission. These findings again substantiate the use of rifaximin alone for the induction of remission in CD (Shafran & Burgunder, 2010).

Several studies on the efficacy of rifaximin in CD have shown that it has a good potential in CD therapy, either as a first or second line treatment. Nevertheless, further research of rifaximin efficacy in patients with CD is required. Among other things, its precise mechanism of action in CD should be clarified.

4.4 Antibiotics in the prevention of post-operative CD

Antibiotics are most frequently applied for the prevention of post-operative recurrence of CD (Doherty et al., 2009; Doherty et al., 2010; Lal & Steinhart, 2006). Rutgeerts and co-workers published two double-blind randomized studies of the efficacy of nitroimidazole antibiotics in the prevention of postoperative CD (Rutgeerts et al., 2005; Rutgeerts et al., 1995). In the first study, one week after resection surgery, 30 patients started to receive antibiotic metronidazole at a dose of 20 mg/kg body weight once a day for a period of three months (Rutgeerts et al., 1995). Another 30 patients received placebo. Nine patients did not finish the study, two in the placebo group and seven in metronidazole group. The reasons for the latter patients were gastrointestinal intolerance, acute paranoia, polyneuropathy, suture leak, and the lack of compliance. After the end of the therapy, patients were observed every 6 month for the period of three years. After a 3 month therapy, 21 of 28 (75%) patients in the placebo group had recurrent lesion in neoterminal ileum, while this only happened to 12 of 23 (52%) patients in the metronidazole group. Metronidazole significantly reduced endoscopic recurrence, which was observed in 3 of 23 (13%) patients in metronidazole group and in 12 of 28 (43%) patients in the placebo group. Statistically significant reduction of clinical recurrence was observed only after one year. The reduction was no longer significant two and three years after surgery, but the benefit of metronidazole treatment was still present. This study showed that metronidazole was effective in preventing early severe recurrence of CD. However, several side effects occurred in the metronidazole group, including gastrointestinal intolerance, metallic taste, leucopenia, paraesthesias of the limbs, abnormal liver function, polyneuropathy, and psychosis. Because of high rates of adverse effects with metronidazole, a second study for the prevention of postoperative CD was performed with antibiotic ornidazole (Rutgeerts et al., 2005). Ornidazole is also a nitroimidazole antibiotic, but supposedly causes fewer side effects than metronidazole. 80 patients after ileocolonic resection were included. Half of the patients received 500 mg of ornidazole twice daily and half received a placebo for 12 months. After the end of the treatment, clinical recurrence manifested in 3 of 38 (7.8%) patients in the ornidazol group and in 15 of 40 (37.5%) patients in the placebo group. Additionally, the results of clinical recurrence were measured two and three years after surgery. After two years, 11 of 37

(29.7%) patients had clinical recurrence in the ornidazol group, and 18 of 40 (45%) patients in placebo group. After 3 years, 17 of 37 (45.9%) patients had clinical recurrence in the ornidazol group and 19 of 40 (45.5%) patients in the placebo group. Similar to metronidazol, ornidazol has shown efficacy in preventing postoperative clinical recurrence of CD, but has also caused numerous side effects. To alleviate these, the authors suggested the use of a smaller dose (500 mg/day) of ornidazol in postoperative therapy of CD.

When antibiotics are used for preventing postoperative recurrence of CD, they are often combined with other therapies for CD, including immunomodulators, probiotics, steroids, and others. The studies of combinations of antibiotics with probiotics were presented in the Chapter 2.2. The combination of antibiotic metronidazole and immunomodulator azathioprine was studied in a placebo-controlled randomized trial to prevent postoperative recurrence of CD (D'Haens et al., 2008). It was performed on 81 CD patients after curative ileal or ileocolonic resection. The first group of 40 patients received 500 mg metronidazole three times per day and 100-150 mg azathioprine once per day for a period of three months. The second group of 41 patients received metronidazole without azathioprine. After three months, the metronidazole treatment was discontinued, but the study continued for another nine months with azathioprine treatment only (the first group received azathioprine and the second group placebo). 32 patients from the first group and 29 patients from the placebo group reached the end of the study. Endoscopic recurrence was measured three and twelve months after the beginning of the study. After 3 months, significant endoscopic recurrence occurred in 12 of 35 (34.3%) patients in the first group, and in 20 of 38 (52.6%) patients in the placebo group. After twelve months, significant endoscopic recurrence occurred in 14 of 32 (43.7%) patients in the first group and in 20 of 29 (69%) patients in the placebo group. Also after twelve months, inflammatory lesions were not observed in seven patients in the first group and only in one patient in the placebo group. There was no clinical recurrence in patients after three months of surgery. Twelve months after surgery, 10 clinical recurrences were observed, three in the first group and seven in the placebo group. Some adverse effects occurred in both groups, but overall the treatment was well tolerated. It can be concluded that the combination of antibiotic with immunomodulator is superior to antibiotic alone in preventing postoperative recurrence of CD. Because of the shorter period of antibiotic treatment, the number of side effects in patients was lower than in previous studies. Nevertheless, further studies on larger number of patients are needed to support this approach.

5. Conclusion

Human intestinal bacteria are an important factor in human health, as well as in the pathogenesis of intestinal disorders, including CD. However, none of the proposed mechanisms of action can alone sufficiently explain the disease occurrence. Bacterial components are undoubtedly involved in the activation of abnormal autoimmune responses which further trigger the disease symptoms. The whole picture is however more complex with more active bacterial involvement.

Probiotics are an obvious choice for influencing the intestinal microbiome. Probiotics have shown some promising initial results in the treatment of CD. However, in general, they were not found to be superior to placebo in increasing the time of remission of CD or reducing post-operative recurrence in controlled clinical trials. Two notable exceptions preserve hope for probiotics in the treatment of CD. Yeast *S. boulardii* was shown to be more effective than melsalazine in maintaining remission of CD (Guslandi et al., 2000) and improving intestinal permeability in CD patients (Van Gossum et al., 2007). Probiotic mixture VSL#3 was successful in the treatment of CD-induced arthralgia (Karimi et al., 2005) and in the prevention of postoperative recurrence of CD (Madsen et al., 2008). These studies offer support for the commonly asserted claim that further trials are justified.

There are several reasons that could explain the failure of other clinical trials and speak in favor of probiotics. The overall number of clinical trials is low, as well as the number of participants. Trials were designed in different ways, had different goals and measured different outcomes. Despite the abundance of bacteria with attributed probiotic properties, just a few were used in clinical trials. Additionally, there were differences in doses and regimens. Future trials should broaden the spectrum of probiotic bacteria in the treatment. Probiotics are not alike and exert effects by different mechanisms. The growing number of probiotic bacteria, however, clearly prevents systematic testing of all of them. To overcome this difficulty two strategies can be foreseen.

The first includes testing of larger combinations of bacterial strains. Individual bacteria in the mixture would have different effects and could well act synergistically. This view can be supported by the success of probiotic mixture VSL#3 relative to individual bacteria *Lb. rhamnosus* GG and *Lb. johnsonii* LA1. The ultimate example of that approach would be a fecal transplant from healthy donors to patients. This has been successfully applied in the treatment of *C. difficile* infection. It was also shown that the changes in the composition of a recipient's intestinal flora were long-lasting. Recipients' intestinal flora resembled the composition of the donor's flora even after 24 weeks (Grehan et al., 2010). This approach is not without risks, as transfer of potential pathogens is difficult to exclude.

The second approach would necessitate better understanding of the disease etiology and modes of action of various bacteria. This would require the use of better animal models of CD. The majority of the studies in mice were performed on models of intestinal inflammation which resemble that of ulcerative colitis, with inflammatory changes limited to the colon. Inflammation was achieved with chemicals or genetic knock-out, which only weakly reflect the origin and course of CD in humans. Two mouse models of CD have been described, TNF ΔARE and SAMP1/YitFc (Pizarro et al., 2003). They should be applied in the search of a single probiotic strain with the desired properties.

Recombinant probiotics have reasonable potential for the treatment of CD in the future. They combine the safety of probiotics with a defined mechanism of action. However, solution of the remaining safety concerns and further human clinical trials will be needed before they can be recommended.

Antibiotics constitute the most straightforward approach for interfering with the intestinal microbiome by lowering the bacterial content in a mostly unspecific fashion. The approach has shown clinical efficacy, but at a price of quite severe adverse effects. Rifaximin could assume greater importance in the future since it is a poorly absorbed, broad-spectrum antibiotic with fewer side effects.

6. Acknowledgment

This work was supported by the Slovenian Research Agency Grant No. P4-0127. The authors are grateful to Prof. Roger Pain for critical reading of the manuscript.

7. References

Barnich, N., & Darfeuille-Michaud, A. (2007). Adherent-invasive *Escherichia coli* and Crohn's disease. *Current Opinion in Gastroenterology*, Vol. 23, No. 1, pp. 16-20, ISSN 1522-8037

Benjamin, J. L., Hedin, C. R. H., Koutsoumpas, A., Ng, S.C., McCarthy, N. E., Hart, A.L., Kamm, M. A., Sanderson, J. D., Knight, S. C., Forbes, A., Stagg, A. J., Whelan, K., & Lindsay, J. O. (2011). Randomised, double-blind, placebo-controlled trial of fructo-oligosaccharides in active Crohn's disease. *Gut*, Vol. 60, No. 7, pp. 923-929, ISSN 0017-5749

Boirivant, M., & Strober, W. (2007). The mechanism of action of probiotics. *Current Opinion in Gastroenterology*, Vol. 23, No. 6, pp. 679-692, ISSN 0267-1379

Borruel, N., Carol, M., Casellas, F., Antolín, M., Lara, F. de, Espín, E., Naval, J., Guarner, F., & Malagelada, J. R. (2002). Increased mucosal tumour necrosis factor alpha production in Crohn's disease can be downregulated *ex vivo* by probiotic bacteria. *Gut*, Vol. 51, No. 5, pp. 659-664, ISSN 0017-5749

Bousvaros, A., Guandalini, S., Baldassano, R. N., Botelho, C., Evans, J., Ferry, G. D., Goldin, B., Hartigan, L., Kugathasan, S., Levy, J., Murray, K. F., Oliva-Hemker, M., Rosh, R. J., Tolia, V., Zholudev, A., Vanderhoof, J. A., & Hibberd, P. L. (2005). A randomized, double-blind trial of *Lactobacillus GG* versus placebo in addition to standard maintenance therapy for children with Crohn's disease. *Inflammatory Bowel Diseases*, Vol. 11, No. 9, pp. 833–839, ISSN 1078-0998

Braat, H., van den Brande, J., van Tol, E., Hommes, D., Peppelenbosch, M., & van Deventer, S. (2004). *Lactobacillus rhamnosus* induces peripheral hyporesponsiveness in stimulated CD4+ T cells via modulation of dendritic cell function. *American Journal of Clinical Nutrition*, Vol. 80, No. 6, pp. 1618-1625, ISSN 0002-9165

Braat, H., Rottiers, P., Hommes, D. W., Huyghebaert, N., Remaut, E., Remon, J. P., van Deventer, S.J.H., Neirynck, S., Peppelenbosch, M.P., & Steidler, L. (2006). A Phase I Trial With Transgenic Bacteria Expressing Interleukin-10 in Crohn's Disease. *Clinical Gastroenterology and Hepatology*, Vol. 4, No. 6, pp. 754-759, ISSN 1542-3565

Campieri, M., Rizzello, F., Venturi, A., Poggioli, G., & Ugolini, F. (2000). Combination of antibiotic and probiotic treatment is efficacious in prophylaxis of post-operative recurrence of Crohn's disease: A randomized controlled study VS mesalamine. *Gastroenterology*, Vol. 118, No. 4, pp. A781, ISSN 0016-5085

Chermesh, I., Tamir, A., Reshef, R., Chowers, Y., Suissa, A., Katz, D., Gelber, M., Halpern, Z., Bengmark, S., & Eliakim, R. (2007). Failure of Synbiotic 2000 to prevent postoperative recurrence of Crohn's disease. *Digestive Diseases and Sciences*, Vol. 52, No. 2, pp. 385-389, ISSN 0163-2116

De Hertogh, G., Aerssens, J., Geboes, K. P., & Geboes, K. (2008). Evidence for the involvement of infectious agents in the pathogenesis of Crohn's disease. *World Journal of Gastroenterology*, Vol. 14, No. 6, pp. 845-852, ISSN 1007-9327

Dharmani, P., & Chadee, K. (2008). Biologic therapies against inflammatory bowel disease: a dysregulated immune system and the cross talk with gastrointestinal mucosa hold the key. *Current molecular pharmacology*, Vol. 1, No. 3, pp. 195-212, ISSN 1874-4702

Doherty, G., Bennett, G., Patil, S., Cheifetz, A., & Moss, A. (2009). Interventions for prevention of post-operative recurrence of Crohn's disease. *Cochrane Database of Systematic Reviews*, No. 4, pp. 1-60, ISSN 1469-493X

Doherty, G. A., Bennett, G. C., Cheifetz, A. S., & Moss, A. (2010). Meta-analysis: targeting the intestinal microbiota in prophylaxis for post-operative Crohn's disease. *Alimentary pharmacology & therapeutics*, Vol. 31, No. 8, pp. 802–809, ISSN 0269-2813

D'Haens, G. R., Vermeire, S., Van Assche, G., Noman, M., Aerden, I., Van Olmen, G., & Rutgeerts, P. (2008). Therapy of metronidazole with azathioprine to prevent postoperative recurrence of Crohn's disease: a controlled randomized trial. *Gastroenterology*, Vol. 135, No. 4, pp. 1123-1129, ISSN 0016-5085

Garcia Vilela, E., De Lourdes De Abreu Ferrari, M., Oswaldo Da Gama Torres, H., Guerra Pinto, A., Carolina Carneiro Aguirre, A., Paiva Martins, F., Marcos Andrade Goulart, E., & Sales Da Cunha, A. (2008). Influence of *Saccharomyces boulardii* on the intestinal permeability of patients with Crohn's disease in remission. *Scandinavian Journal of Gastroenterology*, Vol. 43, No. 7, pp. 842–848, ISSN 0036-5521

Gibson, G. R., Probert, H. M., Loo, J. V., Rastall, R. a, & Roberfroid, M. B. (2004). Dietary modulation of the human colonic microbiota: updating the concept of prebiotics. *Nutrition research reviews*, Vol. 17, No. 2, pp. 259-275, ISSN 0954-4224

Gibson, G. R., & Roberfroid, M. B. (1995). Dietary Modulation of the Human Colonie Microbiota : Introducing the Concept of Prebiotics. *The Journal of Nutrition*, Vol. 125, pp. 1401-1412, ISSN 0022-3166

Greenbloom, S. L., Steinhart, A. H., & Greenberg, G. R. (1998). Combination ciprofloxacin and metronidazole for active Crohn's disease. *Canadian Journal of Gastroenterology*, Vol. 12, No. 1, pp. 53-56, ISSN 0835-7900

Grehan, M. J., Borody, T. J., Leis, S. M., Campbell, J., Mitchell, H., & Wettstein, A. (2010). Durable alteration of the colonic microbiota by the administration of donor fecal flora. *Journal of Clinical Gastroenterology*, Vol. 44, No. 8, pp. 551-561, ISSN 0192-0790

Guandalini, S. (2010). Update on the role of probiotics in the therapy of pediatric inflammatory bowel disease. *Expert Review of Clinical Immunology*, Vol. 6, No. 1, pp. 47–54, ISSN 1744-666X

Gupta, P., Andrew, H., Kirschner, B. S., & Guandalini, S. (2000). Is *Lactobacillus GG* helpful in children with Crohn's disease? Results of a preliminary, open-label study. *Journal of Pediatric Gastroenterology and Nutrition*, Vol. 31, No. 4, pp. 453-457, ISSN 0277-2116

Guslandi, M., Mezzi, G., Sorghi, M., & Testoni, P. A. (2000). *Saccharomyces boulardii* in Maintenance Treatment of Crohn ' s Disease. *Digestive Diseases and Sciences*, Vol. 45, No. 7, pp. 1462-1464, ISSN 0163-2116

Hamady, Z. Z. R., Scott, N., Farrar, M. D., Wadhwa, M., Dilger, P., Whitehead, T. R., Thorpe, R., Holland, K.T., Lodge, J.P.A., & Carding, S.R. (2010). Treatment of colitis with a commensal gut bacterium engineered to secrete human TGF-beta1 under the control of dietary xylan. *Inflammatory Bowel Diseases*, 17: n/a.

Hanauer, S. B. (2006). Inflammatory bowel disease: epidemiology, pathogenesis, and therapeutic opportunities. *Inflammatory Bowel Diseases*, Vol. 12, No. 5, pp. S3–S9, ISSN 1078-0998

Hart, A L, Lammers, K., Brigidi, P., Vitali, B., Rizzello, F, Gionchetti, P., Campieri, M., Kamm, M. A., Knight, S. C., & Stagg, A. J. (2004). Modulation of human dendritic cell phenotype and function by probiotic bacteria. *Gut*, Vol. 53, No. 11, pp. 1602-1609, ISSN 0017-5749

Hugot, J. P., Chamaillard, M, Zouali, H., Lesage, S., Cézard, J. P., Belaiche, J., Almer, S., Tysk, C., O'Morain, C., A., Gassull, M., Binder, V., Finkel, Y., Cortot, A., Modigliani, R., Laurent-Puig, P., Gower-Rousseau, C., Macry, J., Colombel, J. F., Sahbatou, M., & Thomas, G. (2001). Association of NOD2 leucine-rich repeat variants with susceptibility to Crohn's disease. *Nature*, Vol. 411, No. 6837, pp. 599-603, ISSN 0028-0836

Isaacs, K., & Herfarth, H. (2008). Role of probiotic therapy in IBD. *Inflammatory Bowel Diseases*, Vol. 14, No. 11, pp. 1597–1605, ISSN 1078-0998

Karimi, O., Peña, A. S., & Bodegraven, A. A. (2005). Probiotics (VSL# 3) in arthralgia in patients with ulcerative colitis and Crohn's disease: A pilot study. *Drugs of Today*, Vol. 41, No. 7, pp. 453–460, ISSN 0025-7656

Koo, H. L., & DuPont, H. L. (2010). Rifaximin: a unique gastrointestinal-selective antibiotic for enteric diseases. *Current opinion in gastroenterology*, Vol. 26, No. 1, pp. 17-25, ISSN 0267-1379

Lal, S., & Steinhart, A. H. (2006). Antibiotic therapy for Crohn's disease: A review. *Canadian Journal of Gastroenterology*, Vol. 20, No. 10, pp. 651-655, ISSN 0835-7900

Leenen, C. H. M., & Dieleman, L. A. (2007). Inulin and oligofructose in chronic inflammatory bowel disease. *The Journal of Nutrition*, Vol. 137, No. 11, pp. 2572S-2575S, ISSN 0022-3166

Lindsay, J. O., Whelan, K., Stagg, A.J., Gobin, P., Al-Hassi, H. O., Rayment, N., Kamm, M. A., Knight, S. C., & Forbes, A. (2006). Clinical, microbiological, and immunological effects of fructo-oligosaccharide in patients with Crohn's disease. *Gut*, Vol. 55, No. 3, pp. 348-355, ISSN 0017-5749

Liévin-Le Moal, V., Amsellem, R., Servin, A. L., & Coconnier, M. H. (2002). *Lactobacillus acidophilus* (strain LB) from the resident adult human gastrointestinal microflora exerts activity against brush border damage promoted by a diarrhoeagenic *Escherichia coli* in human enterocyte-like cells. *Gut*, Vol. 50, No. 6, pp. 803-811, ISSN 0017-5749

Macfarlane, G., Blackett, K., Nakayama, T., Steed, H., & Macfarlane, S. (2009). The gut microbiota in inflammatory bowel disease. *Current Pharmaceutical Design*, Vol. 15, No. 13, pp. 1528–1536, ISSN 1381-6128

Mack, D. R., Michail, S., Wei, S., Mcdougall, L., & Hollingsworth, A. M. (1999). Probiotics inhibit enteropathogenic *E. coli* adherence in vitro by inducing intestinal mucin gene expression in vitro by inducing intestinal mucin gene expression. *American Journal of Physiology*, Vol. 276, pp. G941-G950, ISSN 0193-1857

Madsen, K., Backer, J., Leddin, D., Dieleman, L., Bitton, A., Feagan, B., Petrunia, D. M., Chiba, N., Enns, R. A., & Fedotak, R. (2008). A randomized controlled trial of VSL#3 for the prevention of endoscopic recurrence following surgery for Crohn's disease. *Gastroenterology*, pp. A-361, ISSN 0016-5085

Madsen, K., Cornish, A., Soper, P., McKaigney, C., Jijon, H., Yachimec, C., Doyle, J., Jewell, L., & De Simone, C. (2001). Probiotic bacteria enhance murine and human intestinal epithelial barrier function. *Gastroenterology*, Vol. 121, No. 3, pp. 580-91, ISSN 0016-5085

Malchow, H. (1997). Crohn's disease and *Escherichia coli*. A new approach in therapy to maintain remission of colonic Crohn's disease? *Journal of Clinical Gastroenterology*, Vol. 25, No. 4, pp. 653-658, ISSN 0192-0790

Manichanh, C, Rigottier-Gois, L., Bonnaud, E., Gloux, K., Pelletier, E., Frangeul, L., Nalin, R., Jarrin, C., Chardon, P., Marteau, P., Roca, J., & Dore, J. (2006). Reduced diversity of faecal microbiota in Crohn's disease revealed by a metagenomic approach. *Gut*, Vol. 55, No. 2, pp. 205-211, ISSN 0017-5749

Marteau, P, Lémann, M., Seksik, P, Laharie, D., Colombel, J. F., Bouhnik, Y., Cadiot, G., Soulé, J. C., Bourreille, A., Metman, E., Lerebours, E., Carbonnel, F., Dupas, J. L., Veyrac, M., Coffin, B., Moreau, J., Abitbol, V., Blum-Sperisen, S., & Mary, J. Y. (2006). Ineffectiveness of *Lactobacillus johnsonii* LA1 for prophylaxis of postoperative recurrence in Crohn's disease: a randomised, double blind, placebo controlled GETAID trial. *Gut*, Vol. 55, No. 6, pp. 842-847, ISSN 0017-5749

Marteau, P, Sokol, H, Dray, X, & Seksik, P. (2009). Bacteriotherapy for inflammatory bowel disease: therapeutic tool and/or pharmacological vectors? *Gastroentérologie clinique et biologique*, Vol. 33, pp. 228–234, ISSN 2210-7401

Mohamadzadeh, M., Olson, S., Kalina, W. V., Ruthel, G., Demmin, G. L., Warfield, K. L., Bavari, S., & Klaenhammer, T. R. (2005). Lactobacilli activate human dendritic cells that skew T cells toward T helper 1 polarization. *Proceedings of the National Academy of Sciences of the United States of America*, Vol. 102, No. 8, pp. 2880-2885, ISSN 0027-8424

Ng, S C, Hart, a L., Kamm, M. a, Stagg, a J., & Knight, S C. (2009). Mechanisms of action of probiotics: Recent advances. *Inflammatory Bowel Diseases*, Vol. 15, No. 2, pp. 300-310, ISSN 1078-0998

Ogura, Y., Bonen, D., Inohara, N., & Nicolae, D. (2001). A frameshift mutation in NOD2 associated with susceptibility to Crohn's disease. *Nature*, Vol. 411, No. 6837, pp. 603-606, ISSN 0028-0836

Otte, J.-M., & Podolsky, Daniel K. (2004). Functional modulation of enterocytes by gram-positive and gram-negative microorganisms. *American Journal of Physiology*, Vol. 286, No. 4, pp. G613-G626, ISSN 01931857

Pizarro, T. T., Arseneau, K. O., Bamias, G., & Cominelli, F. (2003). Mouse models for the study of Crohn's disease. *Trends in Molecular Medicine*, Vol. 9, No. 5, pp. 218–222, ISSN: 1471-4914

Prantera, C. (2009). Antibiotics and probiotics in inflammatory bowel disease: why, when, and how. *Current Opinion in Gastroenterology*, Vol. 25, pp. 329-333, ISSN 0267-1379

Prantera, C., Lochs, H., Campieri, M, Scribano, M. L., Sturniolo, G. C., Castiglione, F., & Cottone, M. (2006). Antibiotic treatment of Crohn's disease: results of a multicentre, double blind, randomized, placebo-controlled trial with rifaximin. *Alimentary Pharmacology & Therapeutics*, Vol. 23, No. 8, pp. 1117-1125, ISSN 0269-2813

Prantera, C., Scribano, M., Falasco, G., Andreoli, A., & Luzi, C. (2002). Ineffectiveness of probiotics in preventing recurrence after curative resection for Crohn's disease: a randomised controlled trial with *Lactobacillus GG*. *Gut*, Vol. 51, No. 3, pp. 405-409, ISSN 0017-5749

Prantera, C., Zannoni, F., Scribano, M., Berto, E., Andreoli, A., Kohn, A., & Luzi, C. (1996). An antibiotic regimen for the treatment of active Crohn's disease: a randomized, controlled clinical trial of metronidazole plus ciprofloxacin. *The American Journal of Gastroenterology*, Vol. 91, No. 2, pp. 328–332, ISSN 0002-9270

Prindiville, T., Cantrell, M., & Wilson, K. H. (2006). Ribosomal DNA sequence analysis of mucosa-associated bacteria in Crohn's disease. *Inflammatory Bowel Diseases*, Vol. 10, No. 6, pp. 824-833, ISSN 1078-0998

Qin, J., Li, R., Raes, J., Arumugam, M., Burgdorf, K. S., Manichanh, C., Nielsen, T., Pons, N., Levenez, F., Yamada, T., Mende, D. R., Li, J., Xu, J., Li, S., Li, D., Cao, J., Wang, B., Liang, H., Zheng, H., Xie, Y., Tap, J., Lepage, P., Bertalan, M., Batto, J. M., Hansen, T., Le Paslier, D., Linneberg, A., Nielsen, H. B., Pelletier, E., Renault, P., Sicheritz-Ponten, T., Turner, K., Zhu, H., Yu, C., Li, S., Jian, M., Zhou, Y., Li, Y., Zhang, X., Li, S., Qin, N., Yang, H., Wang, J., Brunak, S., Doré, J., Guarner, F., Kristiansen, K., Pedersen, O., Parkhill, J., Weissenbach, J., Bork, P., Ehrlich, S. D., & Wang, J. (2010). A human gut microbial gene catalogue established by metagenomic sequencing. *Nature*, Vol. 464, No. 7285, pp. 59-65, ISSN 0028-0836

Ravnikar, M., Strukelj, B., Obermajer, N., Lunder, M., & Berlec, A. (2010). Engineered lactic acid bacterium *Lactococcus lactis* capable of binding antibodies and tumor necrosis factor alpha. *Applied and Environmental Microbiology*, Vol. 76, No. 20, pp. 6928-6932, ISSN 0099-2240

Resta-Lenert, S. C., & Barrett, K. E. (2009). Modulation of intestinal barrier properties by probiotics: role in reversing colitis. *Annals of the New York Academy of Sciences*, Vol. 1165, No. 1, pp. 175–182, ISSN 0077-8923

Roberfroid, M. (2007). Prebiotics: the concept revisited. *The Journal of Nutrition*, Vol. 137, pp. 830S-837S, ISSN 0022-3166

Rolhion, N., & Darfeuille-Michaud, A. (2007). Adherent-invasive *Escherichia coli* in inflammatory bowel disease. *Inflammatory Bowel Diseases*, Vol. 13, No. 10, pp. 1277–1283, ISSN 1078-0998

Rutgeerts, P., Hiele, M., Geboes, K., Peeters, M., Penninckx, F., Aerts, R., & Kerremans, R. (1995). Controlled trial of metronidazole treatment for prevention of Crohn's recurrence after ileal resection. *Gastroenterology*, Vol. 108, No. 6, pp. 1617–1621, ISSN 0016-5085

Rutgeerts, P., Van Assche, G., Vermeire, S., D'Haens, G., Baert, F., Noman, M., & Aerden, I., De Hertogh, G., Geboes, K., Hiele, M., D'Hoore, A., Penninckx, F. (2005). Ornidazole for prophylaxis of postoperative Crohn's disease recurrence: a randomized, double-blind, placebo-controlled trial. *Gastroenterology*, Vol. 128, No. 4, pp. 856–861, ISSN 0016-5085

Schrezenmeir, J., & Vrese, M. de. (2001). Probiotics, prebiotics, and synbiotics-approaching a definition. *The American Journal of Clinical Nutrition*, Vol. 73, No. 2, pp. 361S-364S, ISSN 0002-9165

Schultz, M., Timmer, A., Herfarth, H. H., Sartor, R. B., Vanderhoof, J. A., & Rath, H. C. (2004). *Lactobacillus GG* in inducing and maintaining remission of Crohn's disease. *BMC gastroenterology*, Vol. 4, No. 1, pp. 5, ISSN 1471-230X

Selby, W., Pavli, P., Crotty, B., Florin, T., Radford-Smith, G., Gibson, P., Mitchell, B., Connell, W., Read, R., Merrett, M., Ee, H., & Hetzel, D. (2007). Two-year combination antibiotic therapy with clarithromycin, rifabutin, and clofazimine for Crohn's disease. *Gastroenterology*, Vol. 132, No. 7, pp. 2313–2319, ISSN 0016-5085

Shafran, I., & Burgunder, P. (2008). Rifaximin for the treatment of newly diagnosed Crohn's disease: a case series. *The American Journal of Gastroenterology*, Vol. 103, No. 8, pp. 2158–2160, ISSN 0002-9270

Shafran, Ira, & Burgunder, Patricia. (2010). Adjunctive antibiotic therapy with rifaximin may help reduce Crohn's disease activity. *Digestive Diseases and Sciences*, Vol, 55, No. 4, pp. 1079-1084, ISSN 0163-2116

Smits, H. H., Engering, A., van der Kleij, D., Jong, E. C. de, Schipper, K., van Capel, T. M. M., Zaat, B. A. J., Yazdanbakhsh, M., Wierenga, E. A., & van Kooyk, Y. (2005). Selective probiotic bacteria induce IL-10-producing regulatory T cells in vitro by modulating dendritic cell function through dendritic cell-specific intercellular adhesion molecule 3-grabbing nonintegrin. *The Journal of Allergy and Clinical Immunology*, Vol. 115, No. 6, pp. 1260-1267, ISSN 0091-6749

Sokol, Harry, Pigneur, B., Watterlot, L., Lakhdari, O., Bermúdez-Humarán, L. G., Gratadoux, J. J., Blugeon, S., Bridonneau, C., Furet, J. P., Corthier, G., Grangette, C., Vasquez, N., Pochart, P., Trugnan, G., Thomas, G., Blottière, H. M., Doré, J., Marteau, P., Seksik, P., & Langella, P. (2008). *Faecalibacterium prausnitzii* is an anti-inflammatory commensal bacterium identified by gut microbiota analysis of Crohn disease patients. *Proceedings of the National Academy of Sciences of the United States of America*, Vol 105, No. 43, pp. 16731-16736, ISSN 0027-8424

Steed, H., Macfarlane, G. T., Blackett, K. L., Bahrami, B., Reynolds, N., Walsh, S. V., Cummings, J.H., & Macfarlane, S. (2010). Clinical trial: the microbiological and immunological effects of synbiotic consumption–a randomized double-blind placebo-controlled study in active Crohn's disease. *Alimentary Pharmacology & Therapeutics*, Vol. 32, No. 7, pp. 872–883, ISSN 0269-2813

Steidler, L, Hans, W., Schotte, L., Neirynck, S, Obermeier, F., Falk, W., Fiers, W., & Remaut, E. (2000). Treatment of murine colitis by *Lactococcus lactis* secreting interleukin-10. *Science*, Vol. 289, No. 5483, pp. 1352-1355, ISSN 0036-8075

Steidler, Lothar, Neirynck, Sabine, Huyghebaert, N., Snoeck, V., Vermeire, A., Goddeeris, B., Cox, E., Remon, J. P., & Remaut, E. (2003). Biological containment of genetically modified *Lactococcus lactis* for intestinal delivery of human interleukin 10. *Nature Biotechnology*, Vol. 21, No. 7, pp. 785-789, ISSN 1087-0156

Takesue, Y., Ohge, H., Uemura, K., Imamura, Y., Murakami, Y., Yokoyama, T., Yokoyama, T., Kakehashi, M., & Sueda, T. (2002). Bacterial translocation in patients with

Crohn's disease undergoing surgery. *Diseases of the Colon and Rectum*, Vol 45, No. 12, pp. 1665–1671, ISSN 0012-3706

Tamboli, C., Neut, C., Desreumaux, P., & Colombel, J. (2004). Dysbiosis in inflammatory bowel disease. *Gut*, Vol. 53, pp. 1-4, ISSN 0017-5749

Thomas, D. W., & Greer, F. R. (2010). Probiotics and prebiotics in pediatrics. *Pediatrics*, Vol. 126, No. 6, pp. 1217-1231, ISSN 0031-4005

Van Gossum, A., Dewit, O., Louis, E., Hertogh, G. de, Baert, Filip, Fontaine, F., DeVos, M., Enslen, M., Paintin, M., & Franchimont, D. (2007). Multicenter randomized-controlled clinical trial of probiotics (*Lactobacillus johnsonii*, LA1) on early endoscopic recurrence of Crohn's disease after lleo-caecal resection. *Inflammatory Bowel Diseases*, Vol. 13, No. 2, pp. 135-142, ISSN 1078-0998

Vandenbroucke, K., Haard, H. de, Beirnaert, E., Dreier, T., Lauwereys, M., Huyck, L., Van Huysse, J., Demetter, P., Steidler, L., Remaut, E., Cuvelier, C., & Rottiers, P. (2010). Orally administered L. lactis secreting an anti-TNF Nanobody demonstrate efficacy in chronic colitis. *Mucosal iImunology*, Vol. 3, No. 1, pp. 49-56, ISSN 1933-0219

Vasquez, N., Mangin, I., Lepage, P., Seksik, Philippe, Duong, J.-P., Blum, S., Schiffrin, E., Suau, A., Allez, M., Vernier, G., Tréton, X., Doré, J., Marteau, P., Pochart, P. (2007). Patchy distribution of mucosal lesions in ileal Crohn's disease is not linked to differences in the dominant mucosa-associated bacteria: a study using fluorescence in situ hybridization and temporal temperature gradient gel electrophoresis. *Inflammatory Bowel Diseases*, Vol. 13, No. 6, pp. 684-692, ISSN 1078-0998

Vavricka, S., & Rogler, G. (2009). New insights into the pathogenesis of Crohn's disease: are they relevant for therapeutic options? *Swiss Medical Weekly*, Vol. 139, pp. 527-534, ISSN 1424-7860

Walker, W. A., Goulet, O., Morelli, L., & Antoine, J. M. (2006). Progress in the science of probiotics: from cellular microbiology and applied immunology to clinical nutrition. *European Journal of Nutrition*, Vol. 45, No. S1, pp. 1-18, ISSN 1436-6207

Wehkamp, J., Stange, E., & Fellermann, K. (2009). Defensin-immunology in inflammatory bowel disease. *Gastroentérologie clinique et biologique*, Vol. 33, No. 3, pp. S137–S144, ISSN 2210-7401

Xavier, R. J., & Podolsky, D K. (2007). Unravelling the pathogenesis of inflammatory bowel disease. *Nature*, Vol. 448, No. 7152, pp. 427-434, ISSN 0028-0836

Yan, F., & Polk, D. B. (2002). Probiotic bacterium prevents cytokine-induced apoptosis in intestinal epithelial cells. *The Journal of Biological Chemistry*, Vol. 277, No. 52, pp. 50959-50965, ISSN 0021-9258

Young, S. L., Simon, M. A., Baird, M. A., Tannock, G. W., Bibiloni, R., Spencely, K., Lane, J. M., Fitzharris, P., Crane, J., Town, I., Addo-Yobo, E., Murray, C. S., & Woodcock, A. (2004). Bifidobacterial species differentially affect expression of cell surface markers and cytokines of dendritic cells harvested from cord blood. *Clinical and Diagnostic Laboratory Immunology*, Vol. 11, No. 4, pp. 686-690, ISSN 1071-412X

Zeissig, S., Bürgel, N., Günzel, D., Richter, J., Mankertz, J., Wahnschaffe, U., Kroesen, A. J., Zeitz, M., Fromm, M., Schulzke, J. D. (2007). Changes in expression and distribution of claudin 2, 5 and 8 lead to discontinuous tight junctions and barrier dysfunction in active Crohn's disease. *Gut*, Vol. 56, No. 1, pp. 61-72, ISSN 0017-5749

10

Evidence-Based Evaluation of Biological Treatment in Crohn's Disease

Shiyao Chen and Yuan Zhao
Department of Gastroenterology, Zhongshan Hospital, Fudan University
P.R. China

1. Introduction

Crohn's disease (CD) is a chronic disorder of the gastrointestinal tract, which was characterized by a relapsing–remitting course with trans-mural inflammation of potentially any section of the digestive tract, leading to various intestinal and extra-intestinal manifestations. Although the etiology is currently unknown, inflammation, immunity, genetic and environmental factors have been suggested to predispose to CD.
The precise etiology of CD is not yet elucidated but the mucosal system is the central effector of intestinal inflammation and injury (Fig 1). The dysregulated mucosal immunity of the bowel is contributed by varied factors among which cytokines play a central role in modulating inflammation. Others are gut associated lymphoid tissues (GALT), pathogen recognition receptors (PRRS), professional antigen presenting cells (APCs), epithelial cells of gut and resident microflora, etc.

1.1 Cytokines

There are two types of cytokines: anti-inflammatory cytokines (IL-10, IL-11, etc) and proinflammatory cytokines (IL-1, IL-2, IFNγ, TNFα, IL-12, IL-18, etc). The anti-inflammatory cytokines have some beneficial effects in CD. IL-10 is produced by Th2 cells and suppresses the production of IL-2 and IFNγ by Th1 cells. Evidences showed that IL-10 and IL-11 might be therapeutic agents in CD. IL-10 knockout mice develop severe transmural and granulomatous inflammation of the small and large bowel, reminiscent of CD, and the inflammation can be prevented by the administration of IL-10. IL-11 is derived from mesenchymal cells. Studies showed that IL-11 could attenuate the inflammatory response and enhance the integrity of the intestinal mucosa. Among the proinflammatory cytokines, TNFα is the most important and widely investigated factor. TNFα is secreted into intestinal mucosa by macrophages and monocytes and is bound to T lymphocytes and monocytes. Its biological activity is mediated by cell surface TNFα receptors binding to either membrane-bound or soluble TNFα. TNFα may increase adhesion molecules, allowing for increased cell infiltration and enhanced metalloproteinase and collagenase production, which help form ulcers and fistulas. It can also mediate recruitment of leukocytes from blood vessels into intestinal mucosa through circulating cells interacting with adhesion molecules on the vascular endothelium. TNFα also activates increases the production of IFNγ by mucosal T cells independently of IL-12 and IL-18. It activates CD44 in T cells and enhances intraepithelial lymphocyte proliferation and migration. Multiple antibodies to TNFα have proven effective in both induction and maintenance of remission for CD. TNFα appears to be a determinant in granuloma formation, and, together with IL-6, IL-1 may contribute to the constitutional symptoms of IBD and lead to the generation of acute-phase proteins.

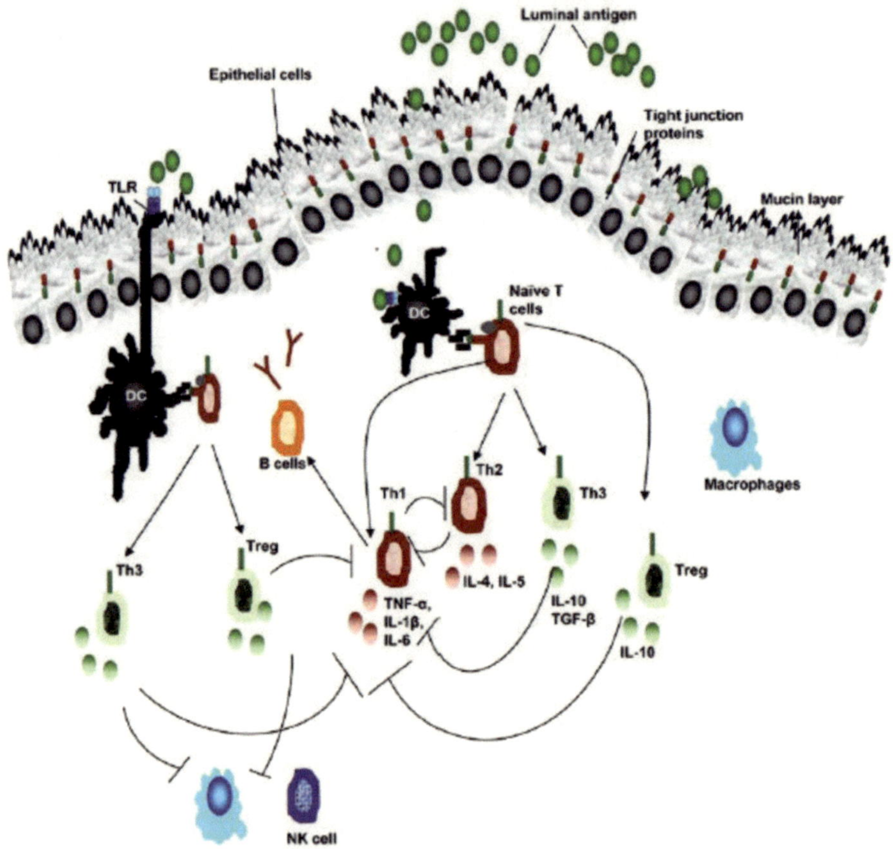

Fig. 1. Intestinal mucosal (immune) homeostasis in healthy state (Dharmani P, 2008)

Mucosal homeostasis is maintained by professional APCs (DC) that differentiate pathogens from commensals through TLRs and leads to balanced differentiation of naive T cells into effector T cells (Th1, Th2 and Th17) against pathogens and Treg and Th3 cells to control the inflammation in absence of pathogens. Epithelial cells lining, tight junction proteins and mucus layer remains intact separating luminal antigen from immune cells.

1.2 PPRs

The recognition, processing and presentation of the luminal antigen is carried out by both dedicated APCs such as dendritic cells (DCs) and macrophages, and non-professional APCs such as epithelial cells. Two PRRs namely Toll-like receptor (TLR) and Nucleotide binding Oligomerization Domans (NOD) proteins are involved in luminal antigen recognition. TLRs are membrane bound receptors while NOD proteins are expressed in the cytosols of APCs. PPRs recognize molecules shared by pathogens but distinguishable from commensal microbes. Such unique microbial components are collectively referred to as pathogen-associated molecular patterns (PAMP), which include CpG regions of methylated DNA, viral specific ssRNA and dsRNA, peptidoglycans, muramyl dipeptide (MDP) and lipo-polysaccharides. Both animal and in vitro studies have shown and exaggerated TLR expression (especially TLR4), that leads to an incorrect immune response (Th1 or Th17 mediated) against resident microflora. NOD2/CARD15 gene is famous as it is the first predisposing gene of CD. Mutations of the NOD2/CARD15 gene have conclusively associated with CD. Both gain and loss of expression of NOD2 gene contributes in disturbing mucosal homeostasis. Loss of NOD2 expression cause change in TLR signaling pathway and thus leads to an increase in Th1 cytokine and defensins. In contrast, gain of expression eventually leads to more Th1 response against the MDP component of microbes.

1.3 T cell polarisation

T helper cells have been classified as either Th1 or Th2 on the basis of function and according to their ability to elaborate specific cytokines. Th1 cells orchestrate cell-mediated immune responses and are characterized by their ability to secrete IL-2, IFNγ and TNFβ. IFNγ activates APCs and macrophages to produce IL-12, thereby driving Th1 cells to produce even larger amounts of Th1 cytokines. In contrast, Th2 cells mediate humoral responses and secrete IL-4, IL-5, IL-6, IL-10 and IL-13. These subsets regulate each other reciprocally through key cytokines. IFNγ, produced by Th1 cells, suppresses the development of Th2, whereas IL-4, IL-10 and IL-13, secreted by Th2 cells, inhibit Th1 responses (Fig 2).CD is thought to be associated with Th1 cell cytokines and inhibition of Th1 responses could represent a significant goal in the treatment of CD. Intestinal Th1 activation and cytokine release are associated with the generation of activated matrix metalloproteinases (MMPs), which are essential mediators of tissue destruction.

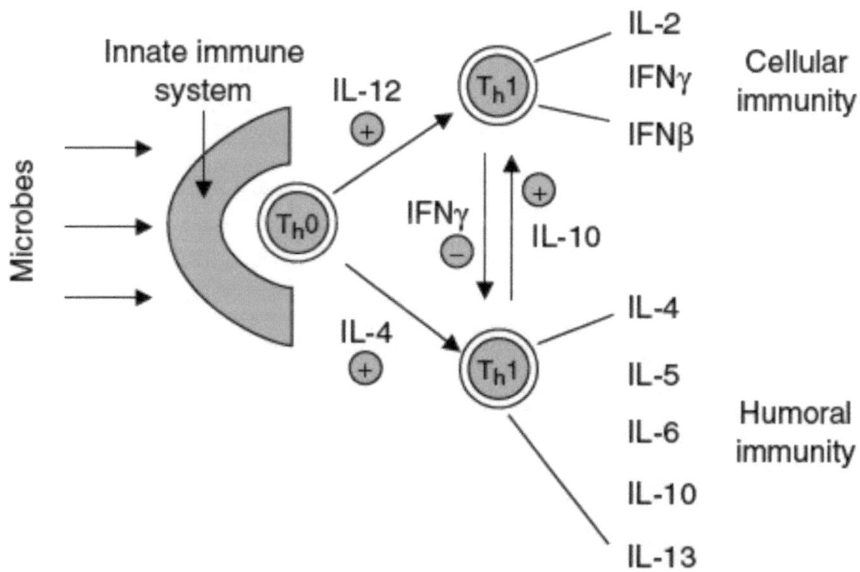

Fig. 2. T-helper (Th)-1 and Th2-mediated cytokine profiles and immune response. IL = interleukin; IFN = interferon (Ardizzone S, 2005).

2. Common categories of biological therapy

Traditionally, the therapeutic goals in CD include i induction of a rapid response, ii maintenance of glucocorticoid-free remission, iii minimization of complications and surgery, iv prevention of disease-related mortality, v improvement in patients' quality of life, vi minimization of the adverse effects of treatment, and vii the so-called 'deep remission' (i.e. simultaneous clinical, biological and endoscopic remission). Both mucosal healing and deep remission need to be evaluated for their prediction of long-term outcome and benefit/risk ratio if treatment escalation becomes necessary.

Existing CD therapies are an amalgamation of pharmacological agents including 5-aminosalicylate compounds, corticosteroids, and immunosuppressors (azathioprines, 6-mercaptopurine, methotrexate, tacrolimus and cyclosporine). Novel biological therapies have been developed in recent years based on better understanding of specific immunopathological processes in intestinal inflammation. There are several categories of biologic therapies that are relevant to CD: 1) antibody-based therapy (monoclonal antibodies, receptor fusion proteins, and soluble receptor antagonists), 2) recombinant cytokines, 3) nucleic acid-based therapies, 4) hormones and growth factors, 5) cell and gene therapy. At present, the biotechnology therapies that are being used in clinical practice or investigated for the treatment of CD are predominantly proteins, usually delivered intravenously or subcutaneously. The types of therapeutic proteins in used include recombinant human proteins with immunoregulatory effects, monoclonal antibodies (chimeric, humanized and fully human) and fusions proteins. Here we chose to focus on therapies that have been used in clinical trials in CD, some of which have been already or may be in the near future approved for commercial daily use (table 1).

Therapy	Target	Origin	Efficacy	Side effects
Inhibition of pro-inflammatory cytokines				
Infliximab	TNFα	Mouse/human chimeric mab	Safe, being used in treatment	Risk of malignancy and infection, infusion site reactions
Adalimumab		Human IgG1 mab	Safe, being used in treatment	Risk of malignancy and infection, infusion site reactions
CDP571		Fusion protein	Still in clinical trial	Risk of malignancy and infection, infusion site reactions
Onercept		Human soluble TNFα p55 receptor	Still in clinical trial	Local reaction
Etanercept		Fusion protein	Safe but ineffective in treatment CD	Itching, pain, swelling and redness at the site of injection
CDP-870		PEGylated anti-TNFα ab	Under clinical trial	No reported major side effects
IL-1 R ab	IL-1 R	Recombinant IL-1 R antagonist	No double placebo control tried yet	Not fully established
Anti-IL-6 R ab	IL-6 R	Human mab	Under clinical trial	Not fully established
Anti-IL-12 p40 ab	IL-12	Human mab	Safe and effective	Possible reactivation of asthma
Fontolizumab	IFNγ	Human mab	Under phase IIclinical trial	Not fully established

Supplementation of regulatory cytokines				
Tenovil	IL-10	Recombinant cytokine	Failed to show efficacy in phase II clinical trial	Reaction at injection site
Turbo probiotics	IL-10	Lactobacillus lactis	Effective in clinical study	Not fully established
IL-11	IL-11	Recombinant cytokine	No efficacy in phase II clinical trials	Not fully established
Inhibition of proliferation of T cells				
Visilizumab	CD3	Human ab	Under clinical trial	Not fully established
Daclizumab	αchain of IL-2R	Human mab	Failed to show efficacy in phase II clinical trial	Hypersensitivity
Basiliximab	α chain of IL-2R	Human mab	Under clinical trail	Mild dizziness, nausea, rashes on skin
Blocking molecule involved in leukocyte adhesion				
Natalizumab	Integrin-α4	Human mab	Approved by FDA	Sometimes causes fatal brain infection (progressive multifocal leukoencephalopathy)
MLN-02	α4β7integrin	Human mab	Under clinical trial	Infusion reaction
Supplementation of growth factor				
somatropin		Recombinant human growth hormone	Under clinical trial	Not intense severe adverse reactions
Nucleic acid based therapies				
alicaforsen	ICAM-1	Antisense phosphorothioat e oligonucleotide	Under phase III clinical trials	Not fully established
Recompositon of intestinal microflora				
Probiotics	Reconstituti on of commensal microbes	Combination of different bacteria	Under clinical trials	
helminthes	Inhibition of excessive immune response	Helminthes	Under clinical trials	Not fully established
Reconstitution of the immune system				
Hematopoietic stem cell transplantation	Replacement of defected hematolymp hatic cells	Infusion of the healthy hematopoietic cells	Under clinical trial	Toxic effects of high dose chemotherapy and post HCT infections

R: receptor; ab: antibody; mab: monoclonal antibody; ICAM-1: intracellular adhesion molecule-1

Table 1. Biological Therapies targeting different factors (Dharmani P, 2008)

3. Evaluations of biological treatment

3.1 Anti-TNF α therapies

Anti-TNFα mAb is the first agent that was approved for patients with persisting signs and symptoms of disease refractory impact in achieving new therapeutic goals. Till now, several anti-TNFα reagents have been developed and used to inhibit TNFα in patients with CD, including the mouse/human chimeric monoclonal antibody (infliximab), the humanized monoclonal antibody CDP571 and D2E7 (adalimumab), the human soluble TNFα p55 receptor (onercept), the p75 soluble TNFα receptor fusion protein (etanercept), and the polyethylene glycol (PEG)ylated anti-TNFα antibody fragment CDP-870 (certolizumab pegol). Peyrin B L and his colleagues performed a meta-analysis including 21 trials to evaluate safety and efficacy of tumor necrosis factor (TNF) antagonists for Crohn's disease (Peyrin-Biroulet L, 2008). They concluded that infliximab, adalimumab, and certolizumab are effective in luminal Crohn's disease. Efficacy of anti-TNF agents other than infliximab in treating fistulizing Crohn's disease requires additional investigations. Longer duration of following-up and larger number of patients are required to better assess the safety profile of TNF antagonists in CD. We also conducted a meta-analysis about anti-TNFα reagents treating CD. As a result, Fifteen RCTs articles with high quality were selected. Compared with placebo, anti-TNF-α agents achieved significantly higher rates of clinical response (44.9% *vs.* 30.0%, RR=1.39, 95% CI: 1.16~1.67, *P*=0.0004) and clinical remission (29.3% *vs.* 18.7%, RR=1.63, 95% CI: 1.26~2.09, *P*=0.0001). We concluded that Anti-TNF-α agents are superior to placebo in the treatment of CD and have similar risks of adverse events and serious adverse events. Long-term trials with large samples are needed for the assessment of its safety and tolerance. Table 2 lists the administrations of some of these agents.

3.1.1 Infliximab

Infliximab is the only biologic agent approved in the China, US and Europe for the treatment of patients with moderate to severe CD unresponsive to conventional therapy or a full and adequate course of corticosteroids and immunosuppressive therapy, and for patients with actively draining fistulas.

The first randomized placebo-controlled trial of infliximab focused on response rates 4 weeks after a single-blind infusion (Targan SR, 1997). All patients presented moderate to severely active disease despite other treatments or had previously been unresponsive to treatment with immunomodulators. A single infusion yielded a decrease in the CDAI of ≥70 points 4 weeks after infusion in 65% of the patients treated with infliximab, compared with a 17% response in the placebo group. The highest response rate was observed in patients receiving infliximab 5mg/kg (81%), with lower response rates in those treated with 10 or 20 mg/kg (50% and 64%, respectively).

Rutgeerts et al conducted a study to find out whether repeated infusions of infliximab could maintain the response (Rutgeerts P, 1999). Seventy-three patients were randomized to receive infliximab or placebo 10 mg/kg every 8 weeks for 36 weeks and were followed up until week 48. At week 44, 52.9% patients received infliximab achieved maintenance of remission, compared with 20% of placebo-treated patients. Quality of life was consistently better (using a inflammatory bowel disease questionnaire) and serum concentrations were maintained at remission levels.

The results were confirmed in the recent multicenter, randomized, placebo-controled, double-blind phase III clinical trial: the ACCENT I (A Crohn's disease Clinical trial Evaluating infliximab in a New long-term Treatment regimen) study (Hanaeur SB, 2002). Five hundred and seventy three patients with active CD received infliximab 5mg/kg at week 0 and were assessed of response at week 2. The responders were then randomized into

3 groups. Group I received placebo at week 2 and 6 and then every 8 weeks until week 46. Group II received 5mg/kg infliximab at the same time points. Group III received 5mg/kg infliximab at week 2 and 6, but followed by 10mg/kg every 8 weeks until week 46. The endpoints were the proportion of patients who responded at week 2 and were in remission (CDAI<150) at week 30, and the time to loss of response up to week 54 in patients who responded. At week 2, 335 patients (58%) responded to infliximab. At week 30, 23 of 110 (21%) patients in group I were in remission, compared with 44 of 113 (39%) in group II (P=0.003) and 50 of 112 (45%) in group III (P=0.0002). The study suggested that patients that were repeatedly administrated with infliximab every 8 weeks are more likely acquiring sustained clinical remission than those with single infusion. The safety was consistent with those in other clinical trials and serious infections were similar across the three groups.

	Infliximab	Adalimumab	Certolizumab pegol
Dosage	5 mg kg^{-1}	40 mg	400 mg
Route of administration	i.v.	s.c.	s.c.
Dosing intervals	8 weeks	2 weeks (e.o.w)	4 weeks
Induction	5 mg kg^{-1} weeks 0, 2, 6	168/80 mg (FDA) or 80/40 mg (EMA)	400 mg weeks 0, 2, 4
Dose escalation	10 mg kg^{-1} or every 4-6 weeks	40 mg e.w.	400 mg e. o. w.

i.v., intra venous; s.c., subcutaneous; e.w., every week; e.o.w., every other week; EMA, European Medicines Agency; FDA, Food and Drug Administration

Table 2. Administrationof biologicalagents in inflammatory bowel disease (Nielsen, 2011)

A study was conducted early in 1999 by Present DH, et al to investigate whether infliximab had the efficacy in healing enterocutaneous fistulas. In their study, 94 adult CD patients with fistulas were randomly assigned to receive placebo, 5mg/kg inflximab or 10mg/kg inflximab at weeks 0, 2 and 6. As a result, 55% patients assigned to receive 5mg/kg infliximab and 38% patients assigned to receive 10mg/kg infliximab had closure of all fistulas, as compared with 13% of the patients assigned to placebo. Adverse events were similar for the 5mg/kg infliximab group and the placebo group, but there was a trend toward more adverse events in the 10mg/kg group.

The multicenter, randomized, placebo-controlled ACCENT II trial further confirmed the efficacy of infliximab as maintenance therapy for fistulas in CD (Sands BE, 2002). After 14-week lead-in period, 195 of 282 (69%) patients responded. The responders were then randomized to receive either 5mg/kg infliximab or placebo every 8 weeks. Forty-eight percent of the infliximab group maintained fistula response at week 30 compared with 27% of the placebo group. At week 54, 36% of the infliximab group had a complete absence of draining fistulas compared with 19% of the placebo group.

Infliximab is also efficacy for patients who are intolerant of, resistant to or dependent on steroids. On study showed that of the first 100 patients administered infliximab, 29 of 40 (73%) were able to completely withdraw from steroids (Ricart E, 2001). At study entry in the ACCENT I, more than half of the patients were taking corticosteroids; one third of the patients receiving maintenance infliximab discontinued steroids and maintained clinical benefit.

There is also evidences that infliximab likely has a role in treating some extraintestinal manifestations, such as ankylosing spondylitism peripheral arthritis, pyoderma gangrenosum and erythema nodosum. CD patients are at increased risk of low bone mineral density (BMD), with reports of prevalence of osteopenia and osteoporosis as high as 50% and 10%, respectively. Infliximab may improve BMD in CD patients. A prospective study was conducted by Abreu et al to evaluate the effect of infliximab on surrogate markers of bone turnover in 38 CD patients. The data obtained demonstrated that bone synthesis markers were increased in the infliximab-treated patients (Abreu MT, 2006). Longer-term studies are needed to clarify the effect of infliximab on BMD.
Although efficacy of infliximab for the treatment of CD has clearly been demonstrated, serious side effects have been reported. In particular, these include acute infusion reactions, delayed hypersensitivity reactions, infections including reactivation of tuberculosis (TB), autoantibody formation, and a Lupus-like syndrome. Acute infusion reactions are adverse events that occur during infusion or within 2 hours after completion of the infusion. According to the manufacturer's drug insert, 22% of patients administered infliximab occurred compared with 9% of patients administered placebo (Lichtenstein GR, 2011). Delayed-hypersensitivity reactions can occur several days after infusion. Symptoms include severe pruritus, headaches, hand, facial or lip swelling, myalgias, rash, sore throat, and dysphagia. In the ACCENT I study, the frequency of delayed hypersensitivity reaction was 2%. Infections have been observed with pathogens, including viral, bacterial, fungal, and protozoal organisms. The majority of infections involved the respiratory and urinary tracts. Reactivation of latent TB after infusion with infliximab has occurred, mandating screening of patients for TB prior to infusion. A purified protein derivative (PPD) should be administered to all patients being considered for treatment with infliximab, with the results interpreted according to the risk atrata adapted from the American Thoracic Society (ATS), patients with a positive PPD should undergo a chest radiograph. Lymphoma has been reported in association with all 3 approved TNFα antagonists. A meta-analysis performed by Siegel et al suggested that the risk of lymphoma was increased in patients receiving infliximab for CD.
Since infliximab contains exogenous proteins, it can prompt the formation of antibodies-to-infliximab (ATIs) and thus may lead to the infusion reaction or loss of response. In ACCENT I trial, 64/442 (14.5%) developed antibodies. Patients administered a single dose of infliximab had higher incidence of ATI formation than those administered scheduled maintenance regiments of 5 or 10 mg/kg (28% vs 9% and 6%, respectively). The clinical response rates were similar in the patients regardless of their ATI status. The infusion reactions were more common in the ATI-positive patients compared with the ATI-negative group (16% vs 8%). The majority of the infusion reactions were mild to moderate.

3.1.2 Adalimumab

Adalimumab (first named D2E7) is a subcutaneously administered, recombinant, fully human, IgG1 monoclonal antibody that binds with high affinity and specificity to human TNFα, thus modulating its biologic functions by blocking the interaction with p55 and p75 cell surface TNF receptors. It is available in a number of countries, including the US and EU countries.
In CD, adalimumab has received both FDA and EMEA approval with the following indications: 1) for reducing the signs and symptoms and inducing and maintaining clinical

remission in adults with moderately to severely active CD who have had an inadequate response to conventional therapy, and 2) for reducing the signs and symptoms and inducing clinical remission in these patients if they have also lost response or are intolerant to IFX.
Therefore, adalimumab is the second biologic therapy approved for the treatment of patients with moderately to severely active CD. Adalimumab is administered by subcutaneous injection, as commercially available prefilled pen (HUMIRA Pen) containing 0.8 mL (40 mg) of drug.
The recommended adalimumab induction dose regimen for adult patients with moderate-severe CD is usually 80 mg at week 0 followed by 40 mg at week 2. In case there is a need for a more rapid response to therapy, the regimen with 160 mg at week 0 (dose can be administered as 4 injections in one day or as 2 injections per day for 2 consecutive days) and 80 mg at week 2 can be used with the awareness that the risk for adverse events is higher during induction. After induction treatment, the recommended dose is 40 mg every other week via subcutaneous injection as maintenance treatment. For induction treatment, adalimumab should be given in combination with corticosteroids. Adalimumab can be given as monotherapy in case of intolerance to corticosteroids or when continued treatment with corticosteroids is inappropriate (Cassinotti A, 2008).
In a phase III, placebo-controlled, dose-ranging induction trial named CLASSIC I (CLinical Assessment of adalimumab Safety and efficacy Studied as Induction therapy in Crohn's disease), 299 patients with moderate to severe CD, naive to anti-TNF therapy were randomized to 4 groups. Patients in group I received adalimumab 40mg at week 0 and 20mg at week 2; patients in group II received adalimumab 80mg at week 0 and 40mg at week 2; patients in group III received adalimumab 160mg at week 0 and 80mg at week 2; patients in group IV received placebo at the same points. All the patients were followed through week 4. A response was defined as a CDAI score reduction of ≥70 points (70-point response) or of ≥100 points (100-point response) from week 0, while remission was defined as a CDAI score <150. At week 4, patients in group II and group III showed a significantly greater remission rate (24% and 36%) than patients in group IV (12%) (P=0.004 among the 3 groups). There was a linear dose response across the 3 adalimumab treatment groups at week 4 for the endpoints of remission and 100-point response, with only the highest dose group demonstrating statistical significance in the pairwise comparisons with placebo: 36% vs 12% for remission (p = 0.001) and 50% vs 25% (p = 0.002) for the 100-point response; the 70-point response was also significantly higher in the adalimumab recipients than placebo, both for the 160/80 mg dosage (59% vs 37%; p = 0.007) and for the 80/40 mg group (59% vs 37%; p = 0.01). The reduction of CDAI from baseline was evident as early as week 1. Only 11% (32/299) of the randomized patients had draining enterocutaneous or perianal fistulas at baseline and were unevenly distributed across the treatment groups. The rates of fistula improvement and remission for the ADA-treated patients and those receiving placebo were not significantly different, but the number of these patients precluded a powered analysis (Hanauer SB, 2006).
A total of 276 patients who completed the 4-week CLASSIC-I trial entered a long-term extension study named CLASSIC-II (Sandborn WJ, 2007). This was a randomized, placebo-controlled, maintenance follow-up trial, demonstrating that adalimumab 40 mg every other week or weekly was superior to placebo in maintaining remission for 1 year in patients with moderate to severe CD naive to anti-TNF agents who achieved remission with adalimumab induction therapy.

Eligible patients (belonging to the pool of CLASSIC-I enrolled patients) were treated with adalimumab 40 mg at week 0 (corresponding to week 4 of CLASSIC-I) and week 2. Those in remission at both week 0 and week 4 (n = 55) were randomized to receive adalimumab 40 mg every other week (n = 19), adalimumab 40 mg weekly (n = 18), or placebo (n = 18), through 56 weeks.
At week 56, remission was maintained in 79%, 83%, and 44% of patients in the respective groups (primary endpoint), with a statistically significant difference between each adalimumab group and placebo ($p< 0.05$). The 100-point response at week 56 was also better in adalimumab recipients (79% vs 89% vs 56%, respectively), as was the 70-point response rates (79% vs 89% vs 72%), although differences between groups were not statistically significant.

3.1.3 CDP571

CDP571 was a humanised monoclonal antibody to human TNF-α. It was constructed by linking the complementarity determining regions (CDR) of a murine antihuman TNF monoclonal antibody to a human IgG4 antibody. A total number of 396 patients with moderate to severe CD were included in a randomized, double blind and placebo controlled trial in 2004. The patients were received intravenous 10mg/kg CDP571 or placebo every 8 weeks to week 24 and were followed up to week 28. Clinical response was defined as a decrease in the CDAI to ≥ 100 points or remission (CDAI score ≤ 150 points) at week 28. Initial clinical response occurred in 90/263 (34.2%) CDP571 patients and 28/32 (21.2%) placebo patients (P=0.011). At week 28, 80/263 (30.4%) CDP571 patients and 31/132 (23.5%) placebo patients achieved clinical response (P=0.102). Adverse events were similar in both groups. A *post hoc* analysis of a subgroup of patients with CRP concentrations ≥ 10mg/L demonstrated significantly increased response rates for CDP571 10mg/kg at both week 2 and 28 (Sandborn WJ, 2004). Two controlled trials failed to demonstrate a steroid-sparing benefit of CDP571 in patients with steroid-dependent CD. Further clinical development of CDP571 for the treatment of CD has been discontinued.

3.1.4 Certolizumab pegol

Certolizumab pegol (CDP870) is a humanized TNFα Fab monoclonal antibody fragment linked to polyethylene glycol that is administered subcutaneously. A phase III, randomized, double-blind, multicenter study that assessed the efficacy and tolerability of certolizumab in patients with moderate to severe CD showed a modest improvement in response rates, as compared with placebo but no significant improvement in remission rates (Sandborn WJ, 2007). In addition, patients who had a response to induction therapy with certolizumab were more likely to have maintained response and remission at 26 weeks with continued treatment compared with a switch to placebo.

3.2 Other novel biological therapies

3.2.1 Natalizumab

Natalizumab is a recombinant humanized monoclonal antibody IgG4, with a molecular weight of 149 kDa. It contains 95% human peptide sequences and only 5% mouse sequences in the complementary determining regions. It inhibits both α4β7-integrin/MAdCAM-1 interaction and α4β1/VCAM-1 binding.
ENACT-1 (Efficacy of Natalizumab as Active Crohn's Therapy) is a randomized double-blind, placebo-controlled Phase III trial (Sandborn WJ, 2005), in which 905 patients were

randomly assigned in a 4:1 ratio to receive an intravenous infusion of 300mg natalizumab or placebo at week 0, 4 and 8. The patients were then followed until week 12. The primary end point was the proportion of patients who had a clinical response (ΔCDAI score ≥70 points). No difference in the response remission (CDAI < 150) rates was seen between the natalizumab group and the placebo group (P=0.051 and P=0.12, respectively). A significant difference of CRP was present in the subgroup of 660 patients who had a baseline CRP level more than 2.87 mg/l compared with the placebo group.

The patients who responded in the ENACT-1 trial were randomly reassigned in a 1:1 ration to receive either natalizumab 300mg intravenously every 4 weeks or placebo and were followed up to 36 weeks (ENACT-2) (Sandborn WJ, 2004). At week 36, 61% of natalizumab patients had a sustained response compared with 28% in the placebo group (P<0.001). The remission rates was also significantly higher in the natalizumab group (44%) than in the placebo group (26%) at week 36 (P=0.003). Forty five percent of patients in the natalizumab group were no longer taking corticosteroids and remained in remission at week 36 compared with 22% of patients in the placebo group (P=0.003).

Natalizumab should not be given with immunomodulators (e.g.6-mercaptopurine, azathioprine, cyclosporine or methotrexate) or inhibitors of TNF-a. Corticosteroids should be tapered.

Natalizumab is not approved in Europe for the treatment of CD. It is available in the USA under a special restricted distribution program called CD-TOUCH (Tysabri® outreach unified commitment for health). Under this program, prescribers, pharmacies, infusion centers and patients are made aware of risks of opportunistic infections, including PML. Patients are evaluated 3 months after the first infusion, 6 months after the first infusion and every 6 months thereafter. Any serious opportunistic or atypical infections are reported (Bickston SJ, 2010).

3.2.2 Fontolizumab

Fontolizumab is a humanized IgG1 antibody with high binding affinity and specificity for IFNγ By inhibiting the binding of IFNγ to its cellular receptor, fontolizumab prevents downstream physiologic effects, such as expression of major histocompatibility complex class II molecules.

In a Phase II, randomized, double-blind, placebo-controlled study, 201 patients with CDAI scores between 250 and 450 were randomized to receive an initial intravenous dose of 1.0 or 4.0 mg/kg fotolizumab or placebo, and then were received 0.1 or 1.0 mg/kg fontolizumab or placebo every 4 weeks. The primary endpoint of efficacy evaluations was the proportion of patients who achieved a clinical response (defined as a decrease in the CDAI of ≥100 points from baseline levels without an accompanying increase in dose of concomitant medications for CD) by day 29. Secondary endpoints were clinical response rates on days 43, 57, 85, 113, and at the 3-month follow-up visit. The response rates were similar in all treatment groups (31%-38%) at day 29. At subsequent timepoints a significantly greater proportion of patients in the 1.0 mg/kg intravenous / 1.0 mg/kg subcutaneous fontolizumab group had clinical response and significantly greater improvement in the CDAI score compared with patients who received placebo. The CRP levels were significantly improved in the fontolizumab groups. The overall frequency of adverse events was similar in all groups (58%-75%) (Reinisch W, 2010). Further clinical studies with fontolizumab for the induction and maintenance of remission in patients with CD are anticipated.

3.2.3 Anti-IL-12 P40 antibody

IL-12 is a heterodimeric molecule composed of IL-12 p40 and IL-12 p35 subunits. The p40 subunit is also a component of IL-23, in which p40 forms a heterodimer with a p19 subunit. IL12/23 is a key cytokine in the Th1/Th17 development and is abundantly produced in the gut of CD patients. IL-12 p40 is, therefore, a pivotal target for the treatment of CD.

A double-blind, placebo controlled randomized study of a humanized IgG1 monoclonal antibody against IL-12 p40 (ABT-874) was performed in 79 patients with active CD (Mannon PJ, 2004). The patients were randomized to receive seven weekly injections of 1 or 3 mg/kg anti-IL-12 or placebo subcutaneously either with or without 4 wk intervals between the first two injections. The patients who received 3 mg/kg anti-IL-12 for 7 wk showed a significantly greater clinical response rate than the patients treated with a placebo (75% *vs* 25%). The production Th1 proinflammatory cytokines from patient's colonic lamina propria mononuclear cells dramatically decreased after the anti IL-12 therapy. The most frequent adverse event was a local reaction at the injection site, which was observed with a greater rate in the anti IL-12 treated group than in the placebo-treated group. No serious side effects were observed during the anti-12 therapy. Anti IL-12 therapy is therefore considered to be a safe and effective treatment for active CD.

4. Conclusion

There are multiple biological therapies based on different targets in addition to those we introduced above. More clinical studies for the efficacy and safety should be conducted. Overall, the biological treatments differ from conventional CD therapy in several aspects: They are usually peptides or proteins; are administered parenterally; target specific molecules, cells, or processes; and their manufacture is more sophisticated and more expensive than the conventional drugs. The development of biological therapies is based on better understanding of mucosal intestinal processes in homeostasis and uncontrolled inflammation and is possible due to great biotechnological progress such as genetic engineering and development of novel vehicles.

5. Acknowledgment

We acknowledge Dr. Jingjing Lian for the efforts of the literature retrieval and the works of meta-analysis of efficacy of anti-TNF reagents in patients with active CD.

6. References

Abreu MT, Kam LY, Vasiliauskas EA, Kam Ly, Vora P, Martyak LA, Yang H, Ju B, Lin YC, Keenan G, Price J, Landers CJ, Adams JS & Targan SR. (2006) Treatment with infliximab is associated with increased markers of bone synthesis in patients with Crohn's disease. *Journal of Clinical Gastroenterology*. Vol.40, No.1, (January, 2006), pp. 55-63, ISSN 0192-0790

Ardizzone S & Porro GB. (2005). Biologic therapy for inflammatory bowel disease. *Drugs*. Vol.65, No.16, pp. 2253-2286

Bickston SJ & Muniyappa K. (2010). Natalizumab for the treatment of Crohn's disease. *Expert Review of Clinical Immunology*. Vol.6, No.4, (July, 2010), pp. 513-519, ISSN 1744-8409

Cassinotti A, Ardizzone S & Porro GB. (2008). Adalimumab for the treatment of Crohn's disease. *Biologics: Targets & Therapy*. Vol.2, No.4, (December, 2008), pp. 763-777, ISSN 1177-5491

Dharmani P & Chadee K. (2008). Biologic therapies against inflammatory bowel disease: a dysregulated immune system and the cross talk with gastrointestinal mucosa hold the key. *Current Molecular Pharmacology*. Vol.1, No.3, (November, 2008), pp. 195-212, ISSN 1874-4702

Hanauer SB, Feagan BG, Lichtenstein GR, Mayer LF, Schreiber S, Colombel JF, Rachmilewitz D, Wolf DC, Olson A, Bao W & Rutgeerts P. (2002). Maintenance infliximab for Crohn's disease: the ACCENT I randomized trial. *Lancet*. Vol.359, No.9317, (May, 2002), pp. 1541-1549, ISSN 1474-547X

Hanauer SB, Sandborn WJ, Rutgeerts P, Fodorak RN, Lukas M, MacIntosh D, Panaccione R, Wolf D & Pollack P. (2006). Human anti-tumor necrosis factor monoclonal antibody (adalimumab) in Crohn's disease: the CLASSIC-I trial. *Gastroenterology*. Vol.130, No.2, (February, 2006), pp. 323-333, ISSN 0016-5085

Lichtenstein GR. (2011) *Crohn's disease: the complete guide to medical management*. SLACK Incorporated. ISBN 978-1-55642-944-6, Thorofare, NJ, USA.

Mannon PJ, Fuss IJ, Mayer L, Elson CO, Sandborn WJ, Present D, Dolin B, Goodman N, Groden C, Hornung RL, Quezado M, Yang Z, Neurath MF, Salfeld J, Veldman GM, Schwertschlag U & Strober W. (2004). Anti-interleukin-12 antibody for active Crohn's disease. *The New England Journal of Medicine*. Vol.352, No.20, (November, 2004), pp. 21-31, ISSN 1533-4406

Nielsen OH, Seidelin JB, Munck LK & Rogler G. (2011). Use of biological molecules in the treatment of inflammatory bowel disease. *Journal of Internal Medicine*. Vol.270, No.1, (July, 2011), pp. 15-28, ISSN 1365-2796

Peyrin-Biroulet L, Deltenre P, Suray ND, et al. Efficacy and safety of tumor necrosis factor antagonists in Crohn's disease: meta-analysis of placebo-controlled trials. *Clinical Gastroenterology & Hepatology*. Vol. 6, No.6, (June 2008): pp. 644-653. ISSN 1542-3565

Present DH, Rutgeerts P, Targan S, Hanauer SB, Mayer L, van Hogezand RA, Podolsky DK, Sands BE, Braakman T, Dewoody KL, Schaible TF, & van Deventer SJ. (1999). Infliximab for the treatment of fistulas in patients with Crohn's disease. *The New England Journal of Medicine*. Vol.340, No.18, (May, 1999), pp. 1398-1405, ISSN 1533-4406

Recart E, Panaccione R, Loftus E, Tremaine W & Sandborn W. (2001). Infliximab for Crohn's disease in clinical practice at the Mayo Clinic: the first 100 patients. *The American Journal of Gastroenterology*. Vol. 86, No.3, (March, 2001), pp. 722-729, ISSN 0002-9270

Reinisch W, Villier W, Bene L, Silmon L, Racz I, Katz S, Altorjay I, Feagan B, Riff D, Bernstein CN, Hommes D, Rutgeerts P, Cortot A, Gaspari M, Cheng M, Pearce T & Sands BE. (2010). Fontolizumab in moderate to severe Crohn's disease: a phase 2, randomized, double-blind, placebo-controlled, multiple-dose study. *Inflammatory Bowel Disease*. Vol.16, No.2, (February, 2010), pp. 233-242 ISSN 1536-4844

Rutgeerts P, D'Haens G, Targan S, Vasiliauskas E, Haunauer SB, Present DH, Mayer L, Van Hogezand RA, Braakman T, Dewoody KL, Schaible TF & van Deventer SJ. (1999). Efficacy and safety of retreatment with anti-tumor necrosis factor antibody (infliximab) to maintain remission in Crohn's disease. *Gastroenterology*. Vol.117, No.4, (October, 1999), pp. 761-769, ISSN 0016-5085

Sandborn WJ, Feagan BG, Radford-Smith G, Kovacs A, Innes A & Patel J. (2004). CDP571, a humanised monoclonal antibody to tumour necrosis factor α, for moderate to severe Crohn's disease: a randomised, double blind, placebo controlled trial. *Gut.* Vol.53, No.10, (October, 2004), pp. 1485-1493, ISSN 1468-3288

Sandborn WJ, Colombel JF, Enns R, Feagan B, Hananer S, Lawrance I, Panaccione R, Sanders M, Schreiber S, Targan S, Deventer SV & Rutgeerts P. (2004). A phase III, double blind, placebo-controlled study of the efficacy, safety, and tolerability of antegren (Natalizumab) in maintaining clinical response and remission in Crohn's disease (ENACT-2). (Abstract). *Gastroenterology.* Vol.127, No.1, (July, 2004), pp. 332, ISSN 0016-5085

Sandborn WJ, Colombel JF, Enns R, Feagan B, Hanauer S, Lawrance IC, Panaccione R, Sanders M, Schreiber S, Targan S, Deventer SV, Goldblum R, Despain D, Hogge GS & Rutgeerts P. (2005). Natalizumab induction and maintenance therapy for Crohn's disease. *The New England Journal of Medicine.* Vol.353, No.3, (November, 2005), pp. 1912-1925, ISSN 1533-4406

Sandborn WJ, Hanauer SB, Rutgeerts P, Fedorak RN, Lukas M, Maclntosh DG, Panaccione R, Wolf D, Kent JD, Bittle B, Li J & Pollack PF. (2007). Adalimumab for maintenance treatment of Crohn's disease: results of the CLASSIC II trial. *Gut.* Vol.56, No.9, (September, 2007), pp. 1232-1239, ISSN 1468-3288

Sandborn WJ, Feagan BG, Stoinov S, Honiball PJ, Rutgeerts P, Mason D, Bloomfield R & Schreiber S. (2007). Certolizumab pegol for the treatment of Crohn's disease. *The New England Journal of Medicine.* Vol.357, No.19, (July, 2007), pp. 228-238, ISSN 1533-4406

Sands BE, Van Deventer S, Bernstein C, et al. (2002). Long-term treatment of fistulizing Crohn's disease: response to infliximab in the ACCENT II trial through 54 weeks. *Gastroenterology.* Vol.122, supplement 4, (April, 2002), pp. A81, ISSN 0016-5085

Schreiber S, Khaliq-Kareemi M, Lawrance IC, Gazelle GS, Sands BE, Thomsen OO, Hanauer SB, McColm J Bloomfield R & Sandborn WJ. (2007). Maintenance therapy with certolizumab pegol for Crohn's disease. *The New England Journal of Medicine.* Vol.357, No.19, (July, 2007), pp. 239-250, ISSN 1533-4406

Siegel CA, Hur C, Korzenik JR, Gazelle GS & Sands BE. (2006). Risks and benefits of infliximab for the treatment of Crohn's disease. *Clinical Gastroenterology and Hepatology.* Vol.4, No.8, (August, 2006), pp. 1017-1024, ISSN 1542-3565

Targan SR, Haunauer SB, van Deventer SJH, Mayer L, Present DH, Braakman J, Dewoody KL, Schaible TF& Rutgeerts PJ. (1997). A short-term study of chimeric monoclonal antibody cA2 to tumor necrosis factor α for Crohn's disease. *The New England Journal of Medicine.* Vol.337, No9, (October, 1997), pp. 1029-1035, ISSN 1533-4406

11

Minimally Invasive Surgical Treatment in Crohn's Disease

Antonino Spinelli, Piero Bazzi, Matteo Sacchi and Marco Montorsi
Dept. and Chair of General Surgery, University of Milano, Istituto Clinico Humanitas IRCCS, Rozzano Milano Italy

1. Introduction

Crohn's disease is a chronic and idiopathic inflammation that can affect any part of the gastrointestinal tract and the terminal ileum is the most frequently involved site; moreover, the first peak of the disease is between 20 and 30 years of age. Surgery plays a very important role in its management: the lifetime risk of surgery is about 70% - 90% [1], for its complications or failure of medical treatment and the reoperation rate is approximately 40% - 50% within 10-15 years after the first operation [2].

Laparoscopic colorectal surgery began in the early 90's; nowadays the equipment development, the surgeons experience and the results of clinical trials lead to affirm the feasibility and safety of laparoscopic surgery, which should be considered as the first line surgical approach in selected patients. In fact, a less surgical trauma should lead to a better preservation of immune response, better cosmetic result, less post-operative pain and faster return of bowel functionality with faster hospital discharge [3].

2. Primary small bowel Crohn's disease

Several studies, including four randomized trials [4-7] and three meta-analyses [8-10], demonstrated the benefits of laparoscopic approach in the surgical path of small bowel Crohn's disease, regarding short-term outcomes like post-operative pain and analgesics use, complication rates, return to normal bowel habitus, hospital stay and cosmesis. For these reasons, laparoscopic procedure in primary Crohn's disease is nowadays worldwide considered the first choice surgical treatment.

Many studies showed laparoscopy is less painful than open surgery and requires less analgesics consumption [11-15].

The reduction of post-operative pain leads to a faster mobilization of patients and to an improvement of pulmonary function [17]: these are very important factors to obtain lower rates of general complications [18] and a smoother recovery.

Benefits of laparoscopic surgery could include lower morbidity, a significantly faster resumption of bowel function and a shorter hospital stay [4,6,19-23]. It is well known that the use of opiate analgesics negatively affects recovery of gastrointestinal function [24]: laparoscopic approach, due to both a limited wound extension and tissue handling, leads to a reduction of post-operative pain, morphine supply and to a quick resolution of paralytic ileus and discharge from hospital, respectively.

Furthermore, laparoscopic surgery improves cosmesis and might induce less adhesions [25]: this is very important, because patients are generally young and the reoperations are common.

It has been demonstrated that the introduction of a fast-track perioperative care program, also referred to as enhanced recovery after surgery (*ERAS*) [26, 27], may reduce hospital stay to 2-3 days after open colorectal surgery [28, 29], even if high readmission rates are reported [28, 30]. Only few studies have evaluated the role of laparoscopic approach combined to fast-track protocols in enhancing recovery after colorectal surgery, obtaining conflicting results: Basse *et al.* [31] found no difference between fast-track patients undergone to laparoscopic or open resection, while King *et al.* [32] found a significant reduction of the hospital stay in fast-track patients after laparoscopic surgery. The only randomized, multicentric clinical trial (LAFA-study) [33] investigating both surgical techniques (laparoscopic and open) combined with fast-track and standard care demonstrated that the best option is laparoscopic resection embedded in a fast-track care; nevertheless, this study focused on colon cancer, so these results have not yet been validated in patients with inflammatory bowel disease.

The mean conversion rate reported in the current literature is 11,2% and it ranges from 4,8% to 29,2% [8] .

As already reported in some studies [6, 34,35] , the duration of laparoscopic ileocolic resection's laparoscopic surgery can be very similar to open surgery after completion of the learning curve by the surgical team.

It has been demonstrated the safety of laparoscopic ileocolectomy also in the long-term outcomes; Eshuis and colleagues [36] showed no differences with open surgery regarding reoperations for disease recurrence and non-disease related complications.

3. Recurrent small bowel Crohn's disease

While for primary laparoscopic ileocolectomy there are many clinical trials demonstrating short and long-term benefits, in the current literature there are only a few studies investigating the feasibility and safety of laparoscopic resection for recurrent disease [37-41] , often considering small sample size. Recently Chaudhray and colleagues [42] reported one of the largest series of patients who underwent laparoscopic ileocolonic resection for recurrent Crohn's disease, demonstrating the same benefits observed after primary resection without increased complication rates or delayed discharge. Although longer operating time, conversion rate was similar to that reported after primary resection.

In conclusion, more contributions with larger sample size are needed to go deeper into this topic, but laparoscopic approach in recurrent Crohn's disease should not be avoided in principle, because despite high technical difficulty in expert hands can be feasible, safe and lead to significant advantages in the postoperative time.

4. Crohn's colitis

Terminal ileitis is the most frequent presentation of Crohn's disease and more rarely, in about 30% of cases, patients have a disease affecting the colon with or without rectal involvement.

While for small bowel Crohn's disease laparoscopic technique has been worldwide adopted and its benefits well established, in the present literature only a few studies investigated the role of laparoscopy in the surgical treatment of Crohn's colitis.
The largest series of laparoscopic colectomies for Crohn's disease has been recently reported by Holubar and colleagues [43] from the Mayo Clinic: 92 patients underwent mini-invasive colectomies with short postoperative length of stay and low morbidity, confirming previous results obtained by other Authors [44,45] . Umanskiy and coworkers [45] also demonstrated reduced operative times: this result can be attributed to the high experience reached by the surgeons, but also to a selection bias of the patients due to non-randomized inclusion criteria of the laparoscopic group.
Ultimately, laparoscopic approach is feasible and safe in patients with Crohn's colitis and can improve surgical outcome when performed by experienced hands in selected cases; however, these findings must be supported by more contributions and are not yet validated by randomized-controlled trials.

5. Gastroduodenal Crohn's disease

It is a rare conditions that affect up to 4% of patients with Crohn'disease; it can be an asyntomatic endoscopic finding or a clinical-radiological disease where obstruction is the most frequent presentation. Medical therapy with PPI and steroids or immunosuppressive agents is the current management but sometimes surgery is necessary because of its failure; gastrojejunal bypass and stricturoplasty are the validated surgical options. Because this type of disease and surgical procedures are very uncommon there is lack of experience in the current literature regarding laparoscopic approach in the surgical treatment of gastroduodenal Crohn's disease; in 2008, Shapiro and coworkers from The Mount Sinai Medical Center [46] published the first experience of 13 laparoscopic gastrojejunal bypass, reporting less morbidity rates and shorter length of stay than after open surgery.
To date, probably due to the rarity of the disease and limited number of operations, no more clinical trials supported these findings and no certain conclusions about benefits of laparoscopic procedures in gastroduodenal Crohn's disease can be drawn.

6. New technical aspects

Single-incision laparoscopic surgery

Single-incision laparoscopic surgery was born in the beginning of the Nineties when the first appendectomy and cholecystectomy were performed with the aim of minimizing the surgical incisions and morbidity rates, improving cosmesis and short term outcomes respect to standard laparoscopic procedures. However, this technique developed slowly and only in the last years it has been kept in attention by the surgeons and started to be applied to the main operations of general, urologic and gynaecologic surgery. Recently has been published the initial experience of single-incision laparoscopic segmental colectomy and ileocolic resection for Crohn's disease [47,48], with longer operative time but similar morbidity rates and length of stay compared to laparoscopic assisted procedures. Single-incision laparoscopic colectomy seems to be feasible and safe when performed by experts laparoscopic surgeons after completion of an additional learning curve, and must be validated by further clinical trial.

Laparoscopic resection with transcolonic specimen extraction

Eshuis and colleagues [49] reported a series of ten patients affected by Crohn's disease who underwent to entirely laparoscopic ileocolic resection with endoscopic transcolonic specimen removal. The procedure was possible only for small inflammatory mass (<7-8 cm) and needed longer operative time; infectious complications were high with 2 intraabdominal abscesses and patients did not perceived benefits in terms of body image respect to conventional laparoscopic surgery. Thus, based on these findings, benefits of laparoscopic resection followed by endoscopic transcolonic specimen extraction are unclear and the technique doesn't seem as safe as conventional laparoscopic surgery.

7. References

[1] Milsom JW. Laparoscopic surgery in the treatment of Crohn's disease. Surg Clin North Am 2005; 85: 25-34.

[2] Hasegawa H, Watanabe M, Nishibori H, Okabayashi K, Hibi T, Kitajima M. Laparoscopic surgery for recurrent Crohn's disease. Br J Surg 2003; 90: 970-973.

[3] Casillas S, Delaney CP. Laparoscopic surgery for inflammatory bowel disease. Dig Surg 2005; 22: 135-142.

[4] Bemelman WA, Slors JF, Dunker MS *et al.* Laparoscopic-assisted vs open ileocolic resection for Crohn's disease – a comparative study. Surg Endosc 2000; 14: 721-725.

[5] Milsom JW, Hammerhofer KA, Bohm B *et al.* Prospective, randomized trial comparing laparoscopic vs conventional surgery for refractory ileocolic Crohn's disease. Dis Colon Rectum 2001; 44: 1-8.

[6] Benoist S, Panis Y, Beaufour A, Bouhnik Y, Matuchansky C, Valleur P. Laparoscopic ileocecal resection in Crohn's disease – a case-matched comparison with open resection. Surg Endosc 2003; 17: 814-818.

[7] Maartense S, Dunker MS, Slors FM *et al.* Laparoscopic-assisted versus open ileocolic resection for Crohn's disease – a randomized trial - . Ann Surg 2006; 243: 143-149.

[8] Tan JJY, Tjandra JJ. Laparoscopic surgery for Crohn's disease: a meta-analysis. Dis Colon Rectum 2007; 50(1): 1-10.

[9] Dosman AS, Melis M, Fichera A. Metaanalysis of trials comparing laparoscopic and open surgery for Crohn's disease. Surg Endosc 2005; 19: 1549-1555.

[10] Tilney HS, Constantinides VA, Heriot AG *et al.* Comparison of laparoscopic and open ileocecal resection for Crohn's disease: a meta analysis. Surg Endosc 2006; 20:1036-1044.

[11] Schwenk W, Bohm B, Muller JM. Postoperative pain and fatigue after laparoscopic or conventional colorectal resections. A prospective randomized trial. Surg Endosc 1998; 12(9): 1131-1136.

[12] Braga M, Vignali A, Zuliani W *et al.* Metabolic and functional results after laparoscopic colorectal surgery: a randomized, controlled trial. Dis Colon Rectum 2002; 45(8): 1070-1077.

[13] Lezoche E, Feliciotti F, Paganini AM, Guerrieri M, Campagnacci R, De Sanctis A. Laparoscopic colonic resections versus open surgery: a prospective non-randomized study on 310 unselected cases. Hepatogastroenterology 2000; 47: 697-708.

[14] Danelli G, Berti M, Perotti V *et al.* Temperature control and recovery of bowel function after laparoscopic or laparotomic colorectal surgery in patients receiving combined epidural/general anesthesia and postoperative epidural analgesia. Anesth Analg 2002; 95(2): 467-71, table of contents.
[15] Schwenk W, Haase O, Neudecker J, Müller JM (2005). Short term benefits for laparoscopic colorectal resection. The Cochrane Database of Systematic Reviews, Issue 2. Art. No.: CD003145. DOI: 10.1002/14651858.CD003145.pub2, April 20, 2005.
[16] Ekstein P, Szold A, Sagie B, Werbin N, Klausner JM, Weinbroum AA. Laparoscopic surgery may be associated with severe pain and high analgesia requirements in the immediate postoperative period. Ann Surg 2006; 243: 41-46.
[17] Schwenk W, Bohm B, Witt C *et al.* Pulmonary function following laparoscopic or conventional colorectal resection: a randomized controlled evaluation. Arch Surg 1999; 134 (1): 6-12.
[18] Boni L, Benevento A, Rovera F *et al.* Infective complications in laparoscopic surgery. Surg Infect (Larchmt) 2006; 7 Suppl 2: S109-111.
[19] Kirat HT, Pokala N, Vogel JD *et al.* Can laparoscopic ileocolic resection be performed with comparable safety to open surgery for regional enteritis: data from National Surgical Quality Improvement Program. Am Surg 2010; 76(12): 1393-1396.
[20] Duepree HJ, Senagore AJ, Delaney CP, Brady KM, Fazio VW. Advantages of laparoscopic resection for ileocecal Crohn's disease. Dis Colon Rectum 2002; 45: 605-610.
[21] Schwenk W, Bohm B, Haase O, Junghans T, Muller JM. Laparoscopic versus conventional colorectal resection: a prospective randomised study of postoperative ileus and early postoperative feeding. Langenbecks Arch Surg 1998; 383(1): 49-55.
[22] Msika S, Iannelli A, Deroide G *et al.* Can laparoscopy reduce hospital stay in the treatment of Crohn's disease? Dis Colon Rectum 2001; 44: 1661-1666.
[23] Salimath J, Jones MW, Hunt DL, Lane MK. Comparison of return of bowel function and length of stay in patients undergoing laparoscopic versus open colectomy. JSLS 2007; 11: 72-75.
[24] Luckey A, Livingston E, Tache Y. Mechanisms and treatment of postoperative ileus. Arch Surg 2003; 138(2): 206-214.
[25] Zmora O. Laparoscopy for Crohn's disease. Semin Laparosc Surg 2003; 10: 159-167.
[26] Wilmore DW, Kehlet H. Management of patients in fast track surgery. BMJ 2001; 322(7284): 473-476.
[27] Fearon KC, Ljungqvist O, Von Meyenfeldt M *et al.* Enhanced recovery after surgery: a consensus review of clinical care for patients undergoing colonic resection. Clin Nutr 2005; 24(3): 466-477.
[28] Basse L, Thorbol JE, Lossl K, Kehlet H. Colonic surgery with accelerated rehabilitation or conventional care. Dis Colon Rectum 2004; 47: 271-278.
[29] Andersen J, Kehlet H. Fast track open ileo-colic resections for Crohn's disease. Colorectal Disease 2005; 7: 394-397.
[30] Kariv Y, Delaney CP, Senagore AJ *et al.* Clinical outcomes and cost analysis of a "fast track" postoperative care pathway for ileal pouch-anal anastomosis. A case control study. Dis Colon Rectum 2006; 50: 137-146.
[31] Basse L, Jakobsen DH, Bardram L *et al.* Functional recovery after open versus laparoscopic colonic resection: a randomized blinded study. Ann Surg 2005; 241: 416-423.

[32] King PM, Blazeby JM, Edwings P *et al.* Randomized clinical trial comparing laparoscopic and open surgery for colorectal cancer within an enhanced recovery programme. Br J Surg 2006; 98: 300-308.
[33] Vlug MS, Wind J, Hollmann MW *et al.* Laparoscopy in combination with fast track multimodal management is the best perioperative strategy in patients undergoing colonic surgery: a randomized clinical trial (LAFA-study). Ann Surg 2011; [Epub ahead of print].
[34] Tabet J, Hong D, Kim CW, Wong J, Goodacre R, Anvari M. Laparoscopic versus open bowel resection for Crohn's disease. Can J Gastroenterol 2001; 15: 237-242.
[35] Luan XJ, Gross E. Laparoscopic assisted surgery for Crohn's disease: an initial experience and results. J Tongji Med Univ 2000; 20: 332-335.
[36] Eshuis EJ, Slors JF, Stokkers PC *et al.* Long-term outcomes following laparoscopically assisted versus open ileocolic resection for Crohn's disease. Br J Surg 2010; 97(4): 563-568.
[37] Heimann TM, Greenstein AJ, Lewis B *et al.* Comparison of primary and reoperative surgery in patients with Crohn's disease. Ann Surg 1998; 227: 492-495.
[38] Hasegawa H, Watanabe M, Nishibori H *et al.* Laparoscopic surgery for recurrent Crohn's disease. Br J Surg 2003; 90: 970-973.
[39] Holubar SD, Dozois EJ, Privitera A *et al.* Laparoscopic surgery for recurrent ileocolic Crohn's disease. Inflamm Bowel Dis 2010;16(8):1382-6.
[40] Broquet A, Bretagnol F, Soprani A *et al.* A laparoscopic approach to iterative ileocolic resection for the recurrence of Crohn's disease. Surg Endosc 2010; 24: 879-887.
[41] Bandyopadhyay D, Sagar PM, Mirnezami A *et al.* Laparoscopic resection for recurrent Crohn's disease: safety, feasibility and short-term outcomes. Colorectal Dis 2011; 13(2): 161-165.
[42] Chaudhray B, Glancy D, Dixon AR. Laparoscopic surgery for recurrent ileocolic Crohn's disease is as safe and effective as primary resection. Colorectal Dis 2010; doi: 10.1111/j.1463-1318.2010.02511.x. [Epub ahead of print].
[43] Holubar SD, Dozois EJ, Privitera A *et al.* Minimally invasive colectomy for Crohn's colitis: a single institution experience. Inflamm Bowel Dis 2010; 16: 1940-1946.
[44] da Luz Moreira A, Stocchi L, Remzi FH *et al.* Laparoscopic surgery for patients with Crohn's colitis: a case-matched study. J Gastrointest Surg 2007; 11: 1529-1533.
[45] Umanskiy K, Malhotra G, Chase A *et al.* Laparoscopic colectomy for Crohn's colitis. A large prospective comparative study. J Gastrintest Surg 2010; 14: 658-663.
[46] Shapiro M, Greenstein AJ, Byrn J et al. Surgical management and outcomes of patients with duodenal Crohn's disease. J Am Coll Surg. 2008;207(1):36-42.
[47] Champagne BJ, Lee EC, Leblanc F *et al.* Single-incision vs straight laparoscopic segmental colectomy: a case-controlled study. Dis Colon Rectum 2011; 54(2): 183-186.
[48] Ross H, Steele S, Whiteford M *et al.* Early multi-institution experience with single-incision laparoscopic colectomy. Dis Colon Rectum 2011; 54(2): 187-192.
[49] Eshuis EJ, Voermans RP, Stokkers PC *et al.* Laparoscopic resection with transcolonic specimen extraction for ileocaecal Crohn's disease. Br J Surg 2010; 97(4): 569-574.

12

Advances in Management of Crohn's Disease

Talha A. Malik
Division of Gastroenterology/Hepatology
University of Alabama at Birmingham, Birmingham, Alabama
USA

1. Introduction

Crohn's disease (CD) is one of two forms of inflammatory bowel diseases (IBD), the other being ulcerative colitis (UC). CD is in fact itself a heterogeneous condition describing a group of closely related disease processes that result from an uncontrolled immune mediated inflammatory response primarily affecting the alimentary tract. CD may affect any part of the gastrointestinal tract and causes transmural intestinal inflammation. It is characterized by flares and remission. CD usually presents with diarrhea, abdominal pain and/or weight loss. Fever, blood in stool, oral ulcers, and/or perianal lesions may also occur. Most patients with CD end up requiring surgery.

In some cases of colitis, the distinction between CD and UC cannot be clearly made despite a detailed evaluation based on a thorough clinical exam, endoscopy, imaging and a biopsy. The term "Indeterminate colitis" is used for these cases. Based on the increasing recognition of the so-called "indeterminate colitis" and the considerable heterogeneity even within the two discrete IBD subtypes, efforts calling for a revisit of IBD classification are under way. In 2000, the Working Party for the World Congresses of Gastroenterology, which had met in Vienna in1998, published their report in the journal Inflammatory Bowel Diseases and proposed the Vienna classification. The Vienna classification attempted to classify CD based on objective variables that included age of onset, disease location, and disease behavior. The Vienna classification classifies CD into 24 disease clusters. Since then however, the Vienna classification has come under criticism due to its lack of clinical applicability, however it is still being used for research purposes. In 2005 Silverberg and colleagues presented the report of the Working Party of the Montreal World Congress of Gastroenterology in which they put forth the Montreal classification of IBD. Montreal classification classified CD largely based on variables chosen by the experts at Vienna except for adding a perianal disease modifier variable. Neither Vienna nor Montreal classification commented on the extra intestinal manifestations of CD though. Extra-intestinal manifestations of CD may include rheumatologic, dermatologic, ocular or hepatobiliary conditions. These have been identified in the Crohn's Disease Activity Index (CDAI) initially introduced as far back as 1979.

It is estimated that approximately 750, 000 people in the United States have CD. There is a lot of variation in data with regard to the incidence and prevalence of CD in the US. For example, incidence in the US of CD is estimated at 1 to 6 per 100, 000 . The prevalence of CD in the US is estimated to be 10-100 per 100,000. There doesn't seem to be a significant difference in the incidence and prevalence of CD between males and females. The peak age of onset for CD is 15-25 years of age. There seems to be another peak between the ages of 45 and 55. Smoking seems to predispose to CD.

2. Etiology and pathogenesis

The most popular theory regarding pathogenesis of CD considers it to be a result of an uncontrolled immune mediated inflammatory response to a still unknown trigger that occurs in genetically predisposed individuals, primarily affecting the alimentary tract and also involving the intestinal flora.

2.1 Intraluminal factors

Different triggers have been implicated, both external and auto-antigens. External antigens include viruses, bacteria and dietary agents. The most common virus implicated in the pathogenesis of CD is the measles virus. The most common external bacterial agent that has been implicated in the pathogenesis of CD is Mycobacterium paratuberculosis. An antigen on a dietary agent may also trigger an uncontrolled immune mediated inflammatory response leading to the development of CD, but no such agent has yet been identified. Auto-antigens that have been implicated in the pathogenesis of CD may be located on non-pathogenic bacteria which constitute the intestinal flora. Similarly it is postulated that a certain antigenic trigger on a yet unknown luminal agent present in the gastrointestinal tract may also trigger an abnormal inflammatory response within the gastrointestinal tract leading to intestinal inflammation.

2.2 Epithelial barrier, innate and acquired immune actors

Despite the lack of definitive knowledge about the potential triggering agents, it is well established that the main mechanism of inflammatory injury is immune mediated and that it occurs in genetically predisposed individuals. There are various mechanisms by which immune mediated injury takes place. It is a combination of the interaction between breakdown in the intestinal epithelial barrier, innate immune system and activation of acquired immune mechanisms. An important factor is abnormal or exaggerated immune response. HLA Class II molecules that are predominantly found on macrophages are considered to be the major mediators of the process of autoimmune injury. They occur in high numbers within the intestinal epithelial cells of patients with active CD. The HLA-Class II molecules are responsible for antigen processing and presentation. HLA-DR molecules seem to play the most active role in this regard. Activated macrophages also secrete pro-inflammatory cytokines including IL-1, IL-6, IL-8 and TNF-alpha within the lamina propria of the intestinal wall. IFN- gamma is also produced and it increases intestinal permeability. There is decreased production of IL-2, IL-10, TNF- beta and TGF-beta, which are down-regulatory cytokines. In patients with IBD, this may explain chronic inflammation. Moreover, direct cell mediated immune mechanisms may also be involved in the immune pathogenesis of IBD. It is postulated that B-cell mediated mechanisms are also important, as there is increased secretion of IgM and IgG classes of antibodies by the intestinal mononuclear cells. Other immune mediators that seem to be involved in the pathogenesis of CD include oxygen radicals, most importantly superoxide molecules. Oxygen radicals are produced by activated neutrophils and they cause further inflammatory injury. Leukotriene Neutrophil Chemotactic Compounds (LNCC) and nitric oxide also enhance the inflammatory process of IBD by causing vasodilatation and vascular leakage. It has been demonstrated in animal models that the inflammatory process of IBD is enhanced by CD-4^+ T helpers. This provides evidence for a dominant role of T-cells in the pathogenesis of IBD. Moreover, the effectiveness of TNF-alpha and IFN-gamma antibodies in counteracting T-cell mediated inflammatory damage lends credence to the belief that both TNF-alpha and IFN-gamma are important mediators of the T-cell induced damage in inflammatory bowel diseases.

2.3 Genetic predisposition

Up to fifteen percent of patients with CD may have a first degree relative who also suffers from IBD. Haplotypes associated with CD are HLA-DR1/DQw5 and HLA-DRB3*0301. IBD1 susceptibility locus on chromosome 16 is associated with CD. The NOD2 gene located on this locus undergoes a mutation leading to abnormality in NOD2 protein, which is an intracellular bacterial lipopolysaccharide receptor in monocytes. This mutation is seen in up to fifteen percent of patients with CD. The IBD2 susceptibility locus on chromosome 12 is also associated with CD.

3. Management

3.1 Goals

The historic goal of treatment of CD was to induce and maintain clinical remission. However, it has now become evident that the natural course of disease progression of CD is not positively impacted if focus is laid only on clinical remission. Therefore the goal of treatment of CD has evolved into a broad stratagem. Current goals of medical management of CD include rapid induction and then maintenance of clinical as well as endoscopic remission. This seeks to minimize bowel damage. Other goals of management that are now actively pursued include decreasing rate of complications, hospitalizations, surgical interventions, infections, steroid use, cancer and overall mortality. Moreover, improving compliance and health related quality of life (HRQL) also figure prominently among current management goals. The goals of CD therapy continue to evolve and eventually will include not just minimizing the impact of the disease but perhaps obliterate it altogether. For this purpose, research is ongoing in search of additional biological modifiers. Genetic studies are also being undertaken.

3.2 Approach

Traditionally, a step up approach was applied that involved starting with corticosteroids and evolving to more invasive and newer modalities. Then there was evidence to suggest that top-down therapy might be the best way to achieve the evolving goals of therapy. However, recently there is more support for the accelerated step-up approach.

3.3 Supportive therapy

In regard to diet, there is not a lot of data that suggests a strong link between diet and CD. However some diets that have been suggested to possibly be related to onset as well as increased disease activity and more severe course include diets consisting of red meats. Moreover, diets high in fats and refined carbohydrates also seem to be risk factors for CD whereas fruits and vegetables are perhaps protective. Patients are also advised to make a list

of others foods that seem to worsen their symptoms and to avoid consuming them. Despite a few studies demonstrating benefits of an elemental diet, the risk of malnutrition in patients on it has caused decrease in enthusiasm.
In regard to behavioral management, regular exercise enhances functional capacity of IBD patients. Smoking is strongly associated with CD exacerbations. There is observational data to suggest that NSAID use may increase CD activity. In patients with CD, behavioral counseling and ways to facilitate daily living needs to be ensured.

3.4 Advances in medical therapy

Traditional Therapies have included systemic corticosteroids. They were and are still used for induction of remission in CD. While 5-Aminosalicylates like mesalamine have traditionally been the primary treatment modality in mild to moderate UC but their effectiveness in CD has largely been marginal if any at all. Antibiotics are considered among the most effective and safe therapies used to treat patients with mild to moderately active CD. The antibiotics most frequently used are metronidazole and ciprofloxacin. The most common traditional immune modulators used to maintain remission in CD as well as UC are azathioprine (AZA) and 6-mercaptopurine (6-MP).The role of methotrexate (MTX) appears to be limited to CD.
Newer Therapies are represented by biological immune modulators. Advances made in understanding the pathogenesis of CD have pushed us into the era of biological agents and beyond. The most important biological agents being used today are the TNF-alpha blockers. However, there is a long list of biologics that work by targeting other areas of the entire spectrum of the pathogenesis of CD.

3.5 TNF blockers

The first biologic agent that was approved for CD treatment was infliximab (Remicade). Infliximab is a half murine half human, chimeric monoclonal antibody consisting of an Fc portion as well as a Fab fragment which is active against TNF-alpha. It is administered intravenously, usually every 8 weeks. Infliximab has been found to be effective in inducing and maintaining remission in moderate to severe inflammatory as well as fistulizing CD disease in several multicenter double-blind, placebo controlled trials. The typical induction regimen of infliximab is 5mg/kg intravenously at 0, 2 and 6 weeks followed by 5mg/kg intravenous infusion every 8 weeks.Infliximab also reduces the requirements for corticosteroids, leads to mucosal healing, and reduces complications such as surgical intervention and hospitalization. It has also demonstrated improved quality of life. Initial response rates to infliximab may be as high as 75% but is generally maintained in approximately one third of patients.
Adalimumab (Humira) is a monoclonal IgG1 antibody against TNF-alpha which is fully humanized and has shown promise in the treatment of CD. Adalimumab is administered subcutaneously. Similar to infliximab, adalimumab works as an induction as well as a maintenance medication. The Classic I trial revealed that induction with 160 mg of adalimumab followed in two weeks by 80 mg of adalimumab resulted in over 35 percent of CD patients achieving remission at 4 weeks follow up.The GAIN (Gauging Response in Infliximab Nonresponders) trial was conducted to evaluate response to induction by adalimumab of patients which also included those who had either failed to respond to infliximab or had developed recurrence of disease after an initial response to infliximab. It

was a placebo controlled double-blind trial which revealed that remission rate with adalimumab induction was about 21 percent, and not as good as what the Classic I trial had revealed. An interesting finding was that those patients who had previously either failed to respond to infliximab or had developed disease recurrence actually had decreased remission rate in response to adalimumab than the initial response to infliximab induction. The Classic II and CHARM trials evaluated the efficacy of maintenance with adalimumab. The CLASSIC II trial was a double-blind, placebo-controlled trial and went on for a year. In this trial the investigators maintained initial responders on 40mg of adalimumab every week or every other week or to placebo. After a year of this trial, 79% of the patients on 40mg every other week and 83% of the patients on 40mg of adalimumab every week had achieved remission compared to 44% of the placebo group.The CHARM trial studied 854 patients with moderate to severe Crohn's disease. In CHARM, the 80/40 mg induction with adalimumab had already taken place. The responders to this induction regimen were then randomized to the two maintenance regimens of adalimumab or placebo. These patients were then followed for a year. Forty one percent of the patients who received adalimumab every week were in remission after about a year, whereas 36 percent of those who were on every other week of adalimumab maintenance were in remission. The CLASSIC II and CHARM trials also showed that adalimumab could be used as a steroid sparing agent in order to maintain remission in patients with CD, as most patients on adalimumab in the CLASSIC II trial were off steroids compared to those on placebo. In the CHARM trial, it was seen that the steroid-free clinical remission rates were significantly higher in those patients who received adalimumab versus those who were on placebo. The CHARM trial also revealed a statistically significant decrease in hospitalization in patients who were on adalimumab versus placebo. Adalimumab also helped heal fistulas in patients with CD. At the end of one year, one third of patients who received adalimumab had achieved closure of fistula compared to 13 percent of those were treated with placebo. The CHARM trial was extended for another one year and the end of the additional year, almost 71 percent of the fistulas had healed in patients who received adalimumab.[14]

Certolizumab pegol (Cimzia) is a humanized monoclonal agent against TNF-alpha that is comprised of just the Fab fragment and does not contain the Fc moiety. Certolizumab is pegylated by the addition of two polyethylene glycol molecules which increases the half-life as well as well its binding affinity to TNF-alpha. Certolizumab pegol is administered once a month subcutaneously at 400 mg dose each time. The induction regimen of Cimzia is 400mg subcutaneously at week 0, 2 and then 4. So far, two placebo controlled, double blind trials have been performed to evaluate certolizumab pegol in CD. PRECISE I (add reference) looked at the effectiveness of induction therapy. Even though a benefit was found in inducing a response with it compared to patients on placebo, the response was not statistically significant. The response to induction was assessed at 2 weeks, 6 weeks and then at 26 weeks. It was noted though that the maximum response occurred in patients who had CRP level higher than 10mg/dl. Patients with high CRP levels were therefore evaluated separately based on a previous post-hoc analysis revealing a greater rate of response in this patient population anyway (add reference). The primary endpoints of this study were the induction of clinical response at weeks 6 and a response at both weeks 6 and 26. In this study, it was demonstrated that 37% of patients with CRP level higher than 10 mg/l experienced response at the end of 6 weeks vs. only 26% in the placebo group. The difference in response at weeks 2 and 26 were not statistically significant

In the PRECISE 2 trial, researchers randomized week 4 responders to certolizumab pegol 400mg every 4 weeks to week 26 or placebo. Randomization was again stratified based on CRP level. It was demonstrated that 64% of the patients responded to induction therapy. This response was maintained in 63% of the intention to treat population up until week 26 vs. 36% who were receiving placebo). In terms of clinical remission at week 26, 48% of the patients on certolizumab pegol achieved it vs. 29% among the placebo group. In the end, stratification by CRP levels did not appear to yield a significant benefit in any of these studies. Moreover, it was noted that the efficacy of certolizumab pegol was not impacted by steroid use or the use of infliximab in the past. But once again, those who had received a TNF blocker in the past had a lower response rate than those who had never received a biologic. The open-label stage of the WELCOME trial was based on CD patients who had been unable to tolerate infliximab or who had developed secondary loss of response to it. The patients received induction with certolizumab 400 mg at weeks 0 and 2. The primary response defined as a decrease in CDAI of 100 was measured at week 6. It was seen that 55% of these patients had responded based on this criterion.

3.6 Adhesion molecule inhibitors

Natalizumab (Tysabri) is a monoclonal antibody against the alpha-4 subunit of integrin molecules which are important mediators of vascular inflammation. Integrin molecules are located on surface of vessels and they play an important role in adhesion and migration of inflammatory cells from the vasculature into inflamed tissue. Natalizumab essentially blocks integrin association with vascular receptors, limiting adhesion and transmigration of leukocytes. Specifically, in CD, natalizumab decreases inflammation by binding to alpha-4 integrin and thus blocking adhesion and migration of inflammatory leukocytes in the gut. Natalizumab has not been studied in patients with UC. Because of the incidence of PML in some cases and in two cases PML leading to death in MS patients who were treated with natalizumab, natalizumab was briefly taken off the market. In order to use natalizumab now in patients with CD, they must be enrolled in the Crohn's disease Tysabri® Outreach Unified Commitment to Health (CD-TOUCH™).Healthcare providers must also register with the program in order to prescribe, dispense or administer natalizumab. Treatment must be reauthorized every 6 months. Natalizumab is available only through infusion centers registered with the TOUCH™ program. Natalizumab is given in a 300 mg dose infused over 1 hour every 4 weeks. It is discontinued if no therapeutic benefit is observed in the first 12 weeks.

Vedolizumab, previously called MLN-0002, MLN-02 or LDP-02, is similar to natalizumab but with some important differences. It is a recombinant humanized anti alpha-2 beta-7 integrin monoclonal antibody, which is undergoing Phase 3 trials to test its efficacy in treatment of UC as well as CD. The alpha-2 beta-7 integrin subunit is relatively specific to the gastrointestinal tract. The Gemini I, II and III (also called the Millennium Trials) are all phase III clinical trials which are being conducted to test efficacy of Vedolizumab in inducing and maintaining remission in patient with UC and CD.

3.7 IL-6 inhibitors

Toclizumab is a humanized monoclonal antibody directed against the receptor of IL-6. An early randomized safety and efficacy trial assessing toclizumab in CD was published in 2004. The trial had 2 treatment arms and one placebo arm with a total accrual of 36 patients. Even though there was a significant difference in serologic and clinical response parameters between those who received toclizumab vs. placebo at assessment of the induction endpoint assessment, the highest response rate was two out of 10(20%) patients who received toclizumab. No difference was seen in terms of mucosal healing between treatment and placebo groups at 12 weeks.. Due to these less than encouraging results in CD, further clinical trials evaluating the efficacy of toclizumab in patients with IBD have not conducted so far. However, recently, there has been more activity in research assessing efficacy of toclizumab in other autoimmune diseases, most importantly rheumatoid arthritis with several phase II and phase III clinical trials underway.

3.8 IFN-γ blockers

Fontolizumab is a humanized monoclonal antibody fragment that possesses potent binding and neutralizing activity against human interferon-γ (IFN-γ). IFN-γ is a prominent pro-inflammatory effector cytokines. Two safety and clinical efficacy trials assessing the ability of fontolizumab in inducing remission in active CD were published in 2006. They did demonstrate a serologic and mucosal response in the patients who received fontolizumab but there was no significant difference seen in clinical remission between patients on fontolizumab vs. place.. In February 2010, results of a placebo controlled Phase 3 trial assessing efficacy of fontolizumab in patients with CD were published. In this trial, a total of 201 patients with Crohn's Disease Activity Index (CDAI) scores between 250 and 450 were randomized to receive an initial intravenous dose of 1.0 or 4.0 mg/kg fontolizumab or placebo, followed by up to 3 subcutaneous doses of 0.1 or 1.0 mg/kg placebo every 4 weeks. At the end of induction phase assessed at 4 weeks, there was no significant improvement in patients who had received fontolizumab. However, during the maintenance period the patient arm that received 1.0 mg/kg intravenous followed by 1.0 mg/kg subcutaneous of fontolizumab group had clinical response and significantly greater improvement in the CDAI score compared with patients who received placebo. But a similar improved response was not seen in the other fontolizumab group. However, all fontolizumab groups had significant improvement in C-reactive protein levels. Adverse event rates were similar in all groups. The significantly low levels of CRP in patients who received fontolizumab suggested a biological effect of fontolizumab on inflammation associated with Crohn's. Further trials are therefore being planned but no trial is currently underway.

3.9 IL-12/23p40 inhibitor

Interleukin-12 (IL-12) and Interleukin-23 (IL-23) are functionally closely associated effector cytokines that seem to play an active role in promoting intestinal inflammation in inflammatory bowel disease. IL-12 and IL-23 are structurally separate but both exist linked to a common subunit p40. IL-12 attaches to the p40 subunit through its unique subunit p35 whereas IL-23 is attached to p40 through its unique subunit p19. Both IL-12 and IL-23 attach to cell surface receptors on T-helper cells to trigger Th1 and Th17 mediated inflammatory cascades respectively. Briakinumab is also a human monoclonal antibody directed against IL-12/23p40 subunit.. Results of a phase II dose ranging and efficacy study published in 2004 demonstrated a significantly higher response in patients on briakinumab (75%) compared to placebo (25%) at the end of 7 weeks (P=0.03). (84)A subsequent phase IIb randomized double blind placebo controlled clinical efficacy trial was started in 2007. The trial sought to test safe dose and efficacy of briakinumab in moderate to severely active CD however it was terminated in April, 2010 without publication of findings. There are no other clinical trials underway testing briakinumab in CD or UC (Abbott ;.Dose Ranging Study Comparing the Efficacy, Safety and Pharmacokinetics of Intravenous Infusions of ABT-874 vs Placebo in Subjects With Active Crohn's Disease . In: ClinicalTrials.gov [Internet]. Bethesda (MD): National Library of Medicine (US). 2000- [cited 2010 Oct 12]. Available from: http://clinicaltrials.gov/show/ NCT00562887).

STA-5326 mesylate (also called apilimod mesylate) is a small molecule that blocks the release of IL-12 from peripheral blood mononuclear cells. In 2006, results of a safety and dose-ranging study with an accrual of 73 that evaluated oral STA-5326 mesylate (apilimod mesylate) in CD were published. They revealed a remission rate of between 15 and 36% at the end of 4 weeks. Approximately half of the patients demonstrated a decrease in mucosal disease activity. A subsequent phase II dose-ranging randomized placebo control clinical trial assessing the efficacy of oral STA-5326 mesylate (apilimod mesylate) in CD was undertaken between 2005 and 2008, but the results have not been published yet (B.Sands; Synta Pharmaceutical Corp. Study of STA-5326 Mesylate in Patients With Moderate to Severe Crohn's Disease In: ClinicalTrials.gov [Internet]. Bethesda (MD): National Library of Medicine (US). 2000- [cited 2010 Oct 12]. Available from: http://clinicaltrials.gov/show/ NCT00138840). Another similar randomized double blind placebo control phase II study that sought to assess peripheral mononuclear and cytokine responses to oral STA-5326 mesylate (apilimod mesylate) was completed in December 2008. The results of this study have not been published yet. There have been no additional studies evaluating STA-5326 mesylate (apilimod mesylate) in CD since then. There are also no studies that have assessed STA-5326 mesylate in UC yet (P.Mannon; Synta Pharmaceutical Corp. Study of STA-5326 Mesylate in Patients With Moderate to Severe Crohn's Disease In: ClinicalTrials.gov [Internet]. Bethesda (MD): National Library of Medicine (US). 2000- [cited 2010 Oct 12]. Available from: http://clinicaltrials.gov/show/NCT00234741).

Ustekinumab, a human monoclonal antibody has specific affinity to the p40 subunit. By doing this, ustekinumab prevents IL-12 and Il-23 from attaching to their cell surface T-helper cell receptors and therefore helps prevent the subsequent inflammatory process. Results of a double blind crossover clinical study assessing efficacy of ustekinumab in moderate to severe CD were published in 2008. They demonstrated a statistically significant difference in clinical response (53%) in patients who received ustekinumab vs. those who were in the placebo arm (30%) (P=0.02) by the end of week 6 but this difference was not maintained at the end of week 8 (49% with ustekinumab vs. 40% with placebo; P=0.34). It was noted however that when the subgroup of previous non-responders to infliximab were evaluated separately, the difference in clinical response to ustekinumab vs. placebo became statistically significant. Consequently, a multicenter double-blind placebo controlled randomized trial testing efficacy and safety of ustekinumab in subjects with moderately to severely active CD previously treated with TNF blockers was started. This trial is still ongoing with no results published so far. (Centocor Inc;. A Study of Safety and Effectiveness of Ustekinumab in Patients With Moderate to Severe Active Crohns Disease Who Have Been Previously Treated With Anti-TNF Therapy. In: ClinicalTrials.gov [Internet]. Bethesda (MD): National Library of Medicine (US). 2000- [cited 2010 Oct 12]. Available from: http://clinicaltrials.gov/show/ NCT 00771667). There are no ongoing trials testing efficacy of ustekinumab involving UC patients.

3.10 Other promising agents affecting cytokines

Thalidomide is a glutamic acid derivative that has historically been notorious for its devastating teratogenic potential, a property most probably linked to it toxic effect on endothelial tissue structures. There is growing evidence that thalidomide in fact also effectively inhibits transcription of TNF among other of its functions that may also be of value in combating intestinal inflammation in IBD. In a retrospective study published in 2007, thalidomide was shown to potentially be an effective in some patients with refractory luminal and fistulizing Crohn's disease. Randomized Controlled Trials testing efficacy of thalidomide in adults with active CD have not begun yet. It is important to note that an RCT conducted in children with CD, testing efficacy OF lenalidomide, an analogue of thalidomide in treatment of active CD did not demonstrate any significant benefit over placebo (94). Similarly, despite pre-clinical evidence to support efficacy of thalidomide and lenalidomide in decreasing intestinal inflammation associated with IBD, no maintenance trials have yet been published to justify its safety for use in humans. However, clinical trials are being planned.

RDP58 is an oral d-amino acid decapeptide that has powerful immunosuppressive activity which includes inhibition of TNF synthesis as well inhibition of IFN-γ, IL-2 and IL-12. It has been demonstrated in murine models that RDP58 is extremely effective in reducing intestinal inflammation including histological scores in colitis. RDP58 has also demonstrated variable efficacy in treatment of several inflammatory and presumably autoimmune conditions that include IBD, interstitial cystitis and autoimmune encephalomyelitis. RDP58 has demonstrated ex vivo anti-inflammatory activity in tissue from patients with CD. It has also demonstrated efficacy in vivo murine models.

3.11 Mucosal barrier enhancement/restoration

The intestinal epithelium is a part of the innate immune system of the intestinal tract. It functions as a protective wall that seeks to maintain a balance between the contents of the lumen and the immune cells and matrix that lie on the other side.

Intestinal epithelial cells are the individual units that give rise to this normally impenetrable intestinal barrier by forming tight junctions. Any insult that results in the failure of the tight junctions to keep the contents of the two environments separate is what heralds intestinal inflammation by activating a hyper-reactive acquired immune system made up primarily of effector cells.

Emerging therapies include therapeutic agents that seeks to enhance or restore this important protective immune play. Teduglitide is a dipeptidyl peptidase IV resistant glucagon-like peptide-2 (GLP-2) analogue. The manner in which GLP-2 repairs the intestinal epithelium is still unclear. However, it is being tested for its ability to restore the intestinal epithelial barrier. Results of a randomized, placebo-controlled, double-blind trial evaluating efficacy of teduglutide in inducing clinical and mucosal remission in moderate to-severe CD were published in 2010. They demonstrated a significant difference in clinical response and therefore more studies have been planned.

Growth hormone has also demonstrated positive effects on enhancing function of neutrophils. Somatropin, growth hormone, has demonstrated efficacy in repairing the intestinal epithelium in pre-clinical studies. Some early studies have demonstrated that somatropin enhances the innate immune system and repairs the intestinal epithelium through its positive impact on protein synthesis. A phase III study evaluating the efficacy of somatropin in induction of histological healing in children with Crohn's Disease (CD) was completed. Publication of the results of this trial is still pending CD (L.Denson; Children's Hospital Medical Center, Cincinnati. Trial of Growth Hormone Therapy in Pediatric Crohn's DiseaseIn: ClinicalTrials.gov [Internet]. Bethesda (MD): National Library of Medicine (US). 2000- [cited 2010 Oct 12]. Available from: http://clinicaltrials.gov/show/NCT00109473).

Another agent that has demonstrated the ability to enhance the innate immune system is the synthetic growth factor Sargramostim. Sargramostim is a granulocyte-macrophage colony stimulating factor (GM-CSF) which specifically stimulates production of neutrophils, monocytes, and epithelial cells. A phase 1 study published in 2009 assessed efficacy of sargramostim in treatment of patients with moderately to severely active CD. The study demonstrated modest benefit with only a few patients experiencing clinical remission. There were no serious reported adverse drug events.

Recently published results of a placebo-control randomized trial that assessed the efficacy of sargramostim in corticosteroid-dependent patients with Crohn's disease demonstrated that it was more effective than placebo in inducing corticosteroid-free remission. It was also demonstrated that treatment with sargramostim was associated with significant improvements in health-related quality of life. Two phase III clinical trials testing efficacy of sargramostim in treatment of moderate to severe CD have recently been completed but results have not been published yet

(Medical Montor; Genzyme. Efficacy (Induction of Response/Remission) and Safety Study in Patients With Moderate to Severe Crohn's Disease In: ClinicalTrials.gov [Internet]. Bethesda (MD): National Library of Medicine (US). 2000- [cited 2010 Oct 12]. Available from: http://clinicaltrials.gov/show/NCT00206674) (Medical Monitor; Genzyme.Study in Patients With Crohn's Disease Who Are Steroid Dependent, Despite Previous Unsuccessful Attempts to Reduce Steroids Due to Worsening of Crohn's Disease In: ClinicalTrials.gov [Internet]. Bethesda (MD): National Library of Medicine (US). 2000- [cited 2010 Oct 12]. Available from: http://clinicaltrials.gov/show/NCT00206596).

There is evidence for granulocyte colony-stimulating factor's (G-CSF) ability to inhibit effects of T helper 1 cells and of its ability to induce IL-10-secreting regulatory T cells. Filgrastim, a synthetic granulocyte colony-stimulating factor (G-CSF) that specifically stimulates production of neutrophils has also shown promise in early safety and efficacy trials. In a recently published early phase study, the clinical benefit of G-CSF therapy in active CD was tested. The results of the study were important as it was demonstrated that clinical benefit from G-CSF treatment was associated with induction of IL-10 secreting T cells as well as a rise in plasmacytoid dendritic cells in the lamina propria of the inflamed intestinal mucosa. Another phase I study assessing the efficacy of G-CSF in inducing an immune and clinical response in CD patients was recently completed but the results of this trial have not been published yet National Institute of Allergy and Infectious Diseases; National Institutes of Health Clinical Center. G-CSF to Treat Crohn's Disease In: ClinicalTrials.gov [Internet]. Bethesda (MD): National Library of Medicine (US). 2000- [cited 2010 Oct 12]. Available from: http://clinicaltrials.gov/show/NCT00025805).

3.12 Intra-luminal targets

While there is no paucity of hypotheses regarding implication of intra-luminal agents as triggers of inflammation, the real advance in devising therapeutic strategies by modulating intra-luminal agents has been the realization that intestinal inflammation seen in CD is actually a result of an imbalance between the intestinal milieu comprising of micobiota, most likely gut commensals on one side and various components of the immune system on the other. This theory receives more credence with the observation of increased inflammation seen in murine models with defects in any of these components.

Based on the sometimes contradictory observations made, it is very plausible that there are indeed competing and opposing effects of microorganisms in the gut. This dilemma is explained well when one notes that intestinal inflammation is not just the net result of the imbalance between intra-luminal antigens and intestinal immune actors but in fact is also related to the imbalance between the so considered commensal and pathogenic strain of bacteria residing within the intestinal lumens.

Another group of intraluminal actors that has recently garnered the interest of researchers comprises the parasitic helminths. It has been postulated that as development and industrialization became harbingers of improved hygiene, intestinal colonization of people with helminths, a fact of life across the entire globe just a hundred years ago, began to subside. Additionally, it was noted that almost precisely around the same period, there began to occur a substantial increase in the incidence of autoimmune conditions such as inflammatory bowel disease among populations residing in these rapidly industrializing nations. The association between the two phenomena became clearer when evidence of the role of helminths in depressing the intestinal immune reaction also began to emerge. It is now being seen that there seems to be a rapidly rising rate of inflammatory bowel disease among the urbanized populations of several rapidly developing countries whereas their rural counterparts continue to largely enjoy protection from this process. Another theory brought to the fore is popularly termed as the "IBD hygiene hypothesis". It theorizes that immune deregulation occurs early in childhood among populations that are brought up in extremely hygienic environments largely devoid of helminthic colonization. It has been postulated that intestinal helminthic colonizers may actually enhance one's immune regulation processes. Through this mechanism, they may prove to be effective weapons against the various effector cells that are the greatest drivers of the inflammatory cascade representative of CD.

There is also evidence based on murine models suggesting that helminths have a protective effect against the development of colitis. There is evidence based on an open-label clinical trial done on patients with CD that supports the therapeutic role of helminths in these patients. These studies used live ova from porcine whipworm as an oral therapeutic intervention.

4. References

B. E. Sands: Inflammatory bowel disease: past, present, and future. J Gastroenterol, 42(1), 16-25 (2007)

E. V. Loftus, Jr.: Clinical epidemiology of inflammatory bowel disease: Incidence, prevalence, and environmental influences. Gastroenterology, 126(6), 1504-17 (2004)

B. E. Sands and S. Grabert: Epidemiology of inflammatory bowel disease and overview of pathogenesis. Med Health R I, 92(3), 73-7 (2009)

J. R. Korzenik and D. K. Podolsky: Evolving knowledge and therapy of inflammatory bowel disease. Nat Rev Drug Discov, 5(3), 197-209 (2006)

L. Peyrin-Biroulet, P. Desreumaux, W. J. Sandborn and J. F. Colombel: Crohn's disease: beyond antagonists of tumour necrosis factor. Lancet, 372(9632), 67-81 (2008)

F. Scaldaferri, C. Correale, A. Gasbarrini and S. Danese: Mucosal biomarkers in inflammatory bowel disease: key pathogenic players or disease predictors? World J Gastroenterol, 16(21), 2616-25 (2010)

W. J. Sandborn: Current directions in IBD therapy: what goals are feasible with biological modifiers? Gastroenterology, 135(5), 1442-7 (2008)

S. B. Hanauer, W. J. Sandborn, P. Rutgeerts, R. N. Fedorak, M. Lukas, D. Macintosh, R. Panaccione, D. Wolf and P. Pollack: Human anti-tumor necrosis factor monoclonal antibody (adalimumab) in Crohn's disease: the CLASSIC-I trial. Gastroenterology, 130(2), 323-33; quiz 591 (2006)

W. J. Sandborn, P. Rutgeerts, R. Enns, S. B. Hanauer, J. F. Colombel, R. Panaccione, G. D'haens, J. Li, M. R. Rosenfeld, J. D. Kent and P. F. Pollack: Adalimumab induction therapy for Crohn disease previously treated with infliximab: a randomized trial. Ann Intern Med, 146(12), 829-38 (2007)

W. J. Sandborn, S. B. Hanauer, P. Rutgeerts, R. N. Fedorak, M. Lukas, D. G. Macintosh, R. Panaccione, D. Wolf, J. D. Kent, B. Bittle, J. Li and P. F. Pollack: Adalimumab for maintenance treatment of Crohn's disease: results of the CLASSIC II trial. Gut, 56(9), 1232-9 (2007)

J. F. Colombel, W. J. Sandborn, P. Rutgeerts, R. Enns, S. B. Hanauer, R. Panaccione, S. Schreiber, D. Byczkowski, J. Li, J. D. Kent and P. F. Pollack: Adalimumab for maintenance of clinical response and remission in patients with Crohn's disease: the CHARM trial. Gastroenterology, 132(1), 52-65 (2007)

P. Rutgeerts, W. J. Sandborn, B. G. Feagan, W. Reinisch, A. Olson, J. Johanns, S. Travers, D. Rachmilewitz, S. B. Hanauer, G. R. Lichtenstein, W. J. De Villiers, D. Present, B. E. Sands and J. F. Colombel: Infliximab for induction and maintenance therapy for ulcerative colitis. N Engl J Med, 353(23), 2462-76 (2005)

M. T. Osterman and G. R. Lichtenstein: Current and Future Anti-TNF Therapy for Inflammatory Bowel Disease. Curr Treat Options Gastroenterol, 10(3), 195-207 (2007)

D. K. Podolsky: Inflammatory bowel disease. N Engl J Med, 347(6), 417-29 (2002)

Laurent Peyrin-Biroulet, Pierre Desreumaux, William J. Sandborn and Jean-Frédéric Colombel: Crohn's disease: beyond antagonists of tumour necrosis factor. The Lancet, 372(9632), 67-81 (2008)

V. Leso, L. Leggio, A. Armuzzi, G. Gasbarrini, A. Gasbarrini and G. Addolorato: Role of the tumor necrosis factor antagonists in the treatment of inflammatory bowel disease: an update. Eur J Gastroenterol Hepatol, 22(7), 779-86 (2010)

D. W. Hommes, T. L. Mikhajlova, S. Stoinov, D. Stimac, B. Vucelic, J. Lonovics, M. Zakuciova, G. D'haens, G. Van Assche, S. Ba, S. Lee and T. Pearce: Fontolizumab, a humanised anti-interferon gamma antibody, demonstrates safety and clinical activity in patients with moderate to severe Crohn's disease. Gut, 55(8), 1131-7 (2006)

M. Gandhi, E. Alwawi and K. B. Gordon: Anti-p40 antibodies ustekinumab and briakinumab: blockade of interleukin-12 and interleukin-23 in the treatment of psoriasis. Semin Cutan Med Surg, 29(1), 48-52 (2010)

P. Rafiee, D. J. Stein, V. M. Nelson, M. F. Otterson, R. Shaker and D. G. Binion: Thalidomide inhibits inflammatory and angiogenic activation of human intestinal microvascular endothelial cells (HIMEC). Am J Physiol Gastrointest Liver Physiol, 298(2), G167-76 (2010)

S. Plamondon, S. C. Ng and M. A. Kamm: Thalidomide in luminal and fistulizing Crohn's disease resistant to standard therapies. Aliment Pharmacol Ther, 25(5), 557-67 (2007)

R. Srinivasan and A. K. Akobeng: Thalidomide and thalidomide analogues for induction of remission in Crohn's disease. Cochrane Database Syst Rev(2), CD007350 (2009)

A. K. Akobeng and P. C. Stokkers: Thalidomide and thalidomide analogues for maintenance of remission in Crohn's disease. Cochrane Database Syst Rev(2), CD007351 (2009)

D. C. Baumgart, S. R. Targan, A. U. Dignass, L. Mayer, G. Van Assche, D. W. Hommes, S. B. Hanauer, U. Mahadevan, W. Reinisch, S. E. Plevy, B. A. Salzberg, A. L. Buchman, G. M. Mechkov, Z. A. Krastev, J. N. Lowder, M. B. Frankel and W. J. Sandborn: Prospective randomized open-label multicenter phase I/II dose escalation trial of visilizumab (HuM291) in severe steroid-refractory ulcerative colitis. Inflamm Bowel Dis, 16(4), 620-9 (2010)

G. D'haens and M. Daperno: Advances in biologic therapy for ulcerative colitis and Crohn's disease. Curr Gastroenterol Rep, 8(6), 506-12 (2006)

T. J. Creed, C. S. Probert, M. N. Norman, M. Moorghen, N. A. Shepherd, S. D. Hearing and C. M. Dayan: Basiliximab for the treatment of steroid-resistant ulcerative colitis: further experience in moderate and severe disease. Aliment Pharmacol Ther, 23(10), 1435-42 (2006)

M. Price, C. S. Probert and T. Creed: Basiliximab and Infliximab for the Treatment of Steroid-Refractory Crohn's Disease. Am J Gastroenterol (2008)

W. J. Sandborn and T. A. Yednock: Novel approaches to treating inflammatory bowel disease: targeting alpha-4 integrin. Am J Gastroenterol, 98(11), 2372-82 (2003)

R. Cianci, G. Cammarota, F. Raducci and F. Pandolfi: The impact of biological agents interfering with receptor/ligand binding in the immune system. Eur Rev Med Pharmacol Sci, 9(6), 305-14 (2005)

S. R. Targan, B. G. Feagan, R. N. Fedorak, B. A. Lashner, R. Panaccione, D. H. Present, M. E. Spehlmann, P. J. Rutgeerts, Z. Tulassay, M. Volfova, D. C. Wolf, C. Hernandez, J. Bornstein and W. J. Sandborn: Natalizumab for the treatment of active Crohn's disease: results of the ENCORE Trial. Gastroenterology, 132(5), 1672-83 (2007)

D. Soler, T. Chapman, L. L. Yang, T. Wyant, R. Egan and E. R. Fedyk: The binding specificity and selective antagonism of vedolizumab, an anti-alpha4beta7 integrin therapeutic antibody in development for inflammatory bowel diseases. J Pharmacol Exp Ther, 330(3), 864-75 (2009)

G. Fiorino, C. Correale, W. Fries, A. Repici, A. Malesci and S. Danese: Leukocyte traffic control: a novel therapeutic strategy for inflammatory bowel disease. Expert Rev Clin Immunol, 6(4), 567-72 (2010)

M. Ismail, R. Morgan, K. Harrington, J. Davies and H. Pandha: Immunoregulatory effects of freeze injured whole tumour cells on human dendritic cells using an in vitro cryotherapy model. Cryobiology (2010)

H. Tilg, A. Moschen and A. Kaser: Mode of function of biological anti-TNF agents in the treatment of inflammatory bowel diseases. Expert Opin Biol Ther, 7(7), 1051-9 (2007)

C. W. Thomas, G. M. Myhre, R. Tschumper, R. Sreekumar, D. Jelinek, D. J. Mckean, J. J. Lipsky, W. J. Sandborn and L. J. Egan: Selective inhibition of inflammatory gene expression in activated T lymphocytes: a mechanism of immune suppression by thiopurines. J Pharmacol Exp Ther, 312(2), 537-45 (2005)

S. Buhner, C. Buning, J. Genschel, K. Kling, D. Herrmann, A. Dignass, I. Kuechler, S. Krueger, H. H. Schmidt and H. Lochs: Genetic basis for increased intestinal permeability in families with Crohn's disease: role of CARD15 3020insC mutation? Gut, 55(3), 342-7 (2006)

E. Cario, G. Gerken and D. K. Podolsky: "For whom the bell tolls!" -- innate defense mechanisms and survival strategies of the intestinal epithelium against lumenal pathogens. Z Gastroenterol, 40(12), 983-90 (2002)

S. T. Walk, A. M. Blum, S. A. Ewing, J. V. Weinstock and V. B. Young: Alteration of the murine gut microbiota during infection with the parasitic helminth Heligmosomoides polygyrus. Inflamm Bowel Dis (2010)

E. Cario, D. Brown, M. Mckee, K. Lynch-Devaney, G. Gerken and D. K. Podolsky: Commensal-associated molecular patterns induce selective toll-like receptor-trafficking from apical membrane to cytoplasmic compartments in polarized intestinal epithelium. Am J Pathol, 160(1), 165-73 (2002)

C. P. Tamboli, C. Neut, P. Desreumaux and J. F. Colombel: Dysbiosis as a prerequisite for IBD. Gut, 53(7), 1057 (2004)

L. J. Egan and W. J. Sandborn: Positioning novel biologic, probiotic, and apheresis therapies for Crohn's disease and ulcerative colitis. Curr Gastroenterol Rep, 7(6), 485-91 (2005)

A. Mathias, M. Duc, L. Favre, J. Benyacoub, S. Blum and B. Corthesy: Potentiation of polarized intestinal Caco-2 cell responsiveness to probiotics complexed with secretory IgA. J Biol Chem (2010)

N. E. Ruyssers, B. Y. De Winter, J. G. De Man, A. Loukas, M. S. Pearson, J. V. Weinstock, R. M. Van Den Bossche, W. Martinet, P. A. Pelckmans and T. G. Moreels: Therapeutic potential of helminth soluble proteins in TNBS-induced colitis in mice. Inflamm Bowel Dis, 15(4), 491-500 (2009)

K. Krishnan, B. Arnone and A. Buchman: Intestinal growth factors: Potential use in the treatment of inflammatory bowel disease and their role in mucosal healing. Inflamm Bowel Dis (2010)

J. Jones and R. Panaccione: Biologic therapy in Crohn's disease: state of the art. Curr Opin Gastroenterol, 24(4), 475-81 (2008)

G. Y. Melmed and S. R. Targan: Future biologic targets for IBD: potentials and pitfalls. Nat Rev Gastroenterol Hepatol, 7(2), 110-7 (2010)

N. Saulnier, M. A. Puglisi, W. Lattanzi, L. Castellini, G. Pani, G. Leone, S. Alfieri, F. Michetti, A. C. Piscaglia and A. Gasbarrini: Gene profiling of bone marrow- and adipose tissue-derived stromal cells: a key role of Kruppel-like factor 4 in cell fate regulation. Cytotherapy (2010)

Y. Oyama, R. M. Craig, A. E. Traynor, K. Quigley, L. Statkute, A. Halverson, M. Brush, L. Verda, B. Kowalska, N. Krosnjar, M. Kletzel, P. F. Whitington and R. K. Burt: Autologous hematopoietic stem cell transplantation in patients with refractory Crohn's disease. Gastroenterology, 128(3), 552-63 (2005)

P. H. Carter and Q. Zhao: Clinically validated approaches to the treatment of autoimmune diseases. Expert Opin Investig Drugs, 19(2), 195-213 (2010)

B. Ngo, C. P. Farrell, M. Barr, K. Wolov, R. Bailey, J. M. Mullin and J. J. Thornton: Tumor Necrosis Factor Blockade for Treatment of Inflammatory Bowel Disease: Efficacy and Safety. Curr Mol Pharmacol (2010)

W. J. Sandborn and S. B. Hanauer: Antitumor necrosis factor therapy for inflammatory bowel disease: a review of agents, pharmacology, clinical results, and safety. Inflamm Bowel Dis, 5(2), 119-33 (1999)

D. W. Claussen: Remicade (infliximab). Gastroenterol Nurs, 21(6), 256-9 (1998)

E. Ricart and W. J. Sandborn: Infliximab for the treatment of fistulas in patients with Crohn'S disease. Gastroenterology, 117(5), 1247-8 (1999)

A. Kornbluth: Infliximab approved for use in Crohn's disease: a report on the FDA GI Advisory Committee conference. Inflamm Bowel Dis, 4(4), 328-9 (1998)

B. G. Feagan, W. Reinisch, P. Rutgeerts, W. J. Sandborn, S. Yan, D. Eisenberg, M. Bala, J. Johanns, A. Olson and S. B. Hanauer: The effects of infliximab therapy on health-related quality of life in ulcerative colitis patients. Am J Gastroenterol, 102(4), 794-802 (2007)

C. R. Selvasekar, R. R. Cima, D. W. Larson, E. J. Dozois, J. R. Harrington, W. S. Harmsen, E. V. Loftus, Jr., W. J. Sandborn, B. G. Wolff and J. H. Pemberton: Effect of infliximab on short-term complications in patients undergoing operation for chronic ulcerative colitis. J Am Coll Surg, 204(5), 956-62; discussion 962-3 (2007)

R. Rau: Adalimumab (a fully human anti-tumour necrosis factor alpha monoclonal antibody) in the treatment of active rheumatoid arthritis: the initial results of five trials. Ann Rheum Dis, 61 Suppl 2, ii70-3 (2002)

S. Schreiber and W. J. Sandborn: CLASSIC-I study the efficacy of adalimumab. Gastroenterology, 130(6), 1929-30 (2006)

L. Peyrin-Biroulet, C. Laclotte, X. Roblin and M. A. Bigard: Adalimumab induction therapy for ulcerative colitis with intolerance or lost response to infliximab: an open-label study. World J Gastroenterol, 13(16), 2328-32 (2007)

W. Afif, E. V. Loftus, Jr., W. A. Faubion, S. V. Kane, D. H. Bruining, K. A. Hanson and W. J. Sandborn: Clinical utility of measuring infliximab and human anti-chimeric antibody concentrations in patients with inflammatory bowel disease. Am J Gastroenterol, 105(5), 1133-9 (2010)

N. Goel and S. Stephens: Certolizumab pegol. MAbs, 2(2) (2010)

T. A. Winter, W. J. Sandborn, W. J. De Villiers and S. Schreiber: Treatment of Crohn's disease with certolizumab pegol. Expert Rev Clin Immunol, 3(5), 683-94 (2007)

W. J. Sandborn, B. G. Feagan, S. Stoinov, P. J. Honiball, P. Rutgeerts, D. Mason, R. Bloomfield and S. Schreiber: Certolizumab pegol for the treatment of Crohn's disease. N Engl J Med, 357(3), 228-38 (2007)

S. Schreiber, M. Khaliq-Kareemi, I. C. Lawrance, O. O. Thomsen, S. B. Hanauer, J. Mccolm, R. Bloomfield and W. J. Sandborn: Maintenance therapy with certolizumab pegol for Crohn's disease. N Engl J Med, 357(3), 239-50 (2007)

W. J. Sandborn, S. Schreiber, S. B. Hanauer, J. F. Colombel, R. Bloomfield and G. R. Lichtenstein: Reinduction with certolizumab pegol in patients with relapsed

Crohn's disease: results from the PRECiSE 4 Study. Clin Gastroenterol Hepatol, 8(8), 696-702 e1 (2010)

G. Hutas: Golimumab as the first monthly subcutaneous fully human anti-TNF-alpha antibody in the treatment of inflammatory arthropathies. Immunotherapy, 2(4), 453-60 (2010)

D. Shealy, A. Cai, K. Staquet, A. Baker, E. R. Lacy, L. Johns, O. Vafa, G. Gunn, 3rd, S. Tam, S. Sague, D. Wang, M. Brigham-Burke, P. Dalmonte, E. Emmell, B. Pikounis, P. J. Bugelski, H. Zhou, B. Scallon and J. Giles-Komar: Characterization of golimumab, a human monoclonal antibody specific for human tumor necrosis factor alpha. MAbs, 2(4) (2010)

S. Mazumdar and D. Greenwald: Golimumab. MAbs, 1(5), 422-31 (2009)

R. D. Inman, J. C. Davis, Jr., D. Heijde, L. Diekman, J. Sieper, S. I. Kim, M. Mack, J. Han, S. Visvanathan, Z. Xu, B. Hsu, A. Beutler and J. Braun: Efficacy and safety of golimumab in patients with ankylosing spondylitis: results of a randomized, double-blind, placebo-controlled, phase III trial. Arthritis Rheum, 58(11), 3402-12 (2008)

G. Hutas: Golimumab, a fully human monoclonal antibody against TNFalpha. Curr Opin Mol Ther, 10(4), 393-406 (2008)

V. Cortez-Retamozo, N. Backmann, P. D. Senter, U. Wernery, P. De Baetselier, S. Muyldermans and H. Revets: Efficient cancer therapy with a nanobody-based conjugate. Cancer Res, 64(8), 2853-7 (2004)

J. J. Hulstein, P. G. De Groot, K. Silence, A. Veyradier, R. Fijnheer and P. J. Lenting: A novel nanobody that detects the gain-of-function phenotype of von Willebrand factor in ADAMTS13 deficiency and von Willebrand disease type 2B. Blood, 106(9), 3035-42 (2005)

N. Deckers, D. Saerens, K. Kanobana, K. Conrath, B. Victor, U. Wernery, J. Vercruysse, S. Muyldermans and P. Dorny: Nanobodies, a promising tool for species-specific diagnosis of Taenia solium cysticercosis. Int J Parasitol, 39(5), 625-33 (2009)

S. H. Bakhtiari, F. Rahbarizadeh, S. Hasannia, D. Ahmadvand, F. J. Iri-Sofla and M. J. Rasaee: Anti-MUC1 nanobody can redirect T-body cytotoxic effector function. Hybridoma (Larchmt), 28(2), 85-92 (2009)

A. Y. Lam, E. Pardon, K. V. Korotkov, W. G. Hol and J. Steyaert: Nanobody-aided structure determination of the EpsI:EpsJ pseudopilin heterodimer from Vibrio vulnificus. J Struct Biol, 166(1), 8-15 (2009)

S. Magez and M. Radwanska: African trypanosomiasis and antibodies: implications for vaccination, therapy and diagnosis. Future Microbiol, 4, 1075-87 (2009)

R. B. Abderrazek, I. Hmila, C. Vincke, Z. Benlasfar, M. Pellis, H. Dabbek, D. Saerens, M. El Ayeb, S. Muyldermans and B. Bouhaouala-Zahar: Identification of potent nanobodies to neutralize the most poisonous polypeptide from scorpion venom. Biochem J, 424(2), 263-72 (2009)

K. Vandenbroucke, H. De Haard, E. Beirnaert, T. Dreier, M. Lauwereys, L. Huyck, J. Van Huysse, P. Demetter, L. Steidler, E. Remaut, C. Cuvelier and P. Rottiers: Orally administered L. lactis secreting an anti-TNF Nanobody demonstrate efficacy in chronic colitis. Mucosal Immunol, 3(1), 49-56 (2010)

N. Nishimoto: [Anti-interleukin-6 receptor antibody therapy--from bedside to bench]. Nihon Rinsho Meneki Gakkai Kaishi, 29(5), 289-94 (2006)

H. Ito, M. Takazoe, Y. Fukuda, T. Hibi, K. Kusugami, A. Andoh, T. Matsumoto, T. Yamamura, J. Azuma, N. Nishimoto, K. Yoshizaki, T. Shimoyama and T. Kishimoto: A pilot randomized trial of a human anti-interleukin-6 receptor monoclonal antibody in active Crohn's disease. Gastroenterology, 126(4), 989-96; discussion 947 (2004)

A. Venkiteshwaran: Tocilizumab. MAbs, 1(5), 432-8 (2009)

J. S. Smolen, D. Aletaha, M. Koeller, M. H. Weisman and P. Emery: New therapies for treatment of rheumatoid arthritis. Lancet, 370(9602), 1861-74 (2007)

R. N. Maini, P. C. Taylor, J. Szechinski, K. Pavelka, J. Broll, G. Balint, P. Emery, F. Raemen, J. Petersen, J. Smolen, D. Thomson and T. Kishimoto: Double-blind randomized controlled clinical trial of the interleukin-6 receptor antagonist, tocilizumab, in European patients with rheumatoid arthritis who had an incomplete response to methotrexate. Arthritis Rheum, 54(9), 2817-29 (2006)

F. J. Dumont: Fontolizumab Protein Design Labs. Curr Opin Investig Drugs, 6(5), 537-44 (2005)

W. Reinisch, D. W. Hommes, G. Van Assche, J. F. Colombel, J. P. Gendre, B. Oldenburg, A. Teml, K. Geboes, H. Ding, L. Zhang, M. Tang, M. Cheng, S. J. Van Deventer, P. Rutgeerts and T. Pearce: A dose escalating, placebo controlled, double blind, single dose and multidose, safety and tolerability study of fontolizumab, a humanised anti-interferon gamma antibody, in patients with moderate to severe Crohn's disease. Gut, 55(8), 1138-44 (2006)

W. Reinisch, W. De Villiers, L. Bene, L. Simon, I. Racz, S. Katz, I. Altorjay, B. Feagan, D. Riff, C. N. Bernstein, D. Hommes, P. Rutgeerts, A. Cortot, M. Gaspari, M. Cheng, T. Pearce and B. E. Sands: Fontolizumab in moderate to severe Crohn's disease: a phase 2, randomized, double-blind, placebo-controlled, multiple-dose study. Inflamm Bowel Dis, 16(2), 233-42 (2010)

P. C. Van De Kerkhof: Novel biologic therapies in development targeting IL-12/IL-23. J Eur Acad Dermatol Venereol, 24 Suppl 6, 5-9 (2010)

X. T. Lima, K. Abuabara, A. B. Kimball and H. C. Lima: Briakinumab. Expert Opin Biol Ther, 9(8), 1107-13 (2009)

P. J. Mannon, I. J. Fuss, L. Mayer, C. O. Elson, W. J. Sandborn, D. Present, B. Dolin, N. Goodman, C. Groden, R. L. Hornung, M. Quezado, Z. Yang, M. F. Neurath, J. Salfeld, G. M. Veldman, U. Schwertschlag and W. Strober: Anti-interleukin-12 antibody for active Crohn's disease. N Engl J Med, 351(20), 2069-79 (2004)

R. Burakoff, C. F. Barish, D. Riff, R. Pruitt, W. Y. Chey, F. A. Farraye, I. Shafran, S. Katz, C. L. Krone, M. Vander Vliet, C. Stevens, M. L. Sherman, E. Jacobson and R. Bleday: A phase 1/2A trial of STA 5326, an oral interleukin-12/23 inhibitor, in patients with active moderate to severe Crohn's disease. Inflamm Bowel Dis, 12(7), 558-65 (2006)

G. G. Krueger, R. G. Langley, C. Leonardi, N. Yeilding, C. Guzzo, Y. Wang, L. T. Dooley and M. Lebwohl: A human interleukin-12/23 monoclonal antibody for the treatment of psoriasis. N Engl J Med, 356(6), 580-92 (2007)

M. Elliott, J. Benson, M. Blank, C. Brodmerkel, D. Baker, K. R. Sharples and P. Szapary: Ustekinumab: lessons learned from targeting interleukin-12/23p40 in immune-mediated diseases. Ann N Y Acad Sci, 1182, 97-110 (2009)

W. J. Sandborn, B. G. Feagan, R. N. Fedorak, E. Scherl, M. R. Fleisher, S. Katz, J. Johanns, M. Blank and P. Rutgeerts: A randomized trial of Ustekinumab, a human interleukin-12/23 monoclonal antibody, in patients with moderate-to-severe Crohn's disease. Gastroenterology, 135(4), 1130-41 (2008)

S. V. Sitaraman, M. Hoteit and A. T. Gewirtz: Semapimod. Cytokine. Curr Opin Investig Drugs, 4(11), 1363-8 (2003)

I. Dotan, D. Rachmilewitz, S. Schreiber, R. Eliakim, C. J. Van Der Woude, A. Kornbluth, A. L. Buchman, S. Bar-Meir, B. Bokemeyer, E. Goldin, C. Maaser, U. Mahadevan, U. Seidler, J. C. Hoffman, D. Homoky, T. Plasse, B. Powers, P. Rutgeerts and D. Hommes: A randomised placebo-controlled multicentre trial of intravenous semapimod HCl for moderate to severe Crohn's disease. Gut, 59(6), 760-6 (2010)

S. Schreiber, B. Feagan, G. D'haens, J. F. Colombel, K. Geboes, M. Yurcov, V. Isakov, O. Golovenko, C. N. Bernstein, D. Ludwig, T. Winter, U. Meier, C. Yong and J. Steffgen: Oral p38 mitogen-activated protein kinase inhibition with BIRB 796 for active Crohn's disease: a randomized, double-blind, placebo-controlled trial. Clin Gastroenterol Hepatol, 4(3), 325-34 (2006)

S. Travis: Advances in therapeutic approaches to ulcerative colitis and Crohn's disease. Curr Gastroenterol Rep, 7(6), 475-84 (2005)

S. Murthy, A. Flanigan, D. Coppola and R. Buelow: RDP58, a locally active TNF inhibitor, is effective in the dextran sulphate mouse model of chronic colitis. Inflamm Res, 51(11), 522-31 (2002)

R. Boismenu, Y. Chen, K. Chou, A. El-Sheikh and R. Buelow: Orally administered RDP58 reduces the severity of dextran sodium sulphate induced colitis. Ann Rheum Dis, 61 Suppl 2, ii19-24 (2002)

C. G. Devry, M. Valdez, L. Gao, J. Wang, K. Kotsch, H. D. Volk, I. Bechmann, R. Buelow and S. Iyer: RDP58, a novel immunomodulatory peptide, ameliorates clinical signs of disease in the Lewis rat model of acute experimental autoimmune encephalomyelitis. J Neuroimmunol, 152(1-2), 33-43 (2004)

S. Travis, L. M. Yap, C. Hawkey, B. Warren, M. Lazarov, T. Fong and R. J. Tesi: RDP58 is a novel and potentially effective oral therapy for ulcerative colitis. Inflamm Bowel Dis, 11(8), 713-9 (2005)

W. Liu, B. R. Deyoung, X. Chen, D. P. Evanoff and Y. Luo: RDP58 inhibits T cell-mediated bladder inflammation in an autoimmune cystitis model. J Autoimmun, 30(4), 257-65 (2008)

A. Bourreille, M. Doubremelle, D. R. De La Bletière, J. P. Segain, C. Toquet, R. Buelow and J. P. Galmiche: RDP58, a novel immunomodulatory peptide with anti-inflammatory effects. A pharmacological study in trinitrobenzene sulphonic acid colitis and Crohn disease. Scand J Gastroenterol, 38(5), 526-32 (2003)

E. Kudlacz, M. Conklyn, C. Andresen, C. Whitney-Pickett and P. Changelian: The JAK-3 inhibitor CP-690550 is a potent anti-inflammatory agent in a murine model of pulmonary eosinophilia. Eur J Pharmacol, 582(1-3), 154-61 (2008)

H. Nagai, Y. S. Kim, K. T. Lee, M. Y. Chu, N. Konishi, J. Fujimoto, M. Baba, K. Matsubara and M. Emi: Inactivation of SSI-1, a JAK/STAT inhibitor, in human hepatocellular carcinomas, as revealed by two-dimensional electrophoresis. J Hepatol, 34(3), 416-21 (2001)

K. Yamaoka and Y. Tanaka: Jak inhibitor ; possibility and mechanism as a new disease modifying anti-rheumatic drug. Nihon Rinsho Meneki Gakkai Kaishi, 32(2), 85-91 (2009)

J. S. Fridman, P. A. Scherle, R. Collins, T. C. Burn, Y. Li, J. Li, M. B. Covington, B. Thomas, P. Collier, M. F. Favata, X. Wen, J. Shi, R. Mcgee, P. J. Haley, S. Shepard, J. D. Rodgers, S. Yeleswaram, G. Hollis, R. C. Newton, B. Metcalf, S. M. Friedman and K. Vaddi: Selective inhibition of JAK1 and JAK2 is efficacious in rodent models of arthritis: preclinical characterization of INCB028050. J Immunol, 184(9), 5298-307 (2010)

S. Cohen, S. H. Zwillich, V. Chow, R. R. Labadie and B. Wilkinson: Co-administration of the JAK inhibitor CP-690,550 and methotrexate is well tolerated in patients with rheumatoid arthritis without need for dose adjustment. Br J Clin Pharmacol, 69(2), 143-51 (2010)

R. J. Riese, S. Krishnaswami and J. Kremer: Inhibition of JAK kinases in patients with rheumatoid arthritis: scientific rationale and clinical outcomes. Best Pract Res Clin Rheumatol, 24(4), 513-26 (2010)

J. H. Coombs, B. J. Bloom, F. C. Breedveld, M. P. Fletcher, D. Gruben, J. M. Kremer, R. Burgos-Vargas, B. Wilkinson, C. A. Zerbini and S. H. Zwillich: Improved pain, physical functioning and health status in patients with rheumatoid arthritis treated with CP-690,550, an orally active Janus kinase (JAK) inhibitor: results from a randomised, double-blind, placebo-controlled trial. Ann Rheum Dis, 69(2), 413-6 (2010)

A. Suzuki, T. Hanada, K. Mitsuyama, T. Yoshida, S. Kamizono, T. Hoshino, M. Kubo, A. Yamashita, M. Okabe, K. Takeda, S. Akira, S. Matsumoto, A. Toyonaga, M. Sata and A. Yoshimura: CIS3/SOCS3/SSI3 plays a negative regulatory role in STAT3 activation and intestinal inflammation. J Exp Med, 193(4), 471-81 (2001)

T. T. Pizarro and F. Cominelli: Cytokine therapy for Crohn's disease: advances in translational research. Annu Rev Med, 58, 433-44 (2007)

P. A. Carpenter, F. R. Appelbaum, L. Corey, H. J. Deeg, K. Doney, T. Gooley, J. Krueger, P. Martin, S. Pavlovic, J. Sanders, J. Slattery, D. Levitt, R. Storb, A. Woolfrey and C. Anasetti: A humanized non-FcR-binding anti-CD3 antibody, visilizumab, for treatment of steroid-refractory acute graft-versus-host disease. Blood, 99(8), 2712-9 (2002)

S. Plevy, B. Salzberg, G. Van Assche, M. Regueiro, D. Hommes, W. Sandborn, S. Hanauer, S. Targan, L. Mayer, U. Mahadevan, M. Frankel and J. Lowder: A phase I study of visilizumab, a humanized anti-CD3 monoclonal antibody, in severe steroid-refractory ulcerative colitis. Gastroenterology, 133(5), 1414-22 (2007)

G. Van Assche, W. J. Sandborn, B. G. Feagan, B. A. Salzberg, D. Silvers, P. S. Monroe, W. M. Pandak, F. H. Anderson, J. F. Valentine, G. E. Wild, D. J. Geenen, R. Sprague, S. R. Targan, P. Rutgeerts, V. Vexler, D. Young and R. S. Shames: Daclizumab, a humanised monoclonal antibody to the interleukin 2 receptor (CD25), for the treatment of moderately to severely active ulcerative colitis: a randomised, double blind, placebo controlled, dose ranging trial. Gut, 55(11), 1568-74 (2006)

G. Van Assche, I. Dalle, M. Noman, I. Aerden, C. Swijsen, K. Asnong, B. Maes, J. Ceuppens, K. Geboes and P. Rutgeerts: A pilot study on the use of the humanized anti-interleukin-2 receptor antibody daclizumab in active ulcerative colitis. Am J Gastroenterol, 98(2), 369-76 (2003)

T. J. Creed, M. R. Norman, C. S. Probert, R. F. Harvey, I. S. Shaw, J. Smithson, J. Anderson, M. Moorghen, J. Gupta, N. A. Shepherd, C. M. Dayan and S. D. Hearing: Basiliximab (anti-CD25) in combination with steroids may be an effective new treatment for steroid-resistant ulcerative colitis. Aliment Pharmacol Ther, 18(1), 65-75 (2003)

F. H. Gordon, C. W. Lai, M. I. Hamilton, M. C. Allison, E. D. Srivastava, M. G. Fouweather, S. Donoghue, C. Greenlees, J. Subhani, P. L. Amlot and R. E. Pounder: A randomized placebo-controlled trial of a humanized monoclonal antibody to alpha4 integrin in active Crohn's disease. Gastroenterology, 121(2), 268-74 (2001)

D. T. Selewski, G. V. Shah, B. M. Segal, P. A. Rajdev and S. K. Mukherji: Natalizumab (Tysabri). AJNR Am J Neuroradiol (2010)

M. Yildiz, B. Tettenborn and N. Putzki: Natalizumab and Beyond. Eur Neurol, 64(4), 236-240 (2010)

L. Gorelik, M. Lerner, S. Bixler, M. Crossman, B. Schlain, K. Simon, A. Pace, A. Cheung, L. L. Chen, M. Berman, F. Zein, E. Wilson, T. Yednock, A. Sandrock, S. E. Goelz and M. Subramanyam: Anti-JC virus antibodies: implications for PML risk stratification. Ann Neurol, 68(3), 295-303 (2010)

R. W. Olaussen, M. R. Karlsson, K. E. Lundin, J. Jahnsen, P. Brandtzaeg and I. N. Farstad: Reduced chemokine receptor 9 on intraepithelial lymphocytes in celiac disease suggests persistent epithelial activation. Gastroenterology, 132(7), 2371-82 (2007)

D. C. Baumgart and W. J. Sandborn: Inflammatory bowel disease: clinical aspects and established and evolving therapies. Lancet, 369(9573), 1641-57 (2007)

M. Bayes, X. Rabasseda and J. R. Prous: Gateways to clinical trials. Methods Find Exp Clin Pharmacol, 28(10), 719-40 (2006)

B. Yacyshyn, W. Y. Chey, M. K. Wedel, R. Z. Yu, D. Paul and E. Chuang: A randomized, double-masked, placebo-controlled study of alicaforsen, an antisense inhibitor of intercellular adhesion molecule 1, for the treatment of subjects with active Crohn's disease. Clin Gastroenterol Hepatol, 5(2), 215-20 (2007)

J. R. Philpott and P. B. Miner, Jr.: Antisense inhibition of ICAM-1 expression as therapy provides insight into basic inflammatory pathways through early experiences in IBD. Expert Opin Biol Ther, 8(10), 1627-32 (2008)

S. O. Lopez-Cubero, K. M. Sullivan and G. B. Mcdonald: Course of Crohn's disease after allogeneic marrow transplantation. Gastroenterology, 114(3), 433-40 (1998)

J. A. Snowden, J. Passweg, J. J. Moore, S. Milliken, P. Cannell, J. Van Laar, R. Verburg, J. Szer, K. Taylor, D. Joske, S. Rule, S. J. Bingham, P. Emery, R. K. Burt, R. M. Lowenthal, P. Durez, R. J. Mckendry, S. Z. Pavletic, I. Espigado, E. Jantunen, A. Kashyap, M. Rabusin, P. Brooks, C. Bredeson and A. Tyndall: Autologous hemopoietic stem cell transplantation in severe rheumatoid arthritis: a report from the EBMT and ABMTR. J Rheumatol, 31(3), 482-8 (2004)

R. K. Burt, D. Patel, J. Thomas, A. Yeager, A. Traynor, F. Heipe, R. Arnold, A. Marmont, D. Collier, E. Glatstein and J. Snowden: The rationale behind autologous autoimmune hematopoietic stem cell transplant conditioning regimens: concerns over the use of total-body irradiation in systemic sclerosis. Bone Marrow Transplant, 34(9), 745-51 (2004)

R. J. Xavier and D. K. Podolsky: Unravelling the pathogenesis of inflammatory bowel disease. Nature, 448(7152), 427-34 (2007)

P. B. Jeppesen, E. L. Sanguinetti, A. Buchman, L. Howard, J. S. Scolapio, T. R. Ziegler, J. Gregory, K. A. Tappenden, J. Holst and P. B. Mortensen: Teduglutide (ALX-0600), a dipeptidyl peptidase IV resistant glucagon-like peptide 2 analogue, improves intestinal function in short bowel syndrome patients. Gut, 54(9), 1224-31 (2005)

A. L. Buchman, S. Katz, J. C. Fang, C. N. Bernstein and S. G. Abou-Assi: Teduglutide, a novel mucosally active analog of glucagon-like peptide-2 (GLP-2) for the treatment of moderate to severe Crohn's disease. Inflamm Bowel Dis, 16(6), 962-73 (2010)

X. Wang, B. Wang, J. Wu and G. Wang: Beneficial effects of growth hormone on bacterial translocation during the course of acute necrotizing pancreatitis in rats. Pancreas, 23(2), 148-56 (2001)

D. Decker, W. Springer, R. Tolba, H. Lauschke, A. Hirner and A. Von Ruecker: Perioperative treatment with human growth hormone down-regulates apoptosis and increases superoxide production in PMN from patients undergoing infrarenal abdominal aortic aneurysm repair. Growth Horm IGF Res, 15(3), 193-9 (2005)

D. I. Shulman: Gastrointestinal effects of growth hormone. Endocrine, 12(2), 147-52 (2000)

Y. Huang, S. R. Wang, C. Yi, M. Y. Ying, Y. Lin and M. H. Zhi: Effects of recombinant human growth hormone on rat septic shock with intraabdominal infection by E. coli. World J Gastroenterol, 8(6), 1134-7 (2002)

J. R. Korzenik and B. K. Dieckgraefe: An open-labelled study of granulocyte colony-stimulating factor in the treatment of active Crohn's disease. Aliment Pharmacol Ther, 21(4), 391-400 (2005)

M. Takazoe, T. Matsui, S. Motoya, T. Matsumoto, T. Hibi and M. Watanabe: Sargramostim in patients with Crohn's disease: results of a phase 1-2 study. J Gastroenterol, 44(6), 535-43 (2009)

J. F. Valentine, R. N. Fedorak, B. Feagan, P. Fredlund, R. Schmitt, P. Ni and T. J. Humphries: Steroid-sparing properties of sargramostim in patients with corticosteroid-dependent Crohn's disease: a randomised, double-blind, placebo-controlled, phase 2 study. Gut, 58(10), 1354-62 (2009)

P. J. Mannon, F. Leon, I. J. Fuss, B. A. Walter, M. Begnami, M. Quezado, Z. Yang, C. Yi, C. Groden, J. Friend, R. L. Hornung, M. Brown, S. Gurprasad, B. Kelsall and W. Strober: Successful granulocyte-colony stimulating factor treatment of Crohn's disease is associated with the appearance of circulating interleukin-10-producing T cells and increased lamina propria plasmacytoid dendritic cells. Clin Exp Immunol, 155(3), 447-56 (2009)

C. Abraham and J. H. Cho: Bugging of the intestinal mucosa. N Engl J Med, 357(7), 708-10 (2007)

N. Barnich, F. A. Carvalho, A. L. Glasser, C. Darcha, P. Jantscheff, M. Allez, H. Peeters, G. Bommelaer, P. Desreumaux, J. F. Colombel and A. Darfeuille-Michaud: CEACAM6 acts as a receptor for adherent-invasive E. coli, supporting ileal mucosa colonization in Crohn disease. J Clin Invest, 117(6), 1566-74 (2007)

C. P. Tamboli, C. Neut, P. Desreumaux and J. F. Colombel: Dysbiosis in inflammatory bowel disease. Gut, 53(1), 1-4 (2004)

D. E. Elliott and J. V. Weinstock: Helminthic therapy: using worms to treat immune-mediated disease. Adv Exp Med Biol, 666, 157-66 (2009)

R. W. Summers, D. E. Elliott, J. F. Urban, Jr., R. Thompson and J. V. Weinstock: Trichuris suis therapy in Crohn's disease. Gut, 54(1), 87-90 (2005)